PLATO'S RIVALRY WITH MEDICINE

Plato's Rivalry with Medicine

A STRUGGLE AND ITS DISSOLUTION

Susan B. Levin

OXFORD
UNIVERSITY PRESS

OXFORD
UNIVERSITY PRESS

Oxford University Press is a department of the University of Oxford.
It furthers the University's objective of excellence in research, scholarship,
and education by publishing worldwide.

Oxford New York
Auckland Cape Town Dar es Salaam Hong Kong Karachi
Kuala Lumpur Madrid Melbourne Mexico City Nairobi
New Delhi Shanghai Taipei Toronto

With offices in
Argentina Austria Brazil Chile Czech Republic France Greece
Guatemala Hungary Italy Japan Poland Portugal Singapore
South Korea Switzerland Thailand Turkey Ukraine Vietnam

Published in the United States of America by
Oxford University Press
198 Madison Avenue, New York, NY 10016

Library of Congress Cataloging-in-Publication Data
Levin, Susan B., 1961–
Plato's rivalry with medicine : a struggle and its dissolution / Susan B. Levin.
p. cm.
Includes bibliographical references and index.
ISBN 978–0–19–991980–2 (hardback) 1. Plato. 2. Medicine—Philosophy. 3. Medical ethics.
4. Bioethics. I. Title.
B398.M38L48 2014
184—dc23
2013042244

Contents

Acknowledgments

I BEGAN WORK on Plato's engagement with medicine eight years ago. Shortly thereafter, I had occasion to start teaching biomedical ethics. At the time, I had no idea that the two pursuits would converge so as to yield this book. That this confluence occurred stems in no small part from the rich environment for research and teaching provided by Smith College, my academic home of twenty years.

Some of the material in the book was presented at annual conferences cosponsored by the Society for Ancient Greek Philosophy and the Society for the Study of Islamic Philosophy and Science. Portions were also presented to the Departments of Philosophy at Loyola University Chicago and Connecticut College. Having the opportunity to present my work in these settings helped to enrich my thinking about topics the book addresses.

I am grateful to Smith College for summer research support from 2008 to the present. Thanks go also to the students who were my research assistants from 2007 to 2013: Ellina Nektalova, Mohini Banerjee, Sofia Walker, Caitlin Liss, Fatinha Santos, Juliana Loughrey, and Katherine Russell. In addition, Banerjee and Nektalova commented on the manuscript in part and whole, respectively. Further, I appreciate the interdisciplinary milieu provided by Smith College's Kahn Liberal Arts Institute, where I was a faculty fellow on the project *Wellness and Disease* during 2009–10.

I am grateful for the kindness and support of Edmund Pellegrino, whom I met in 2007 and with whom I corresponded in the earliest phase of my work involving

Plato and bioethics. Further, I wish to thank John Keown, whom I also met in 2007, for his encouragement at the start of my research in this area.

My deep gratitude goes to Julie Ward, who read an early draft of Chapters 1–2, and to Fatinha Santos and Barry Smith, who commented on the manuscript in its entirety. I also wish to thank the referees for Oxford University Press for very helpful comments on the project. Further, I greatly appreciate the contributions made toward the book's success by Peter Ohlin, my editor at Oxford, and Balasubramanian Shanmugasundram, who oversaw the book's production, including the preparation of indices.

I gratefully acknowledge permission from the following to include previously published material: *Philosophical Inquiry*, for "Is Medicine a *Technê*? Health and End-of-Life Care in Plato's *Republic*," in *Reflections on Bioethics and Ancient Philosophy*, edited by Antonio Chu and Ronald Polansky (2007): 125–53; *Apeiron: A Journal for Ancient Philosophy and Science*, for "Eryximachus' Tale: The *Symposium*'s Role in Plato's Critique of Medicine," 42 (2009): 275–308; *Polis: The Journal for Ancient Greek Political Thought*, for "Philosopher-Rulers and the *Laws*: Thing of the Past or (Un)Expected Return?" 27 (2010): 1–24, and "A Rivalry Dissolved: The Restoration of Medicine's *Technê* Status in the *Laws*," 27 (2010): 193–221, Parts I and II, respectively, of "Politics and Medicine: Plato's Final Word." I also include material that previously appeared in *The Journal of Medicine and Philosophy: A Forum for Bioethics and Philosophy of Medicine*, "The Doctor-Patient Tie in Plato's *Laws*: A Backdrop for Reflection," 37/4 (August 2012): 351–72.

Last but not least, my thanks go to Howard Dupuis for his support throughout my work on the project.

Northampton, Massachusetts *S.B.L.*
August 2013

Terms[1]

adikia: injustice, wrongdoing
(*ta*) *agatha*: (the) things that are good, goods
to agathon: the good; *auto to agathon*: literally, "the good itself" (i.e., Plato's Form of the Good)
agôn (plural *agônes*): rivalry, contest
aischron (plural *aischra*): shameful
aisthêsis: sense-perception
aitia (plural *aitiai*): cause, explanatory factor
akairos: untimely
akolasia: self-indulgence, lack of discipline; *akolastos* (plural *akolastoi*): self-indulgent person
andreia: courage
apeiria: inexperience
to apeiron: the indefinite
apeiros (plural *apeiroi*): inexperienced
archê (plural *archai*): source; explanatory factor

[1] This list concentrates on terms in the main text, omitting those that occur exclusively in the notes. Nouns and adjectives are listed in the nominative case, and verbs in their infinitive forms. As Greek is an inflected language, endings used in particular texts will reflect words' grammatical roles in individual sentences.

aretê (plural *aretai*): virtue, excellence
ateles: imperfect (literally, "incomplete")
barbaroi: foreigners (i.e., non-Greeks)
charizesthai: to show or grant a favor
chronios/*chronon*: chronic
dêmiourgoi: craftsmen
diairesis: Method of Division
dialektikê: dialectic
dianoia: reasoning; mental functioning
didakton: teachable
auto to dikaion: literally, "the just itself" (i.e., Plato's Form of Justice)
dikaiosunê: the *technê* of judging; the virtue of justice
dikastês (plural *dikastai*): a judge
dokimasia: scrutiny
doxa: belief; *orthê doxa*: true belief
dunamis (plural *dunameis*): capacity, power
(*to*) *dunaton* (plural [*ta*] *dunata*): (the) possible, something that is possible
eleutheros (plural *eleutheroi*): a free person
empeiria (plural *empeiriai*): a mere "knack"; experience
empeiros (plural *empeiroi*): experienced
enkrateia: mastery; *enkratês*: a morally strong person
epideixis (plural *epideixeis*): a formal display of rhetorical skill
epikouroi: auxiliaries
epimeleia: care
epistêmê: knowledge, understanding; *epistêmai*: fields of expertise
to epithumêtikon: the appetitive aspect of the soul
epithumia (plural *epithumiai*): desire in the sense of appetite ("desire" and "appetite" will be used interchangeably as translations of *epithumia*)
erastês: lover
ergon: function; deed
eris: strife
erômenos: beloved
erôs: love
êthos: character
eudaimonia: flourishing, thriving
eudaimôn: a flourishing person
euthunos (plural *euthunoi*): examiner; *euthuna*: examination
gnôstikê: theoretical expertise

gumnastês: trainer; *gumnastikê*: physical training
hêdonê (plural *hêdonai*): pleasure
hikanos: adequate; *hikanôs*: adequately
hugieia: health
iatrikê: the *technê* of medicine; *iatros* (plural *iatroi*): doctor
kaein: to perform cautery
kairos: right or favorable moment; right measure
kakon (plural *kaka*): evil
kalon (plural *kala*): beautiful, admirable, fine; *to kalon*: the beautiful, beauty; *auto to kalon*: literally, "the beautiful itself" (i.e., Plato's Form of Beauty)
kolakeia: flattery, pandering
kosmios (plural *kosmioi*): an orderly person
kosmos: cosmos, macrocosm, world order
logismos: rational principle
logistikê: calculation
logon dounai, or *logon didonai*: to provide a reasoned account
logos (plural *logoi*): rational account; verbal account; explanation; speech
makros: long (of illness, "chronic")
mania: madness
mantikê: prophecy
melancholia: melancholy
metabolê (plural *metabolai*): change, pressure
metechôn (plural *metechontes*): a participant in a Platonic Form
metrêtikê: art of measurement
to metrion: due measure
mimêsis: imitation; representation
mousikê: poetry and music
muthos: fictional tale
noêsis: understanding
nomophulakes: guardians of the laws
nomos (plural *nomoi*): law
nomothetikê: legislation
ousia: nature, essence
paideia: education
paidotribês: trainer; *paidotribê*: physical training
pathêmata: "affections" in the sense of things undergone
peri ti: literally, "about what"

pharmaka (plural): drugs, medication
philia: friendship; affection
phronêsis: practical wisdom; *phronimos* (plural *phronimoi*): person of practical wisdom
phusiologoi: pre-Socratic philosophers of nature
phusis (plural *phuseis*): nature; *kata phusin*: according to, or in accordance with, nature; *para phusin*: counter to nature
pistis: belief
politikê: *technê* of politics
politikos: statesman
praktikê: practical, or applied, expertise
pros ti: literally, "toward what"
prostatês: sponsor
proteron: earlier (may be used with *husteron*, later)
psuchê (plural *psuchai*): soul
rhêtorikê: rhetoric
sêma: tomb
sêmeion (plural *sêmeia*): sign
sôma: body
sophia: wisdom; *sophos*: a wise person
sôphrosunê: self-control; *sôphrôn* (plural *sôphrones*): a self-controlled person
sunaitios (plural *sunaitioi*): co-causing or co-responsible for something else
sunesis: understanding
sungenê: close aids, allies
technê (plural *technai*): the term is usually rendered "art" or "craft," but "rational purposive discipline" better captures Plato's meaning in the *Gorgias*
technikos: an expert, practitioner of a *technê*
telos (plural *telê*): goal, end, purpose
temnein: to perform surgery
to theion: the divine; *hoi theoi*: the deities
theôria: insight
to thumoeides: the spirited aspect of the soul
timai: offices
trophê: nurture
tuchê: chance

Introduction

FOR THE FIRST time in the history of bioethics as a discipline, the merits of ancient philosophy are receiving notable attention. Thus far, Aristotle's concept of *phronêsis* (practical wisdom) has dominated the conversation. In contrast, not only is Plato's handling of medicine underappreciated by scholars of ancient philosophy, but bioethicists also leave his rich promise nearly untapped. The present book illuminates Plato's engagement with medicine, which I show is complex and far from uniform across the corpus. Over and above the import of this discovery for ancient philosophical thought and the history of medicine, my inquiry shows that Plato's views of the clinical tie, human nature, and political community are valuable right now as bioethics aims to move forward on issues like medical error, transparency, accountability, and physician incentives. Much is at stake in what occurs here not only for the medical profession but for all of us as citizens and human beings.

Plato's handling of medicine is regularly taken as uniform and largely positive across the corpus. In fact, he pursued a significant rivalry with it for authority on human nature and the best life. Showing this requires not only careful explorations of Plato but also substantial attention to ancient medicine. The Hippocratic Corpus contains much discussion of *phusis* (nature) from the standpoint of medicine, with health taken as the highest good. When advancing their positions, ancient medical authors argue or assume that their field is the preeminent human endeavor. In his thoroughgoing efforts to establish philosophy as the rightful arbiter of *phusis* and *eudaimonia* (flourishing), Plato must and does challenge medicine.

The *Gorgias* sets the course for Plato's rivalry with medicine, which is intertwined with his notion of *technê*. Chapter 1 focuses on the dialogue's launch of Plato's highly normative concept of *technê* (traditionally, "art" or "craft," here "rational purposive discipline"), which reserves the *technê* designation for activities that truly promote human thriving. The *Gorgias* contrasts these with *empeiriai* (mere "knacks") such as rhetoric that appear to benefit people but simply flatter them by catering to their governing sources of pleasure.

The *Gorgias*' praise of medicine as a *technê* is evident when the points of comparison are *empeiriai* like rhetoric and cookery. As I show in Chapter 2, the dialogue's systematic account of *technê* has important ties and debts to Hippocratic writings. Contra works like *Ancient Medicine*, however, the primacy that the *Gorgias* grants to the soul already suggests that medicine cannot be preeminent. On the contrary, restoring an individual to health may be at odds with the promotion of justice, as when psychic corruption is irremediable. Further, the *Gorgias*' account of desire, pleasure, and the soul, when applied to medical writings, shows medicine's deeply inadequate and dangerous handling of nature and flourishing. Thus, the stage is set for Plato's overt rivalry with medicine in subsequent dialogues.

His opposition to medicine unfolds in two phases. As I argue in Chapter 3, the *Symposium* actively debunks medicine's claim to be the preeminent *technê*. It furthers the *Gorgias*' adumbration of critique via Eryximachus' articulation of what he, qua medical professional, views as the nature of all, both the broadly cosmic and the human. Further, through Eryximachus, medicine's unquestioned confidence in its role as arbiter of *phusis* (nature) and *eudaimonia* (flourishing) is taken to its natural extreme. The error of its positions on these topics can be shown only from a vantage point other than medicine's own. What is more, Plato must challenge medicine's ability to handle these matters as he defends philosophy's preeminence.

The *Republic* develops Plato's view of the soul-focused *technê* that the *Gorgias* had identified as preeminent. In Chapter 4, I show that the *Republic* furthers Plato's rivalry with medicine even as it argues at length that philosophers, whose insight and character are unerring, must supervise all endeavors. The *Republic* spells out the implications for medicine of the flaws that the *Symposium* diagnosed in its views of nature and flourishing. In the later dialogue, Plato circumscribes the practice of medicine such that the maintenance of health (i.e., lifestyle), to which right handling of desire is central, becomes a matter for philosophy. Further, he limits in salient ways the domain of medical treatment. As to authority in what remains, philosophers will oversee medical practice to ensure that treatments' provision and withholding occur as justice requires. While medicine thus circumscribed has something to offer Kallipolis, the *Republic*'s ideal city, Plato's critique and philosophy's preeminence commit him to withdraw its *technê* standing.

The *Laws*, Plato's final work, is the focus of Chapters 5 and 6, with attention in the former to the *Statesman*'s transitional role between the *Republic* and *Laws* regarding human nature, sociopolitical structures, and medicine specifically. Chapter 5 argues that in the *Laws*, Plato relinquishes the notion that anyone is infallible in character or understanding. Here, for the first time, human cognitive and ethical abilities truly lie on a single continuum. Plato's provisions for Magnesia, the *Laws*' optimal community, reflect this dramatic upgrading of his confidence in the abilities of ordinary citizens. At the same time, his deep acknowledgment of human fallibility grounds Plato's creation of oversight structures across the spectrum of human activities. Even high officials will be monitored, with no single venue being the arbiter in all cases.

In Chapter 6, I show that by key measures Magnesia's metics (resident aliens) come off better than Kallipolis' producers; as Magnesia's physicians are metics, these enhancements necessarily apply to them. In addition, the *Laws* contains strong evidence of medicine's own upgrading in Plato's eyes, including the restoration of its *technê* standing and allocation to it of duties involving justice and the soul that are distinctive for Magnesia and unique in Plato. Further, Magnesia's web of checks and balances, which strongly fosters justice, takes the weight off the health-care setting as the crossroads where decisions about the whole person must be made. This, along with Plato's confidence in doctors, means that no one disrupts their implementation of the medically feasible on grounds of justice. In the *Laws*, not only is Plato's rivalry with medicine no more, but the *Gorgias*' tension between medicine's lauding and incompleteness is resolved.

Chapters 1–6 show the value of investigating Plato's relation to medicine from the standpoints of ancient philosophical thought and the history of medicine. The book's final chapter concentrates on bioethics. Here I argue that the *Laws*' handling of the clinical tie bears importantly on bioethics' quest for a truly collaborative model that avoids extremes of paternalism and autonomy, the arrival at which has proved surprisingly difficult. Further, and fundamentally, Plato's handling of human nature and political community has much to offer bioethical reflection on the role of medicine and the profession's social embedment. Looking to the future, Daniel Callahan (2012, 169), a prominent bioethicist, warns sharply against our "putting to one side and out of sight fundamental questions of good and evil, right and wrong, virtues and vices—the very stuff at the historical foundation of ethics." As we work toward fresh visions of how medicine is best construed respecting these human matters, Plato deserves a serious look.

I close this introduction with three observations and clarifications about my approach. First, my focus concerning Plato is the unfolding of his engagement with medicine, central to which, I argue, are developments in his political thought.

From this vantage point, I concentrate on the *Gorgias*, which introduces the *technê* theory, along with the *Symposium*, *Republic*, *Statesman*, and *Laws*. On my interpretation, each of these dialogues attends importantly to at least two of the following: Plato's notion of *technê* on the *Gorgias*' highly normative construction; medicine; and his political thought. Although a fuller study of Plato's handling of medicine would include the *Phaedrus* and *Timaeus*, their investigation falls outside my purview here.

Second, as in my previous scholarship on Plato, I follow what is often termed a doctrinal approach. This means that I proceed on the assumption that one may glean Plato's stances on issues from careful study of the dialogues and that the character of Socrates (or his functional equivalent) is the primary avenue through which Plato articulates those positions.

Lastly, while I write this book as a specialist in Greek philosophy, I intend it to be accessible also to medical historians and bioethicists. For this reason, much scholarly engagement, along with further material from primary sources, is reserved for the notes. In addition, I provide a list of Greek terms up front and regularly translate them at first mention and often subsequently in the text itself. Further, translations or paraphrases of Greek passages are provided. This, and all else connected to the book, has been done from a fervent hope that it will contribute usefully to explorations of Plato and the core human topics addressed as they bear on medicine.

1

The *Gorgias*' Innovative Lens on Human Existence

1. INTRODUCTION

Because the *Gorgias* sets the course for Plato's overt rivalry with medicine, the present study devotes substantial attention to it. Chapter 1 focuses on the dialogue's introduction of the key Platonic view of *technê* as a designation reserved for activities that genuinely promote human thriving. Chapter 2 concentrates on its handling of medicine, including a tension that emerges between conduct necessitated by medicine's own occupation with health and what Plato deems requisite on grounds of justice.

Most broadly put, the *Gorgias* features an *agôn* (rivalry) between divergent approaches to *phusis* (nature) and *eudaimonia* (flourishing): one centers on fostering humans' absolute well-being, the other on an unbounded pursuit of whatever one's urges and practical goals happen to be at a given time.[1] The philosophical frame for

[1] For present purposes, I need not defend fixed assumptions about all dialogues' relative dates of composition, regarding which some controversy abides. This investigation operates on the following chronological assumptions, which find reasonable support on thematic grounds: (1) dialogues including the *Apology, Crito, Euthyphro, Laches,* and *Charmides* come before the *Gorgias*; (2) the *Gorgias* also postdates the *Protagoras, Euthydemus, Hippias Major,* and *Hippias Minor* and was composed after or in roughly the same period as the *Lysis* (see Dodds 1959, 18–23; Irwin 1979, 1); (3) the writings listed in (1) and (2) antedate the *Cratylus, Phaedo, Symposium,* and *Republic* (at least Books II–X), all of which belong to the middle period, when Forms are introduced (on the *Cratylus*' placement here, see Levin 2001, 4–5n4, 96–98); (4) the *Phaedrus, Parmenides,* and *Theaetetus* belong after those dialogues listed in (3), lying on the cusp between Plato's middle and late writings; (5) the *Sophist, Statesman,* and *Philebus* postdate these writings and come before the *Laws*; and (6) the *Timaeus* belongs with the late group, as most believe (for confirmation, see Cherniss [1965b] against

Plato's conduct of this dispute is his articulation, debuted there, of a highly normative conception of *technê*. The *Gorgias*' selective notion of *technê*, rooted in three central criteria that qualifying activities will meet, departs strongly from what Plato finds a heedless assimilation under that head of diverse occupations involving skill of whatever kind, such as house-building, metalworking, arithmetic, astronomy, agriculture, the domestication of animals, medicine, and prophecy (Aeschylus, *Prometheus Bound*, lines 442–506).[2]

As Chapter 2 makes clear, Hippocratic writings contain versions of all three criteria for *technê* standing that the *Gorgias* provides. The dialogue's argument not only grants medicine's *technê* status but depends on its having such. This is itself a notable move, because several Hippocratic works target a disparaging contention that medicine, far from being the preeminent endeavor, does not warrant inclusion among *technai* at all (*Ancient Medicine* 4; *The Art* 1; *Regimen in Acute Diseases* 8). At the same time, however, Plato's own *technê* grid provides a lens through which core limitations of medicine's authority are seen, including its illegitimate pretention to an absolute grasp of nature and thriving. What is shown indirectly in the *Gorgias* becomes overt in the *Symposium* and *Republic*.

On the *Gorgias*' account, many so-called *technai* (e.g., rhetoric, cookery) are unmasked as *empeiriai* (mere "knacks"); only those select activities meeting its standards for a genuine *technê* warrant pursuit by human beings. As for its investigation of the two rival stances toward flourishing (i.e., those of Gorgianic rhetoric and true politics), the dialogue lays particular stress on Plato's critique of shoddy, self-serving endeavors that pander to people's unregulated desires and motivations. Substantial depiction of the political *technê*—supreme for its exclusive focus on the optimal welfare of the highest good, namely soul—must await later dialogues. However, core elements of the tack to be taken there are evident in the *Gorgias*, and it will be important to bear these threads in mind when our investigation turns to the *Republic*, *Statesman*, and *Laws*.

Owen's [1953] claim for an earlier position). This study treats the *Gorgias* as lying on the cusp, with the *Meno*, between the early and middle dialogues. Though I endorse the claims in (1)–(6) above, if one deemed the *Gorgias* to antedate certain dialogues proceeding discretely regarding the *technê* conditions that ground its own highly normative account, the position defended here would simply have that dialogue as the place where Plato opted to pull those conditions together expressly into a cogent theoretical grid.

2 On other connections between the *Gorgias* and *Prometheus Bound*, see Sedley (2009, 55–56n8); Fussi (2001, 539–40); Penner (1991, 166n21). On the term *technê*'s broad pre-Platonic application, cf. Dodds (1959, 190). The issue of what qualifies as a *technê* at all must be distinguished from the question of which is supreme when *technai* are hierarchically assessed; the present study concentrates extensively on both.

2. *TECHNAI* VERSUS *EMPEIRIAI*: THE *GORGIAS*' ACCOUNT OF WHAT IS AND IS NOT WORTH DOING

Plato's repudiation of rival claims to authority on *phusis* and *eudaimonia* is abundantly clear prior to his introduction of Forms. Before the *Gorgias*, however, his treatment of those claims is unsystematic. Far from approaching the *Gorgias*' demarcation of *technai* (rational purposive disciplines) from *empeiriai* (knacks),[3] earlier writings use the broadly inclusive notion of *technê* seen in *Prometheus Bound* (e.g., *Charmides* 165c–166b, 173a–174c; *Ion* 537e–540e). Though people's specific priorities varied, many in Plato's time concurred that some activities worth engaging in were better than others. His aim in the *Gorgias* is far-reaching and quite controversial, namely, to systematically defend the rank of *technê* as a marked accomplishment. The dialogue's highly normative concept of *technê* gives Plato, at a stroke, a philosophical lens through which to (1) delineate what activities do and do not merit pursuit (*technai* and *empeiriai*, respectively) and (2) defend hierarchical claims about *technai* vis-à-vis one another. Further, the *Gorgias*' notion of *technê* serves as a platform for his later critiques of rivals, salient among them medicine, and defense, in the *Republic*, of philosophy's preeminence. Plato's execution of this two-pronged agenda necessitates the articulation and defense of his own views of *phusis* (nature) and *eudaimonia* (flourishing), central to which is souls' complex structure with tiered loci of motivation.[4]

At *Gorgias* 458a8–b1, Socrates proclaims, "Nothing is worse for a human being than false belief about the matters we're discussing right now [i.e., the just and unjust]" (*ouden gar oimai tosouton kakon einai anthrôpôi, hoson doxa pseudês peri hôn tunchanei nun hêmin ho logos ôn*).[5] This brief assertion alludes to all three core conditions that a genuine *technê* must meet.[6] First, "about the matters we're discussing right now" gestures toward Plato's insistence that genuine *technai*—henceforth interchangeable, unless otherwise noted, with "a *technê*/*technai*"—revolve around

[3] Cf. my earlier claim (Levin 2001, 82n6) that this is a more semantically accurate rendering of *technê* for the *Gorgias*' notion than the standard translations, "art" and "craft."

[4] Singpurwalla (2010, 890) calls the *Republic*'s account of the soul its "tripartite theory of motivation" and construes the soul's dimensions as "distinct, deeply embedded ways of responding to the world." On the notion of motivation apropos of the *Republic*, see also Annas (1981, 124): "We will not understand an individual's actions unless we see that actions do not come from a single motivational source. There is more than one origin of behaviour within a person, and the way the person lives and acts indicates how these sources of behaviour are related." While the *Gorgias* does not treat the soul at this level of complexity, it makes strongly evident that there exist categorically better and worse views of pleasure and thriving.

[5] Unless otherwise noted, translations of Plato are from Cooper (1997), with adjustments. Citations of Plato are from the OCT editions. Those of vol. 1 are from the edition of Duke et al. (1995), and the edition of Slings (2003) has been used for the *Republic*. Remaining references are to the edition of Burnet, 5 vols. (1900–1907).

[6] On these requirements see also Levin (2001, 82–84), on which the present discussion draws.

an ordered and stable domain of objects. One may call this the *peri ti* (subject-matter; literally, "about what") requirement. It is captured in the dialogue by Socrates' persistent requests that Gorgias provide a tenable response to the question, "What is your so-called *technê*, namely rhetoric, about?"[7]

The phrase "false belief" alludes to the second requirement, that practitioners of a *technê* operate with *epistêmê* (knowledge, or understanding) rather than mere belief (*doxa* at 458a8; *pistis* in 454c–d). The possession of understanding is demonstrated by agents' ability to provide a reasoned account (*logon dounai*) of the nature of their subject matter and of why given measures were chosen to maximally attain the practice's aim (465a, 501a).[8] *Gorgias* 458a8–b1 alludes to the "understanding condition" on genuine *technai* by showcasing the defective condition of those who, practicing knacks (*empeiriai*), operate with destructively false views about justice (457b–c); more generally, the latter are at best haphazard, opportunistic combinations of true and false beliefs. This suffices to make clear that epistemological considerations (i.e., agents' cognitive states) are key when one assesses the merit of their activities.[9]

---

[7] The present study uses "rhetoric"/"rhetorician" synonymously with "oratory"/"orator." Moreover, unless otherwise noted, "rhetoric" is used interchangeably with both "sophistry" and "rhetoric/sophistry": though the *Gorgias* gestures toward a split between rhetoric and sophistry qua psychic *empeiriai* (520a–b), that divide is never clearly made out and is perhaps included largely or entirely for purposes of symmetry with Plato's dual psychic *technai*. If so, the situation here would be broadly similar to the Divided Line's provision of an unconvincing break within the figure's lower half at least in part to mirror that within its higher portion (see Annas 1981, 249). See Harrison (1964), who persuasively defends the view that the *Gorgias*' alleged division of sophists from orators is "wholly artificial" (190) and not seriously intended by Plato (186).

[8] See also 505c–d, where the beneficial *logos* is said to be an organic unity (versus a mereological sum); the tight unity of *logoi* here reflects that of the subject matters to which they pertain. Franklin (2005) identifies rhetoric's inability to offer a *logos* as "the central justification" for its lack of *technê* standing (230). While Franklin seems initially to view *logoi* as cognitive items, as when claiming that a *technê*'s *logos* "*grounds* the explanations given by the craft" (231; emphasis added), he also treats them as linguistic items ("The *logos* of a *technê* says what the product is," 248; cf. 237, 239). Though the term *logos* has both cognitive and linguistic referents, a clearer distinction between the two planes is needed here. Unlike the cognitive element, which anchors a *technê* requirement in its own right, the linguistic items that suitably convey one's understanding do not themselves ground a condition. That said, if one takes cognition as the crux, then linguistic formulations' role as necessary external markers of one's insight should be noted expressly. The present study's characterizations of the *technê* theory's epistemological criterion use "understanding," "insight," and "knowledge" interchangeably. On the distinctive features of Plato's notion of understanding, see Moravcsik (1992, 11–45).

[9] On the centrality to the *Gorgias* of what I dub the understanding condition on *technai*, see Segvic (2000, 8). According to Levy (2005), Socrates' exchange with Gorgias shows that rhetoric "fails to satisfy the special knowledge criterion" (199, see also 197–98), which formulation conflates ontological and epistemological considerations. On Levy's account, when Polus takes over, Socrates' ground of disapproval shifts to rhetoric's inability to offer a *logos* of "the activities that make up the practice . . . [including] how each step involved in the performance of the characteristic activities contributes to the achievement of the good at which the overall activity aims" (199). While this is certainly important, Levy treats rhetoric's explanatory failure as a self-contained ground of censure (see also Jaeger 1986a, 131) rather than locating it under a broader epistemological head, i.e., what I call the understanding requirement.

Third and finally, the statement's opening, "Nothing is worse for a human being (*ouden gar oimai tosouton kakon einai anthrôpôi*) than false belief"—reinforced by the fact that at stake is justice, a core value—suggests that the matter of detriment versus benefit (i.e., what is fleshed out later in the dialogue as the "goodness requirement" on *technai*) motivates the entire claim at 458a8–b1. Far from being fortuitous, this suggestion fits with Plato's deployment of the *technê* grid in the *Gorgias* and subsequently (*Cratylus*, *Symposium*, *Republic*), where the three criteria are intertwined but inspired by this last-named requirement that whatever we undertake must offer demonstrable benefit to our existence as individuals and more generally.[10]

Through its cogent presentation of these three core *technê* requirements, the *Gorgias* achieves in unified, concentrated form what had emerged indirectly and in a scattered fashion across earlier dialogues' critiques of rhetoric/sophistry and poetry. The *Gorgias*' "subject-matter condition" is suggested at *Ion* 541e (cf. 539d–540b), where Socrates chastises the dialogue's eponymous rhapsode: this individual, far from providing an *epideixis* (formal display) of his *technê*, has declined "even to tell me what it is that you're so wonderfully clever about though I've been begging you for ages to do so." While previous dialogues indicate that *technai* require clearly specifiable domains, and that practitioners' inability to supply the subject matter of their favored endeavor might jeopardize its "elevated" standing, those discussions lack the *Gorgias*' cogency and decisiveness.

As noted, the requirement that *technê* practitioners' cognitive state be knowledge, not mere belief, includes the evincing of that understanding through experts' reasoned defenses of procedures and their pertinence to the *technê*'s end. This epistemic criterion is intimated at *Charmides* 170e, which demarcates genuine from specious agents of medicine due to the former's understanding as shown by their ability to provide reasoned accounts; this same capacity also permits them to assess one another's words and deeds involving health (171a–c).

Finally, what officially becomes the *Gorgias*' "goodness requirement" on *technai* is adumbrated at *Protagoras* 313d, where, likening sophistry to vending, Socrates observes that "those who market provisions don't know what is good or bad for the body (*oute autoi isasin hoti chrêston ê ponêron peri to sôma*)—they just recommend everything they sell—nor do those who buy (unless the buyer happens to be a trainer or a doctor)." Doctors, in contrast, truly concerned for the welfare of those around whom their efforts revolve, decline to gratify patients' requests for fleeting appetitive indulgence at health's expense (*Laches* 192e–193a).[11]

---

[10] Thus, Levy's (2005, 199n27) claim that the *Gorgias* lacks a distinct goodness condition underplays the salience of that factor to the dialogue's critique of rhetoric.

[11] Cf. Woodruff (1990, 73), who finds an implication of *technai*'s concern with the good at *Laches* 185c–d and *Euthyphro* 14e.

The *Gorgias* works up to its announcement of the *technê-empeiria* split, opening with a sustained treatment of the subject-matter requirement. The dialogue aligns itself here with Socrates' critical stance elsewhere toward sophistry/rhetoric in particular and with his broad insistence that one cannot know whether a value or practice has any attribute (e.g., provides benefit or is teachable) before one is acquainted with its nature, or essence (*ousia*). Socrates' investigation of the natures of values through his renowned "what is *F*-ness?" queries are typically linked to activities featuring those values (e.g., courage to generalship in the *Laches*, and piety to theological praxis in the *Euthyphro*).[12] These inquiries' lack of success (as measured by an absence of tenable responses to their guiding queries)[13] and Socrates' unfulfilled requests for specification of rival practices' subject matter—sophistry in the *Protagoras* and poetry (via rhapsody) in the *Ion*—make fitting indeed the *Gorgias*' launch via protracted examination of the "what is it?" query involving rhetoric. By the end of this dialogue, however, one possesses, if not rich accounts of values themselves, a powerful grid for delineating and ranking practices both across the *technai-empeiriai* boundary and within the already select class of *technai* itself.

At the *Gorgias*' start, the dialogue's eponymous sophist has just completed a formal display that apparently left his auditors in awe (447a). Straightaway, Socrates foregrounds the subject-matter requirement on *technai*—just the start of what will become a prolonged, relentless occupation on his part with this particular *technê* condition.[14] What can Gorgias' *technê* achieve (447b–d)? Framing his query on the model of familiar, mundane crafts like cobblery, Socrates asks, what is it that Gorgias teaches (*didaskei*, c3)? What, most fundamentally, *is* Gorgias? Up front, we see a distinction between the elder, more courteous Gorgias and Polus, an arrogant youth itching to make his mark.[15] Plato signals his lesser regard for Polus,

[12] On the *Gorgias*' tie to the Socratic elenchus as practiced in earlier dialogues, see also Levy (2005, 185); Franklin (2005, 237n21); Dodds (1959, 1).

[13] As is well known, these discussions lack closure because Socrates reduces interlocutors to *aporia* (intellectual perplexity) without discussions' also yielding tenable responses to their governing queries; for instance, "what is piety?" would be answered successfully by a specification, not provided, of the essential feature that all things pious shared (*Euthyphro* 5d, 6d–e). For stress on the philosophical merit of those inquiries, nonetheless, see Robinson (1984, 15–18).

[14] The *Gorgias*' arguments involving one or more interlocutors have been viewed as ad hominem (e.g., Kahn 1983, 76; Weiss 1992, 299). Though arguing the matter falls outside my purview here, I note my broad concurrence with Irwin (1995), who stresses that "in his choice of interlocutors and the views they put forward, Plato wants to show that he is not leaving reasonable objections unheard" (122). The two approaches need not be as far apart as Wolfsdorf (2008, 112) suggests, since an argument's being in some way ad hominem does not suffice straightaway to render it inapplicable or fundamentally problematic.

[15] On the figures of Gorgias and Polus, see further Dodds (1959, 6–12).

Gorgias' self-appointed protector, by having him condescend without hesitation to Chaerephon, Socrates' friend, when seeking to shield Gorgias from having to address Socrates' query (448a–b).

According to Polus, *technê* depends on *empeiria* (here, "experience"), and individuals' caliber reflects the merit of their *technai*, with rhetoric being the best (448c). Polus' attempt here to specify rhetoric's subject matter thus comprises an empty assertion of (1) how *technê* and *empeiria* as such interrelate and (2) the preeminent standing of rhetoric, hence of its practitioners. As to (1), *empeiria* allegedly generates *technê* in every case,[16] while its lack renders agents dependent on *tuchê* (chance); regarding (2), Polus baldly asserts that Gorgias, practitioner of rhetoric, pursues the *technê* par excellence (*metechei tês kallistês tôn technôn*, 448c9). Socrates' response (448e) foregrounds two points: Polus addressed the question as though rhetoric were under attack. Further, as in previous dialogues' inquiries into values, Socrates' query was, what is rhetoric? It was not a request for specification of qualities (e.g., how rhetoric stacks up against other activities) that could be handled only on that foundation.

Gorgias himself now takes over. I am an orator, he proclaims, "if you really want to call me 'what I boast myself to be' as Homer puts it" (449a)—a pronouncement calling to mind Protagoras' own declaration in the eponymous dialogue (317b). Moreover, and crucial to our dialogue's unfolding, Gorgias assures Socrates that he not only functions quite well as an orator but also instructs others (449b). The claim is rife with presumption. Gorgias takes for granted both his grasp of what teaching, in its essence, is and that the province of rhetoric is *didakton* (teachable)—which claims are shattered at 454c–455a, where rhetoric is deemed strictly an agent of persuasion that does not also teach (454e9–455a1). Further, Gorgias assumes at 449a–b that his proficiency in rhetoric equips him to instruct others in the field with utmost effectiveness.[17] While the passage foregrounds Gorgias' own marked self-assurance, it fails to answer the question of what precisely rhetoric's subject matter *is*. From here, Socrates guides the discussion through a series of attempted specifications yielding the outcome that what Gorgias finally concedes rhetoric to do, namely flatter and please the masses, (1) still does not depict it uniquely since

[16] Plato's revisions of medical presentations of what become his core *technê* conditions—including his ontological stress on order and unity, which paves the way for Forms (Moravcsik 1992, 20, 24), sole objects of knowledge—necessarily lead away from a Hippocratic view, represented by Polus, that *technê* and *empeiria* are thus intertwined.

[17] Epistemologically speaking, in Plato's dialogue and Gorgias' own *Encomium of Helen* (see especially secs. 10–14), Gorgias as expert practitioner operates not with knowledge but strictly via belief, with express awareness of so doing (Kahn 1983, 85n16). Notably, from the *Gorgias*' standpoint, in *Encomium of Helen* Gorgias sees no incompatibility between secs. 10–14 on belief and earlier claims that he will provide *logismon tina* (sec. 2) and *tas aitias* of Helen's leaving for Troy (sec. 5).

other *empeiriai* (e.g., cookery), as impersonators of their corresponding *technai*, do this too; and (2) would not qualify, in any case, as a structured and knowable, hence teachable, domain of the kind that *technai* possess.[18]

Socrates' immediate analogies are with weaving and *mousikê*, endeavors that generate clothing and tunes, respectively (449d). Gorgias now posits as rhetoric's distinctiveness its producing effects via *logoi*—here, "verbal accounts" versus reasoned ones in the *Gorgias*' technical sense—which are thus, he submits, its own *peri ti* (subject matter). Socrates rightly rejoins, however, that all activities involve *logoi* about their own subject matters (450a–b). For instance, doctors' *logoi* directed toward patients address treatments' use to aid their recovery, and medical instruction of aspiring physicians fosters their expertise in health, medicine's subject matter (449e–450a).[19] As all *technai* necessarily involve *logoi* pertaining to their own subject matters, why, Socrates asks, are they not all called "rhetoric" (450b)?

Gorgias' adjusted claim is that rhetoric's uniqueness stems from its entire impact's being the outcome of *logoi*-deployment (450b–c). As arithmetic, geometry, and astronomy ostensibly share this distinction with rhetoric (450d–451c), Gorgias is, however, forced again to assay further specification of its domain: rhetoric's purview now becomes "the greatest of human concerns . . . and the best" (*ta megista tôn anthrôpeiôn pragmatôn . . . kai arista*, 451d7–8). This response is crucial for directing the *Gorgias* to the topic of goods (*ta agatha*, literally, "the things that are good"), on whose relative positioning people radically disagree. If those at drinking parties may be trusted, health is supreme (*ariston*), followed by physical attractiveness (with strength, the province of *paidotribê* [physical training]) and wealth (451e–452c).[20] All is about physicality/materiality here, with the items mentioned falling on the two subordinate tiers of goods noted elsewhere in the dialogue (511d).

From the standpoint of goods-promotion, rhetoric is supreme for Gorgias because its sway over others' *psuchai* (souls) through persuasion of large groups on political

---

[18] For the *Gorgias* as not precluding a *technê* of *hêdonê*, see Carone (2004, 87); Berman (1991, 134); Gosling and Taylor (1982, 75, 290). For discussion of why, on the *Gorgias*' account, *technai* cannot revolve around pleasure, see Franklin (2005), who notes that it lacks the stability required of *telê* (249–50), having instead a context-determined merit not unlike that of CPR (251).

[19] Likewise with *gumnastikê* (physical training), which directs the maintenance of health as distinct from its restoration. The proximity of the Greek term *gumnastikê* to the English "gymnastics" might lead one to underestimate the extent of difference between their referents. The scope of contemporary gymnastics, as reflected by the category at Olympic events, is narrower and rather different, including the balance beam, horizontal bar, parallel bars, pommel horse, rings, uneven bars, and vault (http://www.olympic.org/gymnastics-artistic). Ancient *gumnastikê* covered activities such as wrestling, archery, and throwing the javelin; see further Marrou (1982, 70).

[20] On the deeply ingrained Greek view of health as among the highest goods if not atop that list, see Edelstein (1952, 308), who notes a widespread acquaintance with medicine in antiquity (311–12). On health's preeminence, see also Dodds (1959, 200).

and judicial occasions maximizes expert deployers' possession of cherished assets like wealth: if one has this ability to persuade effectively, "[the] financial expert will end up making more money for somebody else instead of himself—for you, in fact, if you've got the ability to speak and to persuade the crowds" (452e).[21] Yet again rhetoric is not unique, for when addressing others, all experts seek to instill persuasion in auditors' souls regarding the content of their own domains (453d–454a).[22] We reach here a key point in the unfolding of Socrates' exchanges with Gorgias. Since Gorgias has singled out political gatherings and the courts, both replete with talk of justice,[23] as the venues where rhetoric's persuasive genius shines, he is compelled by the argument to identify justice and injustice as the objects of rhetoric's linguistic efforts (454b). This verbal compulsion of Gorgias is notable, as he had used the concepts of freedom and slavery to foreground rhetoricians' bending of others to their will (452d–e)—a view also suggested in the orator's own *Encomium of Helen* (see especially sec. 12).[24]

Plato's ensuing, pointed epistemological distinction (454c–d) between belief (*pistis*) and knowledge (*epistêmê*)—heretofore unprecedented in the dialogues (Dodds 1959, 206)—grounds the understanding condition on *technai*. Understanding, which must be taught, is always true, while belief may be true or false (454d). Seen through this lens, what rhetoric (or any other *empeiria*) conveys is mere opinion-based persuasion about the just and unjust, not the insight that genuine instruction alone provides (454e–455a). Any knack that impersonates a *technê* (e.g., rhetoric as opposed to judging, cookery versus medicine) "lacks an account of the nature of whatever things it applies by which it applies them, so that it's unable to

---

[21] Though not all Hippocratic works are scrupulous in their declination of rhetorical techniques, *Precepts* (12) warns doctors against lecturing to crowds; if they cannot bring themselves to refrain, poets must not be cited. Cf. *On Joints* (42, 44), where the author repudiates the notion of "treatment" as theater, favored by dabblers (70), which performers are indifferent to whether they aid or harm.

[22] Gorgias has effectively said that rhetoric is not valuable in its own right but to be favored—at most and contingently—as a tool to foster one's maximal acquisition of whatever he actually values independently of its use: if force promised greater effectiveness, it would presumably be chosen instead.

[23] On citizens' alleged qualification, by virtue of being such, to pronounce on justice, see *Apology* 24e–25c; *Protagoras* 322c–323c, 327a–e.

[24] The *Gorgias* recurs to these concepts at 483e–484b, where Callicles contends that some who are free *phusei* find themselves enslaved *nomôi*; conversely, those whose sheer bulk gives them precedence *nomôi*, with latitude to impose their collective will, may actually be slaves *phusei* (483a–c, 489c). According to 492c, "wantonness, *akolasia*, and freedom, if abundantly available, are *aretê* and *eudaimonia*" (see more generally 491d–492e)—precisely the reverse of Plato's views on freedom, virtue, and flourishing. Notwithstanding these salient differences, Callicles' condemnation of physical strength on its own as a sign of vast deficiency is not unlike Plato's own critical stance toward an occupation with physicality, including fitness, particularly in the *Republic* (410b, 591c–d). On common ground, albeit limited, between Callicles' approach and that of Plato, see further Woolf (2000, 1), who defends "a certain deeper affinity" between Callicles' and Socrates' accounts; Irwin (1979, 176–77); Dodds (1959, 291–92); Tenkku (1956, 89); Klosko (1984a, 134).

state the cause of each thing" (*ouk echei logon oudena hôi prospherei ha prospherei hopoi atta tên phusin estin, hôste tên aitian hekastou mê echein eipein*, 465a).[25] The understanding condition is closely tied to the subject-matter criterion because a practice's having unstable objects, among which are the psychological states fixed on by impersonators' efforts to persuade, necessarily renders un*know*able the contents of its domain.

The *Gorgias*' account of understanding, whose application to the *technê* of medicine is stressed (see especially 501a), meshes well with the Hippocratic Corpus. As will become evident in Chapters 2 and 3, medical accounts are replete not just with prescriptions but with *logoi* specifying ailments' causality. These accounts, in turn, are tightly linked to treatments and amply provided rationales for their selection. In fact, one becomes so accustomed to medical writings' inclusion of explanations and justifications that it is notable when they are not proffered either directly or by implication based on an author's overarching cosmological vision.

When demarcating worthwhile practices from the deleterious, Plato sets great store by the goodness condition (464c–465b).[26] Gorgias' lengthy involvement with Socrates is bookended by Polus' presumption: boasting initially that he could substitute for Gorgias in defense of rhetoric, obviously the *technê* par excellence (448a–e), Polus engineers Gorgias' supplanting by judging his effectiveness blunted through an admission that he teaches "what is just, what is admirable, and what is good" (*ta dikaia . . . kai ta kala kai ta agatha*, 461b6) if students of rhetoric arrive at his door unequipped regarding them. Though the *technai-empeiriai* grid is not elaborated for a few pages yet, Polus' intrusion at 461b–c marks the beginning of the end of Gorgias' substantive assays. His concession that if a pupil did not know the just and unjust, his instruction would include them (460a) is what leads to trouble: Gorgias had earlier hastened to absolve teachers of blame if their pupils, later functioning as experts themselves, deployed their rhetorical training unjustly (456e–457a). Now, however, he claims (460b–e) that no practitioners of *technai*, including rhetoric, will be motivated to act unjustly.

For Polus, Gorgias' concession at 460a stemmed from the prospect of shame if he refused to grant that a pupil would either know the politically central concepts

---

[25] The ignorance of those practicing *empeiriai* when it comes to *phuseis* and *aitiai* also pervades their large groups of auditors (459a–b, cf. 519a). Due to its role as a specious aid to patients' diets across the board, *opsopoiikê* in Plato is fittingly rendered "cookery" with Irwin (1979) rather than by Zeyl's (Cooper 1997) narrower locution "pastry baking." Moss's (2007) useful observation that the closest medical counterpart to cookery is its occupation with regimen (238) is inconsistent with her narrow rendering of one pursuing *opsopoiikê* as a "pastry chef" (239).

[26] I thus diverge from Franklin (2005, 251–52), who takes the "ethical and methodological critiques"—the latter being the "charge that Rhetoric is not a *technê*"—to be closely related but distinct.

of justice and injustice before his instruction by the famous orator or learn those things at his feet (461b). With this provocative contention, young Polus, a self-proclaimed oratorical expert (462a), becomes Socrates' interlocutor as he now disentangles *technê* and *empeiria*, which Polus himself had interlinked (448c), albeit imprecisely. Harking back to the unbreakable tie forged there (and allegedly in Polus' own writing)[27] between *empeiria* and *technê* on the one side and between *apeiria* (inexperience) and *tuchê* (chance) on the other, Socrates drops a bombshell (462b–c): prying *empeiria* and *technê* apart, he claims that far from the latter's depending on the former (qua "experience") as its foundation, the two are antithetically opposed.[28] It is not merely that all activities deemed *technai* and those dubbed *empeiriai* are mutually exclusive. This claim could be read simply as rejecting the view that the historical emergence of *technai* and individuals' mastery thereof is tied to experience, all the while leaving rhetoric's standing as a *technê* intact. Instead, Socrates shifts rhetoric's own classification from the domain of *technai* to that of *empeiriai* (i.e., knacks, 462c). Since Gorgias and Polus (presumably like all others gathered save Socrates) have operated with an unquestioned assumption that rhetoric is a *technê*, with defense needed if at all of its preeminence among such endeavors, its demotion here is radical.

Socrates' specification of the telos of *empeiriai* as "producing a certain gratification and pleasure" (*charitos tinos kai hêdonês apergasias*, 462c7) involves the deleterious opposite to what is stipulated as the goodness condition on *technai*. Polus' reaction at c8–9—"Don't you think that rhetoric's an admirable thing . . . for being able to provide people with gratification (*charizesthai hoion te einai anthrôpois*)?"—evinces his commitment to a second prejudgment, namely, that gratification is itself a good.[29] The

[27] The level of proximity to Polus' treatise is unknown (see Irwin 1979, 112; Dodds 1959, 11, 223). Perhaps the closest Hippocratic comment to that of Polus in the *Gorgias* appears in *Epidemics* VI (3.12, cf. 8.17), though it is hard to be sure since Polus does not specify the nature of the priority that *empeiria* has, and the medical passage does not state that doctors' recognizing patterns of likeness and divergence among phenomena itself yields a *technê*.

[28] This leaves open the question of how Plato would classify medical experience enabling doctors' application of abstract truths to specific ills. It is likely that he does not discount it but would wish to distinguish between a practice's *being* an *empeiria* and physicians' being *empeiroi* (experienced) in all key health-related matters. While controversy obtained in Hippocratic writings about the role of *empeiria* and its relation to understanding and *technê*, generally speaking the *Gorgias*' sharp distinction between the two goes against the grain of what one finds in medical treatises. For this *technê-empeiria* demarcation as originating with Plato, see also Capelle (1922, 262–65); Dodds (1959, 229); Heinimann (1976, 144–45); Allen (1994, 83). Given the evidence from medical writings, I find unwarranted Irwin's (1979, 130) claim that it is unclear how far the divide is inherited by Plato as opposed to stemming from him.

[29] Cf. this view's attribution to ordinary folk at *Protagoras* 353c–354b. In the *Hippias Major*, Socrates notes as *kalon*, by popular conception, what pleases *aisthêsis*, specifically, "food and drink, what attends sex, and the remainder of that kind of thing" (298e). With Woodruff (1982) and Dodds (1959, 7n2), I treat the *Hippias Major* as authentic.

bearing of this stance on medicine will be discussed in Chapter 2. While the subject-matter requirement on *technai* was front and center at the dialogue's start, the goodness criterion dominates from 462c forward.

Although the discussion thus far has focused on rhetoric, which targets the soul, cookery now comes to light as its bodily directed counterpart (462d–e). Cookery's emergence, in turn, will shortly yield (464b–465d) a more concerted handling of medicine beyond its earlier, subordinating invocation by Gorgias, and the content of those remarks will shed important light on what is, on balance, Plato's positive construction of it at this juncture in the corpus. In addition, that discussion gives retroactive bite to 455a–c, where Socrates suggests that far from rhetoric's being useful across the board, when notable topics (e.g., doctors' civic appointment) are publicly discussed, orators should not preside. Instead, if people wish their decisions to offer a boon, they should look directly and solely to experts in the pertinent fields.[30]

In all, the systematic *technê-empeiria* demarcation in 463a–465d foregrounds eight pursuits, four *technai* and their corresponding knacks. In each quartet, one pair addresses the body, while the other duo focuses on the soul; within each pair, one activity concentrates on prevention, that is, maintenance of a salutary state, the other on that state's restoration. The two bodily *technai* are gymnastics and medicine, while those presiding over soul, joined under the *technê* of politics (*politikê*), are legislation (*nomothetikê*) and justice (*dikaiosunê*). *Dikaiosunê* directly signifies here not the character trait but the *technê* of judging. Corresponding bodily charlatans are cosmetics and cookery. Finally, to preserve symmetry with his fourfold distinction of *technai*, Plato splits *empeiriai* involving soul into sophistry and rhetoric.

The crux of *empeiriai* is the fraternal twins flattery (*kolakeia*) and pleasure (*hêdonê*)—the latter's deep link to *epithumia* (desire) garnering special emphasis in Socrates' exchanges with Callicles (491d–494e).[31] Plato illustrates the relevant contrast with *technai* via cookery and medicine (464d–465b): contra the latter, whose practitioners have the requisite insight, the former masquerades as an expert practice, with operators feigning knowledge of what foods benefit the body. In the case of each *empeiria* (i.e., its practitioners), the key epistemological distinction is between knowledge and conjecture (*stochasamenê*, 464c6). At bottom, cookery—and by extension every *empeiria*—is *kolakeia* (flattery), hence *aischron* (shameful), "because it guesses at what is pleasant with no consideration for what is best" (*hoti tou hêdeos stochazetai aneu tou beltistou*, 465a).[32] While "flattery," or "pandering,"

---

[30] These comments recall the *Apology*'s castigation (e.g., 25a–c) of the free-for-all of Athenian politics at the expense of real expertise; see also Xenophon, *Memorabilia* I.2.9.

[31] See Irwin (1979, 193); Gosling and Taylor (1982, 70).

[32] This remark deepens the comment at 462c, where rhetoric, placeholder anticipatorily for all endeavors of its ilk, is a knack *charitos tinos kai hêdonês apergasias*.

may suffice as a one-word rendering, *kolakeia* in the *Gorgias*' discussion bears instead a strong "implication of moral baseness" (Dodds 1959, 225). If—in the vein of Anaxagoras—everything were mixed indiscriminately, there would be no difference "between matters of medicine and health on the one side, and those of cookery on the other" (*Gorgias* 465d). Plato stakes everything on the contention that all is not mingled in a random way.

Callicles picks up the encomium of pleasure, lauded by Polus (462c), in most dramatic terms. That encomium is paired with Socrates' equally dramatic reduction to absurdity, through the examples of scratching and the catamite, of a view privileging the maximal influx of pleasure irrespective of its content and source (494a–e). Even when faced with that extremity, however, Callicles' stubborn refusal to embrace the evident conclusion that pleasures are not equally choiceworthy, being instead divisible into better and worse varieties, endures for several more pages, until 499b. Genuine benefit, the sole telos of *technai*, is, as we saw, vigorously opposed to pleasure and flattery in Socrates' exchanges with Polus. It is from their elaboration of Plato's demarcation of *technai* from *empeiriai* via the goodness condition that Socrates' two arguments against hedonism in his exchange with Callicles (494e–499b) gain their significance.[33] At the same time, these arguments are central to Socrates' support for the philosophical life. For one concentrating on *eudaimonia*, as does Plato across the corpus, much hinges on rightly apprehending pleasure. That understanding, instilled through *paideia* (education) as he construes it, yields an ability and motivation to cultivate what is allowed and to properly restrict what is harmful.[34]

One may also note rhetoric's grave inadequacies vis-à-vis goodness from another vantage point. As Gorgias stresses, rhetoric is at bottom a competitive endeavor, similar in this regard to athletics (456c–d, cf. 457b).[35] In addition to vying with one another (e.g., for pupils able to afford their services),[36] orators must be ready to compete as needed with experts in other fields. In Gorgias' view, it is a badge of honor for the field of rhetoric that accomplished orators can outpersuade physicians, for instance, in getting people to undertake treatments that doctors themselves commend

---

[33] As Gosling and Taylor (1982) observe, Callicles is not first and foremost a hedonist (77); rather, "the dominant theme here is the ideal of success in rising above the need to submit to laws" (78), i.e., power maximization.

[34] Though the *Philebus* is salient to an inquiry focused on Plato's overall handling of pleasure, neither it nor the *Gorgias*' tie to the *Protagoras* on hedonism will receive sustained attention here. For extensive treatment of pleasure in Plato, see Russell (2005); Gosling and Taylor (1982).

[35] Rhetoric's standing as such figures importantly elsewhere, too, especially in the *Protagoras* and *Hippias Major*.

[36] For Gorgias as clearly motivated in the dialogue "to expand his following of students," see Stauffer (2006, 27).

for patients' benefit. This scenario is illustrated at 456b–c (cf. 448b), where Gorgias boastfully touts his successful persuasion of his own brother Herodicus' patients to do what is genuinely best in the way of drugs (*pharmaka*), surgery (*temnein*), or cautery (*kaein*), where the doctor's own persuasive attempts had failed.[37]

While this might look like a saving grace for rhetoric, for Plato it assuredly is not. From the fact that orators might use their abilities in the service of genuine benefit in one situation, nothing follows necessarily about the next—except that their rationales will shift with the winds due to what conquest, contextually determined, requires. In Plato's view, rhetoricians lack an inner compass ensuring that their prime, unremitting concern is the benefit of those toward whom their activity is directed. Thus, in the medical scenario, Gorgias would be equally equipped and ready to foster (1) what is beneficial; (2) patients' refusal of treatment even if its declining pleased them merely in the short term; or (3) patients' following of measures that, though less burdensome (e.g., less painful), either offer little benefit or are outright deleterious.

Individuals' dealings with their doctors are not an entirely private matter. As physicians are well aware, interactions with patients affect their reputations, hence impact their success in acquiring private patients and civic roles. Having boasted of rhetoric's prowess at individuals' bedsides, Gorgias turns to Athens' conduct of its work as a polis, making his point, once again, through medicine. By Gorgias' lights, if an orator and a physician had to contend before a public gathering over the selection of one as a municipal doctor, the medical expert will always fall to "the one with the ability to speak," who "would be appointed, if he so wished" (456c)—and so on with all other craftsmen (cf. 459a–b).[38]

The *Gorgias* argues persistently that orators' activity, steered by their practical goals, is governed by vanity and greed. Expertise in a legitimate sphere, in contrast, entails the use of one's mastery strictly to further the good, as obtains with physicians, whom the *Gorgias* presents as occupied with patients' welfare.[39] Albeit strictly for appearances' sake according to Polus (461b) and Callicles (482d), Gorgias

---

[37] This Herodicus, like Gorgias, hails from Leontini. One named "Herodicus," who relocated from Megara to Selymbria (*Protagoras* 316e1), is identified as a trainer (*Protagoras* 316d9–e1; *Republic* 406a7–8; *Phaedrus* 227d3–5). Pace Cooper (1997, 508n5) and Dodds (1959, ad loc.), though he handled his own chronic illness (*Republic* 406a–b), this individual is clearly a trainer not a doctor by profession (*paidotribês ôn kai nosôdês genomenos*, *Republic* 406a8; an expert in *gumnastikê*, *Protagoras* 316d9). Following Golden (2008, 148n74), I view "trainer" as a suitable rendering of *paidotribês* and *gumnastês* (whose occupation, *gumnastikê*, or physical training, is the *Gorgias*' bodily *technê* occupied with health's preserving).

[38] On doctors' public and private roles, including that of itinerant physician, see Jouanna (1999, 25–26, 29, 52); regarding nonexperts' choice of municipal doctors, including reference to the *Gorgias*, see ibid. (78–80).

[39] This is, of course, a normative claim about the enterprise at its best, not a descriptive one about how all doctors already function.

concedes that, despite rhetoric's being throughout a competitive endeavor, practitioners should not deploy their skill "to rob doctors or other craftsmen of their reputations" just because they can (457b, cf. 456c–d). There is, however, no built-in hedge against this. Moral relativism, the ethical correlate to rhetorical/sophistic technique, militates against practitioners' self-restraint.[40] Key here is that nothing intrinsic tethers rhetoric's ventures involving *logoi*—whether public displays or private tutelage—to the necessity that the outcome of those efforts be a genuine boon. The situation is all the more urgent and pernicious since orators' direct impact is on the highest of *agatha* (goods), namely the soul. For Plato, therefore, the moral neutrality in this sense of rhetorical praxis initially conceded by Gorgias (456e–457a), and prominent in the orator's own writing (*Encomium of Helen*, secs. 8–14), is an irrefutable sign of its inherent immorality.[41]

The *Gorgias*' goodness condition, supported by the ontological and epistemological columns of the *technê* theory (i.e., the subject-matter and understanding criteria), decimates the alleged value-neutrality undergirding rhetorical/sophistic practice, which rejects the natures of justice and injustice as fixed reference points for decision making in favor of one's negotiating the just and unjust, or good and bad, on each occasion. At the same time, the *Gorgias*' goodness criterion formalizes Plato's attention in earlier dialogues to the idea that discipline-specific benefit is intrinsic to expertise, including the grim results of one's embracing the notion that expertise prepares one equally to do well or ill by those on whom one's activity focuses.[42]

---

[40] On Gorgias' "value-free," or "amoral," notion of rhetoric, see Kahn (1983, 84). On Polus' free admission of this feature, see Anton (1980, 54).

[41] On this feature of Gorgianic rhetoric, see also Murray (2001).

[42] See *Euthydemus* 279a–b, 281a–b; *Hippias Major* 295d–e; *Hippias Minor* 375b–c; *Lysis* 209d–210a; *Republic* 345e–346c. As Chapters 1 and 2 make evident, in giving much weight to their favored practices' being intrinsically value laden, Plato and Hippocratic writings broadly concur. From early on the dialogues make evident that Plato knows much about what doctors typically do and refrain from, and that he is confident in his qualifications to pronounce on medical knowledge and praxis. For stress on Plato's familiarity with medicine within, however, an account that treats his attitude as strictly laudatory, see Jouanna (1999, 5–6, 24, 110, 120, 161–62, 216, 256–58 [mention of a difference involving *empeiria* notwithstanding], 348); despite his claim that "the debate over medicine and philosophy is at the very heart of the Hippocratic Collection as a whole" (259), Jouanna does not expand his notion of this *agôn* to cover Plato's own position. While Plato evinces much awareness of medical views and practices throughout the corpus, he only rarely identifies Hippocrates or other specific medical practitioners by name. For exceptions regarding Hippocrates, see *Protagoras* 311b; *Phaedrus* 270c. *Charmides* 156d mentions no names, with Socrates instead describing his source as "one of the Thracian doctors of Zalmoxis"; it is beyond the scope of the present inquiry to speculate on whether a single person is meant and, if so, who. Notably, Hippocratic authors afford philosophers the same "courtesy" as Plato does medical figures by citing them by name on just three occasions across the corpus (see further Chapter 3)—this despite their extensive engagement with philosophical views and approaches; for this restraint's grounding in "a quite admirable custom of scientific debate . . . in the Periclean Age," see Jouanna (1999, 280).

While the superiority of *technai* to *empeiriai* in the *Gorgias* is absolute, not all *technai* are equal. In Plato's view, it is better to maintain good conditions than to need expert contributions toward their restoration. This state of affairs puts one psychic and one bodily *technê* above the other two. More fundamentally, however, psychic *technai* trump the bodily due to the relative merits of their subject matters, *psuchê* (soul) and *sôma* (body). To unpack the soul's preeminence and set the stage for addressing the relative merits of *technai* later in the chapter, let us now turn to the dialogue's presentation of the soul-body relation and the notion that the soul itself is complex.

3. THE *GORGIAS*' SOUL-BODY DIVISION

Before the *Republic*, including the *Gorgias* (463e–464a, 477b–c, 496e, 501c, 513e), Plato emphasizes a distinction between soul and body. The *Gorgias*' juxtaposition of *technai* and *empeiriai* (463a–465d) foregrounds a soul-body division by partitioning activities into those promoting the good and harm of each. Of subsequent note is 504a–e, where a sound bodily condition is clearly separated from psychic *aretê* (virtue, or excellence) qua justice and self-control. Further, at 505a–b defective states of body and soul—illness on the one side, and injustice and a lack of discipline on the other—are kept quite distinct. Such comments elaborate territory opened to view earlier via the goodness condition on *technai* and the soul-body split.

Built into the divide between *technê* and *empeiria* at its introduction is Plato's contention (464a) that (1) body and soul exist and that (2) each has a good condition of its own. Regarding the latter, there is marked divergence between reality and misleading semblance: "The sort of thing I mean is this. There are many people who appear to be physically fit, and unless one is a doctor or a trainer, one wouldn't readily notice that they are not" (ibid.). Care of the soul (i.e., the *technê* of politics), in turn (464b–465c), splits into legislation and justice, with the latter, qua restorative, being the psychic counterpart of medicine.

It is evident from the start in Plato that while bodily health is significant, psychic welfare exceeds it incomparably given the soul's own immeasurable superiority (*Crito* 47d–e; *Charmides* 156b–158e; *Hippias Minor* 372e–373a).[43] At *Gorgias* 465c–d, soul is said to govern body, and this comment about soul and body's distinctness, with

[43] Both the *Laches* (184d–e) and the *Charmides* (155b–e) concentrate initially on the bodily plane, moving from there to emphasize psychic welfare. In the former, directly succeeding an occupation with the battlefield as traditionally the core milieu of courage, the question becomes "whether anyone present has expertise in the soul's care . . . and has been well taught in this regard" (185e). One also finds movement from a stage-setting focus on bodily matters to a concerted occupation with soul in the *Lysis* (207c–210c) and *Protagoras* (313a–314b).

the former as natural ruler,[44] helps to ground the precedence of the *technê* of judging (*dikaiosunê*, 464b–c) over medicine.

Such talk of a soul-body division in the *Gorgias* might seem to assume that the superior element of this duo is a unidimensional, indivisible ruler. Indeed, this view was often front and center in Socrates' conduct of the elenchus (i.e., his philosophical method of cross-examination and refutation),[45] which focused on the soul as the source of beliefs and on guiding convictions such as "virtue suffices for flourishing." However, the *Gorgias* both maintains a strong soul-body binary and shows Plato trying to combine that with the notion of a complex soul. Though core features of our stances differ, I concur with Cooper (1999b, 75) that the *Gorgias* represents a central juncture in Plato's moral psychology. The soul is complex for its housing of divergent motivational strivings toward what is viewed as but may not actually be a boon. Therefore, before zeroing in on *psuchê*, we must take a closer look at the dialogue's handling of goods (*agatha*).

The requirement that *technai* provide genuine benefit to body or soul as the case may be also necessitates that we further consider the topic of goods. Plato's handling of the *technê-empeiria* divide leads inescapably to the conclusion that, apart from things like *kolakeia* (flattery) that are never salutary, items commonly and unreflectively taken as goods, among them wealth[46]—and even health—are not always good in our hands or for us more generally. As *agatha* means literally "things that are good," they include but range far beyond "goods" in our sense of "tangible items." Plato's aim here is to determine what among things spoken of as good are truly boons, not liabilities, and how the former rank when compared against one another.

4. GOODS SET APART FROM THE GOOD

Many in Plato's time regarded power, especially political and military varieties, as an unqualified good. In fact, "the view that the best good is power over others and the best man the man with this power has deep-seated Greek sources" going back to Homer (Irwin 1979, 116). *Gorgias* 466b inaugurates the dialogue's attempt

---

[44] Cf. Dodds (1959, 231), who finds here the advent in Plato of soul and body as ruler and ruled, respectively.

[45] There has been much scholarly debate over Socrates' vintage philosophical method, including whether he saw himself as appealing to an aspect of us distinct from reason, notably affect. Though investigation of the issue falls outside my purview here, in brief my view is that while Socrates was unlikely to have seen the method thus, to succeed in making interlocutors receptive to the need for further inquiry into relevant values, its use must allow one to disentangle reason from at least one other guiding psychic motivation. Further, the *Gorgias* is where Plato takes his first significant steps toward remedying this insufficiency in Socratic psychology and method.

[46] See Penner (1991, 181); Weiss (1992, 307n18).

to redefine power by reference to the provision of genuine benefit.[47] This effort, launched on the heels of the dialogue's voicing of the *technê-empeiria* grid, links the nature of power thus disclosed to the goodness condition on *technai*. Polus misses the point entirely, likening orators encomiastically to tyrants due to their ability to dominate others through radical constrictions of their agency (466b–c). The view here is Gorgias' in the *Encomium of Helen*, where rhetoric's means, being verbal, are no less compelling than sheer force: "Speech is a powerful ruler (*logos dunastês megas estin*) . . . [whose] achievements are superhuman" (sec. 8); while persuasion lacks "an appearance of compulsion, it has the same power (*tên de dunamin tên autên echei*)" (sec. 12).[48] Plato links his transmutation of power as a necessary boon to its possessor with authoritative figures' grasp of what unqualifiedly benefits us, namely virtue (467a, 468e, 470c).[49] From his standpoint, the tyrant—whose raw authority and indulgence are unchecked, and who does willy-nilly what he finds best but never what would really improve him—is the most miserable of all (473e; cf. *Republic* 587d–e).

When Plato normatively addresses goods' identification and relation to *aretê*, he must consider what existents belong in the discussion and how they ought to be hierarchically arranged. The *Euthydemus* helps set the stage by taking further a firm hierarchical distinction in the dialogues between bodily good and that of the soul. The dialogue's initial list of goods (*agatha*) comprises (1) wealth; (2) health, good looks, and enough of other things the body needs; (3) a noble lineage, power, and honor in one's home country; and (4) being self-controlled, just, and courageous

[47] Cf. Dodds (1959, 232), who rightly observes that "the problem of power-politics" comes to the fore at 466a–467c. In no small part, one may tie the antithetical visions of *eudaimonia* foregrounded in Socrates' dealings with Callicles to different views of power or authority. On the dialogue's mutually incompatible notions of power, see also Tschemplik (2008, 79, 81); Bentley (2003, 102); Segvic (2000, 18–19); Penner (1991, 150, 170, 197); Jaeger (1986a, 129, 132–34, 138). A similar divide obtains in the *Republic*, where Thrasymachus' insistence that the brute force of tyrannical power is the sheer pinnacle of human attainment is fundamentally contested and (Plato hopes) supplanted. According to Annas (1981, 49), Thrasymachus' "ideal is the same as Callicles', but expressed in terms of political power." Their views' distinctness is stressed by Irwin (1979) on 488a–489a, 490a; Dodds (1959, 14–15); Weiss (2007, 93–96). For further comparative discussion, see Fussi (2000, 51); Nehamas (1999, 35–36); Woolf (2000, 33); Tschemplik (2008, 83); Berman (1991, 136n35); Kahn (1983, 100nn46–47); Tenkku (1956, 68n3, 69n1).

[48] Later making his point by reference to medicine, Gorgias contends that "the power of speech bears the same relation to the ordering of the mind as the ordering of drugs bears to the constitution of bodies" (*ton auton de logon echei hê te tou logou dunamis pros tên tês psuchês taxin hê te tôn pharmakôn taxis pros tên tôn sômatôn phusin*, sec. 14). Gorgias' claim for the efficacy of language here is strong indeed. This is not to say that he views soul and body as strictly separate, at least according to sec. 17: "Some people before now, on seeing frightful things, have also lost their presence of mind. . . . And many have fallen into groundless distress and terrible illness and incurable madness." The text and translation of *Encomium of Helen* are those of MacDowell (1993).

[49] Cf. Dodds (1959) on 470a9: Plato's point "is not that power is sometimes bad, but that unprincipled politicians do not really exercise power (since what they do is not *ôphelimon* in Socrates' sense)."

(279a–b). To this list are added (5) wisdom and (6) good luck (279c). Not only does the best fortune attend the work of knowledgeable practitioners (279e–280a), but "if a man has wisdom, he has no need of good fortune in addition" (*sophias parousês, hôi an parêi, mêden prosdeisthai eutuchias*, 280b2–3).[50] Building on this claim about insight, Plato stresses that the fruitful deployment of physical and material goods hinges on psychic determinations. In fact, *agatha* under (1)–(2) above are not valuable intrinsically but precisely insofar as knowledge (*epistêmê*) determines their right usage (281a8–b1). *Gorgias* 467e condenses the *Euthydemus*' list into wealth, health, and wisdom, thus incorporating (1), (2)—exclusively health (soon linked with strength, 468a–b)—and (5) on the foregoing list. While the trio of wealth, health, and knowledge at 467e is apparently different from the body-soul binary used to forge subgroups of *technai* and *empeiriai*, the passage does not conflict with, let alone jeopardize, the dialogue's parsing of the relevant terrain in terms of that bifurcation. Given the tie of wealth to bodily comforts and luxuries on the one side and to psychic inflation via honor on the other, the threefold list at 467e reduces fundamentally to a split between body and soul.

The *Gorgias* addresses not only the *technê-empeiria* divide but also mutual relations among *technai* themselves. Apropos of the latter, at 478b the query is, which of the following activities is the finest (*kalliston*): financial management, medicine, or judging? The answer, of course, will depend on what type of good is taken as supreme. Since possessions and health are not intrinsically good but are useful strictly in virtuous hands, whatever *technê* presides over the soul to maximize its excellence will be preeminent (478d–e). As we shall see, references to medicine figure importantly in Plato's making of this point even as they gesture ahead to its nonsupremacy among *technai* insofar as the soul and its well-being categorically trump *sôma* and its benefit.

The *Gorgias*' account of the best psychic condition, namely *aretê*, places special weight on *sôphrosunê*, a virtue that features the right disciplining of one's desires, and *dikaiosunê*—in this case the virtue of justice (504d–e, 507d–508a, 519a) as distinct from the term's use elsewhere for the *technê* of judging. In the *Gorgias*, having understanding (*epistêmê*) is not directly identified with possessing a third psychic virtue, wisdom (*sophia*), but instead represents the epistemological dimension of Plato's *technê* theory. Monitoring how individuals fare regarding *sôphrosunê* (self-control) and *dikaiosunê* (justice) falls under the *technê* of judging, whose practitioners must apprehend the soul's nature and exemplary condition to weigh rightly punishments and individuals' prospects for psychic restoration. A key link between

[50] Cf. the more abbreviated list at *Hippias Major* 291d, which features wealth, health, and honor from one's fellow Greeks. The illustration involving doctors at *Euthydemus* 280a calls to mind Hippocratic discussions of the relation between *technê* and *tuchê*, including whether they are mutually exclusive (*Ancient Medicine* 12; *Diseases* I 1; *Places in Man* 24, 46; *The Art* 4). On *tuchê* and *to automaton*, see *Diseases* I 7; *Prorrhetic* II 9.

these two *aretai* is that both are accessible only to those whose *epithumiai* (desires) are rightly controlled (507d–e, cf. 504d–e).[51] The dialogue's emphasis on such regulation comes to light in tandem with its rejection of hedonism and closer scrutiny of the soul itself.

5. HEDONISM AND ANTITHETICAL WAYS OF LIFE

While a fuller account of the soul and the virtues must await the *Republic*, to the extent that it touches on the nature of *epithumiai* (desires) and their relation to *akolasia* (self-indulgence), the *Gorgias* contributes importantly to Plato's formation of that account. We are told, for instance, that one wishing to flourish must foster *sôphrosunê* (self-control), whose cultivation requires his "flee[ing] away from lack of discipline (*akolasia*) as fast as his feet will carry him" (507d2). The message here is that one cannot indulge inappropriate desires at all without capitulating to badness within. At 507e–508a we learn that one seeking to be good

> should not allow his appetites to be undisciplined or undertake to fill them up (*ouk epithumias eônta akolastous einai kai tautas epicheirounta plêroun*)—a never-ending evil—and live the life of a marauder. Such a man could not be dear to another man or to a god. . . . Wise men claim that partnership and friendship, orderliness, self-control, and justice (*kosmiotêta kai sôphrosunên kai dikaiotêta*) hold together heaven and earth, and gods and men, and that is why they call this universe a world order (*kosmon*) . . . and not an undisciplined world-disorder (*ouk akosmian oude akolasian*). . . . You [i.e., Callicles] have failed to notice that proportionate equality has great power (*mega dunatai*) among gods and men.

This central passage adumbrates Plato's post-*Gorgias* articulation of Forms, in the *Phaedo*, *Symposium*, and *Republic*, as embodiments of consummate stability, with human (i.e., microcosmic) thriving hinging directly on our successful installation of order within.[52] Further, as we will see in Chapter 3, Eryximachus' take on virtue (*Symposium* 188d), offered through a medical lens on *phusis* (nature) and *eudaimonia* (flourishing), harks back to *Gorgias* 507e–508a in a fashion that helps us pinpoint key differences between his and Plato's approaches.

As we have seen, the *Gorgias* is at pains to keep externals (introduced at 451d–452d) sharply distinct from the good of the virtuous life: the pinnacle of flourishing,

[51] On the close tie between these virtues in the *Gorgias*, see Irwin (1979, 220–21).

[52] Cf. Hall (1971, 215–16).

Plato insists, is attained by one whose soul contains no badness (*eudaimonestatos men ara ho mê echôn kakian en psuchêi*, 478d7–8; see more generally 477a–478e). In addition, *Gorgias* 507e–508a weds excellence and well-being to order, prefacing its observations on *aretê* (virtue) with a reminder that self-control and justice are accessible only to those whose desires are rightly controlled (507d6–e3).

The *Gorgias*' clash, voiced a number of times (487e–488a, 492d, 493d–494a, 497c–d, 499e–500d), between rhetoric and philosophy as anchoring modes of existence—the former, qua *empeiria*, built around pleasure (*hêdonê*) and flattery (*kolakeia*)—is a powerful crystallization of the fact that, most fundamentally, antithetical models of *eudaimonia* are at stake, only one of which captures true flourishing. Their competition on rhetoric's side is particularly evident in Callicles' comments in 484c–486d, whose gist is that while it is charming, even admirable, to pursue philosophy when young, if one wants to succeed as a man—and who in his right mind would not?—one must eventually relinquish philosophy for rhetoric. Such is conduct befitting a free man as opposed to a slave (485b).[53] In contrast, one who pursues philosophy much past childhood

> can't help but turn out inexperienced in everything that a man who's to be admirable and good and esteemed should be experienced in (*anankê pantôn apeiron gegonenai estin hôn chrê empeiron einai ton mellonta kalon k'agathon kai eudokimon esesthai andra*).[54] Such people turn out to be inexperienced (*apeiroi*) in their city's laws and in the kind of speech needed for business dealings, public or private, inexperienced also in human pleasures and appetites (*kai tôn hêdonôn te kai epithumiôn tôn anthrôpeiôn*); in short, inexperienced (*apeiroi*) in the ways of human beings altogether. So, when such folk venture into private or political activity, they become laughingstocks. (484c9–e1)[55]

Elaborating later on what he means by "inexperienced also in human pleasures and appetites," Callicles contends that "in truth . . . wantonness, lack of discipline, and

[53] Cf. Pericles' insistence that political involvement broadly speaking lies at the heart of citizenship in Thucydides' Funeral Oration (*History of the Peloponnesian War* 2.40). From the standpoint of one like Callicles, rhetoric is laudable precisely to the degree that it aids the acquisition and exercise of authority over others. Pace Dodds (1959, 272), Plato takes a page from Isocrates' book here (see *Antidosis*, secs. 263–85) both through his foregrounding of oratory's own *agôn* with him and in Callicles' particular line of attack. That said, Callicles does not follow Isocrates' contention that abstract theorizing is mere stage-setting for his own favored praxis, itself viewed as genuine philosophy (secs. 265, 270–71, 285). On the tie to Isocrates, see also Irwin (1995, 95, 368n2).

[54] Callicles foregrounds here a concern with reputation, i.e., with appearance versus reality.

[55] Note the different construction of *empeiria* from that relied upon by Polus at 448c when tracing the evolutionary trajectory from *empeiria* to *technê*.

freedom, if abundantly available, are virtue and thriving" (*têi alêtheiai . . . truphê kai akolasia kai eleutheria, ean epikourian echêi, tout' estin aretê te kai eudaimonia*, 492c3–6; cf. 492d–e).

The position touted by Callicles here is the antithesis of Platonic self-rule—a notion that anchors Socrates' response and is the psychic or individual counterpart to Plato's emphasis on order and harmony in the subject matter of genuine *technai*. What matters is "being self-controlled and master of oneself, ruling the pleasures and appetites within oneself" (491d10–e1). Against this, Callicles juxtaposes his own view of "what's admirable and just according to nature (*kata phusin*)," namely, "one living rightly must allow his own appetites to intensify as far as possible and not restrain them" (*dei ton orthôs biôsomenon tas . . . epithumias tas heautou ean hôs megistas einai kai mê kolazein*, 491e). The exchange at 491d–e crystallizes the psychic and ethical core of what is disputed. Socrates' response, therefore, is to reiterate (492d) that the point of contention between them is whether the best life revolves around appetites (*epithumiai*) or virtue (*aretê*). Such exchanges make clear that one's views of *eudaimonia* and *phusis* are deeply intertwined, with Callicles' stances on both fundamentally opposed to Plato's own.

At this juncture, Plato complicates the *Gorgias*' picture of the soul.[56] Reference to a *sôma-sêma* split[57] by which "our bodies are our [i.e., our souls'] tombs" (493a2–3) is directly followed by the claim that "the part of our souls in which our appetites reside is the sort of thing that's liable to be persuaded and to shift back and forth" (*tês de psuchês touto en hôi epithumiai eisi tunchanei on hoion anapeithesthai kai metapiptein anô katô*, a3–5).[58] In the point's (albeit minimal) elaboration here, we

---

[56] See also Kurihara (2002, 109); Woolf (2000, 30–31); Cooper (1999b, 63); Irwin (1995, 109, 114); Kahn (1987, 92); Tenkku (1956, 73n1). According to Kurihara, the *Gorgias* contains dual psychologies: though its treatment of unhappiness presents the soul as a "composite of reason and desire," its handling of self-contradiction presumes its indivisibility (115). Although Cooper supports the presence in the *Gorgias* of psychic complexity, he takes the notion to stem from Callicles: while Plato "the author . . . is drawing attention to these novel ideas . . . Socrates does not adopt them as he constructs his own ideal of an 'orderly' life" (63). Though the *Gorgias* enriches Plato's view of *psuchê*, it does not show that he has already "developed the moral psychology of the middle dialogues" (Klosko 1984a, 139n23); Klosko (1993, 34) contends, more cautiously, that there "the beginnings of the doctrine of the multipartite soul appear . . . and so clear intimations of the moral psychology of the middle dialogues."

[57] The source here could be Pythagorean. On that link see Gosling and Taylor (1982, 79); Dodds (1959, ad loc.).

[58] As 493a–b does not speak literally of parts, Irwin's (1979) rendering of *tês . . . psuchês touto* as "that of our soul" is more strictly correct. While for present purposes I follow Zeyl in using the term "part," I do not endorse Dorion's (2012, 41) view that the soul here contains "several 'places,'" favoring instead Irwin's (195) broader "aspects." On the passage's evincing both a soul-body split and appetites' lodging within the former, see Gosling and Taylor (1982, 79–80). For this divide and a complex soul as present in the *Phaedo*, too—this despite the dialogue's well-nigh universal reputation as sharply dualistic due to its harsh words for the body (e.g., 66b5–6)—see Tenkku (1956, 105–7); cf. Kahn (1987, 95n27).

learn that the psychic domain under the spotlight "is souls' undisciplined part, one not tightly closed, a leaking jar, as it were, because it couldn't be filled" (*touto tês psuchês hou hai epithumiai eisi, to akolaston autou kai ou steganon, hôs tetrêmenos eiê pithos, dia tên aplêstian apeikasas*, b1–3).[59]

This image of the leaky jar (elaborated at 493d–494a) is a powerful conjurer of (at least certain) desires' continual lack of satiation—a salient point in the *Republic*'s account of the appetitive aspect of the soul (*to epithumêtikon*) when Plato defends the soul's tripartition (see further Chapter 4). The *Gorgias*' image of the leaky jar—reinforced by that of a sieve (493b–c)—is tantamount to a comment, if not on desire as such, at least on the nature of those yearnings (and their associated pleasure) referenced at 493a. Irwin (1995, 109) rightly deems these appetites "unruly and insatiable,"[60] over against those claiming that desires, particularly for food, drink, and sex, are value-neutral or that in the *Gorgias*, "all human desire aims at 'the [genuine versus apparent] good'" (Lorenz 2006, 28).[61] I concentrate on the aforementioned appetites, which I sometimes reference in aggregate as the Big Three, for their prominence not only in Plato but also in Hippocratic discussions of regimen, diagnosis, and treatment (see Chapter 2). The image of a leaky jar, along with that of a sieve whose contents are steadily dripping out, conveys insatiability wherein a lack of discipline sanctions an existence founded on obsession, self-deceptively experienced as need.

Amid Socrates' contesting of hedonism, when Callicles has finally acknowledged the existence of better and worse pleasures (499b), Plato stresses that a *technê* practitioner is needed to distinguish good pleasures from bad (*Ar' oun pantos andros estin eklexasthai poia agatha tôn hêdeôn estin kai hopoia kaka, ê technikou dei eis hekaston*? 500a4–6; cf. b2–3). On this concession, pleasures are justifiably pursued precisely to the extent that they promote an independently specified good; the illustration is food and drink's deployment with a view toward health and strength (499d4–e1).

---

[59] In modifying the rendering of Zeyl here and in the preceding quotation of 493a, I draw on the translation of Irwin (1979). There is linguistic "play" at 493a–b (with quotation marks used to indicate that it is not merely such) involving terms' descriptive content; on etymology in Plato, see Levin (2001, chaps. 2–3).

[60] See also Irwin (1979, ad loc.); Moss (2007, 238).

[61] On desire's aiming at the actual good—versus whatever we take as such (Singpurwalla 2010, 885)—see also Carone (2004): "One should treat the *epithumiai* of 493a, however blind and raw they may seem, as responding to one's basic desire for the good" (65, cf. 78). For Carone, therefore, the *Gorgias* operates with "a monistic psychology, understood not as one where the mind is a merely cognitive entity devoid of affect, but one where affect itself has become foundational" (70); cf. Parry (1996, 38–39, 65n25). Kamtekar (2006, 148) appeals here to recollection: "As people latently believe truths, so they latently want good things." According to Russell (2005), pleasure in the *Gorgias* and *Phaedo* taken together emerges as a "conditional good" (10–11, 76), hence as "extrinsic" (21–22), i.e., as inherently value-neutral. Cf. Bentley (2003, 100), according to whom the *Gorgias* opposes not acting on *epithumiai* as such but merely "pursuing one's desires in an appetitive manner." For *erôs* in the *Gorgias*, *Symposium*, and *Republic* as "value-neutral," see Woolf (2000, 32n44).

Once pleasures' hierarchical arrangement is conceded, rhetoric's essential subordination to the sphere of expertise that masters this becomes inescapable.[62]

At 500b Plato recurs yet again to the *technê-empeiria* distinction of 464b–465d, instantiated there via medicine's categorical surpassing of cookery: while the latter's sights are set on pleasure alone, the former concentrates on the good (*kai etithên tôn men peri tas hêdonas tên mageirikên empeirian alla ou technên, tôn de peri to agathon tên iatrikên technên*, 500b3–5; see also 513d–e). Though the passage accurately reprises what transpired in Socrates' exchange with Polus, the earlier binary of pleasure and the good is not integrated with the distinction now being made between pleasures that are better and worse. Rather, in the course of 500b, the rubric of "better and worse" moves silently from the newly introduced distinction between good and bad pleasures (*hêdonai*) back to the earlier focus on good (i.e., benefit) versus bad (i.e., harm), the latter stemming from a focus on gratification through *kolakeia* (flattery). One may now readily deem the latter to involve bad pleasures (e.g., those associated with drunkenness). What, however, constitute good *hêdonai*?

As most scholars rightly contend, the *Gorgias* rejects hedonism.[63] This, the dialogue makes clear, is compatible with there being certain pleasures that are good. According to Gosling and Taylor (1982, 80), in the *Gorgias* "at least *some* bodily pleasures [i.e., those conducive to health] make *some* contribution to the overall good" (italics in original). In the *Gorgias*' framework centered on virtue, it seems odd to call the pleasure associated with moderate eating a good one, since it does not directly promote or reflect *aretê*. Taken in isolation, 499d, on which Gosling and Taylor rely, seems to support their interpretation, for Callicles answers "yes" to the queries, "Beneficial [pleasures] are the ones that produce something good, while the bad ones are those that give rise to something bad?" and "Now, do you mean pleasures like the ones we were just now mentioning in connection with the body, those of eating and drinking?"

At 503c–d, however, Socrates elaborates on these remarks, claiming emphatically that "a man should satisfy those of his appetites that, when they are filled up, make us better human beings (*hai men tôn epithumiôn plêroumenai beltiô poiousi ton anthrôpon*), not those that make us worse (*hai de cheirô, mê*), and this is a matter of *technê*."[64] Gosling and Taylor (1982, 61) implausibly view Plato's focus in 503d–508c

[62] The claim at 499b that *hêdonai* qualitatively diverge helps pave the way for the *Republic* (580d), where each psychic dimension has its pleasures and the most elevated kind attend *aretê*.

[63] Though I do not further address the issue here, I concur with the balance of scholars that the *Protagoras* supports hedonism: see, e.g., Moss (2006, 509); Irwin (1995, 111, 114); Tenkku (1956, 23, 37–40, 57). For a view according to which Plato rejects hedonism in both dialogues, see Jaeger (1986a, 141–43).

[64] Zeyl's translations, "make him better" and "make him worse," are vague in a way that is philosophically detrimental here.

as the plane of bodily desires—this despite the passage's substantial occupation with soul. Virtue, the province of soul, is the sole unqualified good. As such, it is the one thing whose acquisition renders each of us a better *person* (*beltiô . . . ton anthrôpon*). Most likely, then, Plato has in mind as "good" those pleasures that directly promote a virtuous existence.[65] Moreover, 503d1–2 states that determinations of pleasures' caliber are the province of *technê*, hence a demanding endeavor, which is hard to reconcile with Gosling and Taylor's interpretation.

As Kahn (1987, 91) observes, the *Gorgias* is the first dialogue to include "any systematic discussion of desire."[66] Much, however, remains unclear regarding desire and pleasure. A notable example is the dialogue's lacking an account of reason (92)—this being a needed step for any specification of it as possessing desires and pleasures of its own, as occurs in the *Republic* (580d). Plato's post-*Gorgias* clarification of such matters unfolds in tandem with further inquiry into desire and pleasure.[67]

6. ORDER AS THE KEY TO VIRTUE AND THE GOOD

Respecting the *Gorgias*' condition that *technai* offer boons, at 503c–504a Plato closely ties goodness to order and harmony.[68] As we will see in Chapter 4, this link—including (1) a macrocosm-microcosm analogy centered on Forms' ordered perfection and (2) maximal human assimilation thereto—becomes key to the *Republic*'s handling of *auto to agathon* (literally, "the good itself").[69] Such a tie, intimated in the *Gorgias*, between harmonious organization and the good renders the good wholly incompatible with a pleasure-based approach to *eudaimonia*. In the *Symposium*, Eryximachus claims to have mastered the demarcation of appetites that improve one from those that harm, folding it into his cosmological story, which is itself substantially a defense of an existing aristocratic model of male homosexual ties between *erastês* (lover) and *erômenos* (beloved). As it turns out (see Chapter 3), however, he lacks the *technê* that alone enables those determinations.

The notion that all *technai* orbit around order and organization provides a hint that the subject matter whose right structuring occupies the political *technê* (i.e.,

---

[65] Cf. Irwin (1995, 109–10), for whom the *Gorgias* accommodates "rational and non-rational desires" that naturally diverge.

[66] See also North (1966, 159).

[67] On the *Gorgias*' incompleteness regarding desire, see Irwin (1995, 117). Russell (2005, 48–76) ends his account of the dialogue by claiming that additional work is requisite on the nature and merit of *hêdonê* (76). On the need for further investigation of "organic" and "non-organic" pleasures, which transpires after the *Gorgias*, see Dodds (1959, 309).

[68] Cf. Berman (1991, 135).

[69] See, e.g., *Republic* 508e.

legislation and justice taken together) is the soul based on its having multiple aspects that can be configured for better or worse, namely, in a more or less orderly fashion. *Gorgias* 503c–504e, which expressly ties pleasure to the soul, makes evident that a deeper inquiry into pleasure must be embedded in the same caliber of inquiry into the soul. While the *Gorgias* does not concertedly explore the psychic plane, Plato works up to such comments as he does provide by reference, once again, to medicine, noting that practitioners of medicine and gymnastics "doubtless give order and organization to the body" (504a). Bodies are grouped together here with artifacts (e.g., dwellings and ships) and are set apart from souls in a fashion underscoring soul and body's distinctness and soul's incalculable superiority (504a–b). The term for rightly structured bodily states is "healthy, due to which health and remaining bodily excellences [in particular strength, 504b9] arise in it" (504c). By analogy, "organized and orderly conditions of soul are called 'lawful' and 'law,' from which people become law-abiding and orderly. The conditions themselves are justice and self-control" (*tais de ge tês psuchês taxesi kai kosmêsesin nomimon te kai nomos, hothen kai nomimoi gignontai kai kosmioi; tauta d' estin dikaiosunê te kai sôphrosunê*, 504d1–3). The *technê* presiding over psychic remediation must pull out all the stops to supplant *adikia* (injustice) and *akolasia* (self-indulgence) with *dikaiosunê* (justice) and *sôphrosunê* (self-control) (504d–e).[70] Importantly—for both the *Gorgias* and later dialogues—the claim that "organized and orderly conditions of soul are called 'lawful' and 'law'" (504d1–2), with its attention to self-governance, clearly suggests that while a soul-body divide is foundational to the *Gorgias*' account of *technai* and its *technai-empeiriai* grid, the dialogue's coverage of psychic terrain is more complex than meets the eye.

Plato's contrast between the *sôphrôn* (self-controlled one) and the *akolastos* (self-indulgent person) at *Gorgias* 493d7 represents the clash between philosophy and rhetoric as reflecting two categorically opposed views of *eudaimonia*. Tellingly, *kosmioi* (literally, "orderly ones") stands for *sôphrones* (self-controlled people) in his framing of the same contrast at d2, which adumbrates the *Republic*'s unrelenting espousal of the orderly soul as good.[71] On this foundation—and continuing the *Gorgias*' stress on *sôphrosunê*, which sets the stage for the *Symposium*—506d–e notes the integral tie between order and organization on the one side and *aretê* on the other:

---

[70] At 504d (cf. 511b–c), Plato identifies that ability as the province of "the orator who is skilled and good (*technikos te kai agathos*)." How persuasive speech of this caliber should be construed is not clarified until the *Phaedrus*, with sociopolitical contextualization in the *Statesman*.

[71] For stress on order, see more generally *Gorgias* 493c–494a.

the orderly soul is self-controlled, and the self-controlled soul is good (506e–507a).[72] Plato's expressly connecting order, self-control, and the good represents a step forward, which is deepened by his further claim (507c) that the *sôphrôn* (self-controlled one), being unqualifiedly good, is therefore *eudaimôn* (a flourishing person). The grasp of desire and pleasure that would fuel the *technê* par excellence of politics is identical with the insight steering practitioners' own self-control.[73]

Insofar as insatiable desires under the Big Three have their motivational origin in the soul (493a–d), bodily consumption—including the lead-up thereto via sensory location of promising objects—does not impact *sôma* (body) alone. It also gratifies and nurtures this dimension of *psuchê* (soul), which, being insatiable and blind to all else, aims solely at these desires' "fulfillment." The *Gorgias*' strong pointers to a more complex view of *psuchê* notwithstanding, further defense of the primacy of self-rule, with *eudaimonia* built thereon, must await the *Republic*'s argument for a tripartite soul whose aspects are rightly configured from an absolute vantage point.

7. THE *GORGIAS* ON PUNISHMENT

Although the soul is the *Gorgias*' ultimate concern, the body, in particular its sound condition, is not irrelevant. Plato has nothing against health per se. Indeed, since physical well-being is distinctly preferable to deficient conditions, health's restoration should be pursued all things equal; however, this caveat kicks in for Plato, particularly in the *Republic*, more often than most then and now would concede. Those aiming to address deficiencies in material attainment (i.e., poverty) and the physical defect of disease rush to experts in financial management and medicine respectively (477e–478a). At 478c–d we find that while patients' withholding themselves from medical care through fear of pain might have more passing enjoyment, in the long run medical treatment maximizes the good of health, with the one neglecting it

[72] On Plato's occupation with "psychological structure" as emerging for the first time in the *Gorgias*, with soul's good condition tied to correctness of organization, see Gosling and Taylor (1982, 80–81; cf. 61). As Sedley (2009, 63) observes, 506c–508b makes clear "why appetite control is itself the basis of the whole of virtue: it is from moderation, the control of the appetites, that justice, reverence and the other virtues directly follow. In short, progress from vice to virtue proceeds via the painful appetite-denial that is punishment, to moderation of appetites and thereby on to the rest of virtue." On the *Gorgias*' account, one who reliably behaves justly can do so only if he is already *sôphrôn*. On *sôphrosunê* as primary there, see also Russell (2005, 67); Irwin (1979, 221); Hall (1971, 213); White (1990, 123–25; though he later claims merely that "if a man wants to be happy . . . he must pursue temperance," 126). North (1966) at once bases virtues' unity in the *Gorgias* on *sôphrosunê*—"the *sôphrôn* person does what is fitting in every situation and is therefore pious, just, and brave" (164n29)—which conveys the priority of this *aretê*, and states that it and *dikaiosunê* are interchangeable or nearly so (161n19).

[73] See also the reference at 510a to the *technê* allowing one to keep injustice far from oneself.

steeped in misery. Ordinarily, medical treatment is unpleasant but beneficial (i.e., it satisfies the goodness criterion for that *technê*, 478b), since patients rid themselves of something deleterious in the service of health, a bodily boon. Though it is preferable not to be ailing such that treatment, with its attendant pain, is requisite, people accept this pain for the sake of health's restoration. Applying the same point to *eudaimonia* proper, one who suffers no psychic corruption is best off (478d7–e1). In the runner-up scenario, an unjust person throws himself into eliminating his depravity, tolerating all attendant discomfort for virtue's sake (478e1–4).

Inasmuch as soul trumps body in merit, rendering far more important its good and bad conditions, the *Gorgias* is concerned not only with the virtue of justice, closely joined to self-control, but also with the restorative *technê* of judging should psychic conditions need redressing. If souls' good standing is all that ultimately counts, the question becomes, where does one bring "those who conduct themselves unjustly and self-indulgently" (*tous adikountas kai tous akolastainontas*, 478a4) for the elimination of their corruption? Syntactic parity with the case of medicine, where the ailing are brought to doctors, requires that the proper answer here be not "the courts" but "judges," and it is indeed to judges (*para tous dikastas*, a5) that the depraved are conveyed. Recurring to the point shortly thereafter, Plato asserts that one who has acted unjustly should, of his own accord, "head straight to a judge as though he were going to a doctor, anxious that the disease of injustice shouldn't be protracted and cause his soul to fester incurably" (480a7–b2)—the goal being to "pay his due and get well" (c4–5).[74] One whose soul is corrupt must not capitulate to fear but rather "present himself for remediation with grace and courage as to a doctor for cautery and surgery, pursuing what's good and admirable with no heed at all to the pain" (480c6–8).

Though being unjust is "the worst thing of all for the wrongdoer" (509b1–2, cf. 468e–469c), the vicious individual's situation becomes graver still if he should happen to avoid "paying what's due" (509b2–3).[75] Regarding health and physicality, agents of servile practices aim to gratify whatever *epithumiai* (appetites) their targets happen to have. Abetted by appetites' own tending to insatiability (*dia tên aplêstian apeikasas*, 493b3)—illustrated by the sieve and the leaky jar (493a–c)—these efforts cause illness. Excess consumption of food, for instance, at once increases people's girth and "destroy[s] their original flesh" (518c).[76] If and when such

---

[74] Positive medical terminology here contrasts with the fusing of legal language to that of disease at 480a8–b1.

[75] Socrates had said at 458a8–b1 that worst of all was false belief about the just and unjust; given judgments' tie to character, his focus at 509b, there is no real inconsistency. On this issue see also Moss (2007, 233).

[76] Cf. *Protagoras* 353c–354b. Although we diverge on the issue of appetitive desires' intrinsic nature, on the broad "causal relation" at issue here, cf. Parry (1996, 39–40).

people drag themselves to doctors, either the needed measures are painful (contra the enjoyment, albeit short-term, of their earlier indulgences) or their conditions have become incurable. Rather than taking responsibility for their own self-indulgence (*akolasia*) and gleaning the defects of those who had previously catered to them, people regularly blame the "messenger," namely the physician now attending them (518c–d).[77] Applying this point to the soul (518e–519b), Plato contends that due to a temporal gap between corruption's sowing and its most virulent manifestation, politician-orators' actual responsibility for the city's psychic ills is wrongly allocated to figures who genuinely seek their amelioration. One cannot help thinking, as Plato doubtless was, of Socrates' having been wrongly held to account by his native Athens for corruption well sown by others before he came to prominence.

On the plane of illness, when plying folk with food and drink would be harmful or fail to aid, these should not be provided, since existence with a markedly ailing body is not worthy of prolongation (504e–505a). Continuations of existence are unmerited all the more in cases of irreparable psychic flaws. Key here is that not all unjust and self-indulgent folk can be brought or restored to virtue. Due to soul's fundamental superiority over body, combined with the fact that not all psychic flaws are remediable, under certain conditions a life would not be worth continuing—a truth that obtains irrespective of one's health standing (511d–512d). Unlike the *Republic*, however, where the judge's role is to proclaim souls remediable or not as the case may be (409e–410a), the *Gorgias* stresses that those functioning as judges will concentrate first and foremost on the amelioration of psychic defects, with incurability the determination only after that effort has failed. As we will see, in this respect among others, the *Gorgias* is closer to the *Laws* than to the *Republic*.

As to the content of punishments, the *Gorgias*' account concentrates on familiar penalties ranging from fines and the seizing of property to flogging, imprisonment, banishment, and death (480c–d), all of which involve the material/physical plane.[78] Although the soul is far more valuable than the body, the worst punishment for psychic offenders (execution), like the least severe (whipping), involves physical pain. From the standpoint of the present inquiry, this is a salient pointer to soul-body complexity in that penalties that may appear physical in their very nature are intended to help reshape pertinent psychic inclinations.

Proportionality between the level of defect and punishment will be observed, with execution reserved, as in the *Republic* and *Laws*, for those whose injustice is

---

[77] The Hippocratic Corpus distinguishes cases where the author, naturally an exemplary practitioner, is on the scene right away from those where he follows an inferior, making a similar point to the *Gorgias* about patients' wrongly blaming true experts for the lousy states that they have reached (*Regimen* III 70).

[78] Cf. Brickhouse and Smith (2002, 30–31; 1997, 102–4).

severe and unremitting. Late in the *Gorgias*, the setting of punishment (523a–526d) allegedly shifts to the afterlife in what is typically called its closing "myth." While this section contains mythological material, including those named as judges (Rhadamanthus, Aeacus, Minos; 523e–524a), Socrates pointedly introduces the account to Callicles as a *logos* (rational account), not a *muthos* (fictional tale): "Listen . . . to a very fine account. You'll consider it a mere tale, I believe, but I think it's an account, for what I'm about to say I will tell you as true" (*Akoue . . . mala kalou logou, hon su men hêgêsêi muthon, hôs egô oimai, egô de logon; hôs alêthê gar onta soi lexô ha mellô legein*, 523a1–3).[79]

In keeping with the discussion's status as nonfictional, the sequel contains allusions to key features of embodied, communal life, including assessments grounded in law (*nomos*, 523a5) and made by judges (*dikastas*, e7; cf. 478a, 480a–c), with punishments tailored—as before (511d–512d)—to offenders' prospects for psychic repair (i.e., curability or incurability, 525b). Further, though their names hail from mythology, the judicial personages are described as a select few whose capacity for right assessment is not unqualified but rather surpasses existing practice by penetrating beyond appearances to psychic realities (523e–526c). This is precisely what one would hope for from exemplary human judges, whose essential role the dialogue previously stressed. In fact, this portion of the *Gorgias* reads rather like a statement of wish on Plato's part, regarding this life, that judges' assessments not be steered off course by nonpsychic goods of offenders like "attractive bodies, good stock, and wealth" (523c5–6). The dialogue's concluding remarks, too, focus squarely on this life (527b1–2) and secondarily (if at all) on the hereafter.[80]

Presaging the *Republic*'s integral linkage of *phusis* (nature) and *trophê* (nurture)/*paideia* (education), Plato lodges the causation of psychic defects with *phusis* and people's habitual involvements: "All that's in the soul is evident after it has been stripped naked of the body, both things that are natural to it and things that have happened to it, things that the person came to have in his soul due to his pursuit

---

[79] While some recent accounts continue to see this portion of the dialogue as genuinely focused on the afterlife (see Moss 2007, 232n9; Tschemplik 2008, 80–81, 93; Brickhouse and Smith 2002, 35), other discussions, such as Fussi's (2001; cf. 2000, 51), concentrate on its role vis-à-vis embodiment. As Sedley (2009) maintains, it is indisputable that "the myth and the main body of the dialogue are meant to be read in the light of each other" (53); in fact, the myth on punishment of the psychically incurable "fills a gap . . . left" in the dialogue's earlier account of this salient topic (60). In Sedley's view, the myth's tight philosophical link to what precedes (particularly the segment involving Polus, 53–54), combined with its possible standing as an illustration of the genuine rhetoric for which the *Gorgias* calls (66n23), sheds light on why Socrates dubs the account a *logos* rather than a *muthos*.

[80] I must therefore diverge from Irwin (1979), for whom the myth contends that "we can justifiably treat someone as incurable only after his death" (245) and that "the incurables are examples, not to those on earth, but only to the dead" (246).

of each objective (*ta te tês phuseôs kai ta pathêmata ha dia tên epitêdeusin hekastou pragmatos eschen en têi psuchêi ho anthrôpos*)" (524d4–7). As at 480c–d, but more explicitly in this later *logos*, the goal of punishment is specified as psychic improvement. If substantive enhancement is not a viable option, execution (in the dialogue's earlier terms, 480d) or souls' interminable punishment (as the point is framed at 525a–526b) is required for deterrence's sake. Rightly gauged punishment of the unjust falls to the supreme human endeavor—in the *Gorgias*, *politikê*, which itself remains to be forged (527b–d)—and so it will in the *Republic*, where philosophers who rule and exact justice practice the *technê* par excellence.[81] The *Gorgias* thus inaugurates Plato's lifelong concern not simply with the virtue of justice but with the nature, content, and outcomes of punishment (i.e., judging, along with penalties' implementation).

8. *GORGIAS* 517D–518A AND THE DIALOGUE'S FINAL HIERARCHY OF HUMAN ENDEAVORS

The final two sections of this chapter both tie together what we have learned thus far about human activities' arrangement in the *Gorgias* and incorporate further variables so that we gain a more comprehensive picture of their reciprocal ties. This exercise will also give us a baseline for approaching Plato's assessments and rankings of human pursuits in later dialogues. With this twofold goal in mind, let us consider the *Gorgias*' final hierarchy among *technai* specifically and endeavors generally, including the picture, albeit sketchy, that one obtains of the preeminent *technê* of politics, which 464b–465c introduces as comprising both legislation and justice. Since most of the dialogue's handling of psychic *technai* concentrates directly on judging alone,[82] this reminder of politics' twofold composition is advised.

By the dialogue's close we have learned a number of things about practices' mutual rankings. Above all, we see that the fundamental divide is between *technai* (rational purposive disciplines) and *empeiriai* (knacks). Among knacks, those catering to the soul are more harmful than those occupied with the body due to the soul's vast superiority in merit. The class of *technai*, too, demarcates activities devoted to soul, namely legislation and justice, from those occupied with the body. Respecting *technai* of bodily welfare, though the *Gorgias* concentrates more on medicine than

[81] Though justice alone and not also self-control is singled out at the dialogue's close (527e), there is no reason to think that the two *aretai* remain anything other than closely aligned.

[82] According to Moss (2007, 234n14), while the *Gorgias* itself does not treat legislation, 521d may allude to Socrates' practice of *nomothetikê* insofar as he "aims to instill or maintain virtue in people's souls." Sedley (2009, 65) views the *Gorgias*' use of the Socratic elenchus as spanning the two psychic *technai* of judging and legislation.

gymnastics, the latter surpasses the former (520b) to the extent that a good condition's preservation is preferable to its needing post-disturbance restoration. On this general principle, which applies to the soul as well, the *technê* of gymnastics benefits indirectly at medicine's expense instead of emerging as superior from head-to-head comparisons of their content. Further, with the *Symposium* and *Republic* in view, it is worth noting that the *Gorgias* subordinates medicine expressly to gymnastics but not directly to medicine's psychic counterpart, the *technê* presiding over justice.

When Plato considers endeavors occupied with the physical/material sphere, gymnastics and medicine govern the rest in aggregate (517d–518a). This last

> is the subservient part that enables us to provide our bodies with food whenever they're hungry or with drink whenever they're thirsty, and whenever they're cold, with clothes, wraps, shoes, and other things our bodies come to have an appetite for (*all' hôn erchetai sômata eis epithumian*). . . . It's not at all surprising that one doing such work should think himself a caretaker of the body and be considered such by all others who don't know that over and above all these practices there's a *technê*, that of gymnastics and medicine, that really does care for the body and is entitled to rule all these crafts and use their products because of its knowledge of what food or drink is good or bad for bodily excellence (*tis para tautas hapasas technê gumnastikê te kai iatrikê, hê dê tôi onti ge estin sômatos therapeia, hênper kai prosêkei toutôn archein pasôn tôn technôn kai chrêsthai tois toutôn ergois dia to eidenai hoti chrêston kai ponêron tôn sitiôn ê potôn estin eis aretên sômatos*), a knowledge that all the others lack. That is why the other crafts are slavish, subservient, and ill-bred, and why gymnastics and medicine are rightly mistresses over them.

In addition to the new point made about medicine and gymnastics' co-governance of other activities occupied with material/physical existence, this relatively late passage in the dialogue brings together several of its key themes. On the tie between soul and body, Plato had earlier referenced "the part of our souls in which our appetites reside," which "is the sort of thing that's liable to be persuaded and to shift back and forth" (493a3–5). He then identified this element as "souls' undisciplined part, one not tightly closed, a leaking jar, as it were" (493b1–3). In the *Gorgias*, this psychic complexity is not steadily maintained, as 517d4–5 identifies the body, not an element of soul, as that from which appetite stems (*all' hôn erchetai sômata eis epithumian*). This remark suggests that while Plato is strongly drawn to a more complex picture of *psuchê*, he has yet to commit to it decisively.

Second, the repetition of "whenever" (*ean*, appearing thrice at 517d3–4) points to a lack of discrimination in the identity, amount, and timing of what subordinate activities provide when unsupervised by gymnastics or medicine.[83] This heedlessness meshes with Plato's opposition of benefit to pleasure and pandering throughout the *Gorgias*. That medicine, as a bodily *technê*, can be no final human arbiter the dialogue makes evident through the primacy it grants to soul and what cares for it. The attention to context dependency in 517d is a useful reference point as we consider Plato's handling of medicine's limitations in subsequent chapters. As the Hippocratic Corpus makes clear, doctors' contextual assessments of what is needed in particular situations are key. When the *Gorgias*' account of desire and pleasure is applied to medical writings (see Chapter 2), it becomes crystal clear that medicine's context dependency is itself no panacea even within its own domain of bodily care.

Third, 517d–518a emphasizes an appearance-reality divide insofar as those practicing and admiring servile pursuits wrongly believe their favored activities to foster bodily well-being independently (517e2–518a1). The *Gorgias*' opposing at 517e2–518a1 of ignorance and *doxa* to genuine knowledge—cognitive states occupied with appearance and reality, respectively—harks back to the understanding condition on *technai* previously introduced (see especially 454c–d, 464a–465d). Unlike Gorgianic rhetoricians, craftspeople like weavers, cobblers, and tanners make non-illusory positive contributions. They fail to grasp, however, that their highly circumscribed expertise is necessarily subordinate to *gumnastikê* (physical training) and *iatrikê* (medicine), which preserve and restore, respectively, a sound bodily condition.[84] Regarding an awareness of limitations, as with context dependency, we will subsequently see that medicine itself is also rightfully subject to critique.

Finally, 517d–518a represents a notable break from earlier dialogues' regular presentation of medicine as one craft among many, hence positioned alongside manual endeavors like shoemaking.[85] While there is equalizing material in the *Gorgias* as well (455a–c, 456c, 490b–491a, 504a–b), the overall trend, reprised at 517d–518a, is decisively toward medicine's resting above ordinary crafts. Not even the praxis of

---

[83] Cf. 518c.

[84] Though the term *technê* appears twice in 517d–518a in the loose, inherited sense (517e4, 7) noted when this chapter began, it is evident that Plato is thinking of *empeiriai* in the sense of 463a–465d: (a) these activities' servile standing is emphasized; (b) cookery, whose pursuer is mentioned at 517e1, was pointedly subsumed under *empeiriai* at the earlier juncture; (c) the understanding condition on *technai* is at the fore (517e4, 7, 518a1); and (d) whether, when, and in what respects benefit occurs (i.e., the goodness condition) is also central (517d3–5). Thus, Stauffer's (2006, 156) claim that Plato makes here "significant changes in the [earlier] schema" involving *technai* and *empeiriai* is unfounded, and Tenkku's (1956, 81n1) interpretive gloss (cookery is "included [at 517e among] inferior arts") is insufficiently precise. In fact, such semantic coexistence is the rule when Plato gives existing terms new senses in keeping with his own philosophical ends; examples besides *technê* include *metechein* and *temnein*. Thus, Plato's deployment of *technê* at *Gorgias* 517e typifies a pattern in his deployment of select terms whose referents come to play central roles in his own philosophical theories. See further Levin (2008; 2001).

[85] See *Charmides* 161e–162a; *Laches* 185c–d, 195b–196a, 198d–199a; *Protagoras* 322c–e; *Ion* 537c–540e.

medicine thus elevated, however, has self-control and justice lodged under its subject matter (*peri ti*). These crucial virtues (*aretai*) belong instead under the aegis of politics (*politikê*).

9. THE *GORGIAS*' PREEMINENT *TECHNÊ* OF POLITICS

While previous dialogues reference the notion of an overarching *technê*,[86] the *Gorgias*' conception of the *technê* of politics is an innovation. Since the *Gorgias*' political *technê* is occupied with the highest good, namely soul and its optimal functioning, we must take stock of where the dialogue leaves us regarding this preeminent *technê*, said to encompass legislation—a shadowy activity here—and judging with its concomitant, punishment (464b–c, 517a).[87]

At 513e, we learn that the terrain of *politikê*, in general terms, is "care for the city and its citizens with the goal of making citizens as good as possible." Plato's focus on politics' meeting the goodness condition is subsequently reinforced (515c, 516b). In addition, he foregrounds expressly that to promote citizens' own goodness, the goal of *politikê*, one must be good (i.e., virtuous) oneself (515c5). Further, a mention of doctors' acting in both private and public roles (514d–e)[88] aids Plato in making his point that private work with individuals is the prerequisite and foundation for working on the "big jar" that is the community (514e).[89] Interestingly, while the medical analogy here speaks of efforts as directed to all, irrespective of sociopolitical standing (i.e., "slave or free . . . visitors or townspeople," 514d8–e2; cf. 515a7),[90] *politikê* itself is said to work on citizens alone (515c).[91] As we will see in Chapter 6, Plato's handling of citizens, metics (resident aliens), and slaves in the *Laws* shows this gap start to close between the scope of those treated by doctors and the range of those targeted by positive sociopolitical efforts, with salutary effects on his ability to make a case for the genuine unity of Magnesia, that dialogue's optimal community.

Featuring once again the goodness condition on *technai* applied to psychic welfare on a sociopolitical scale, but framing the point more closely in the terms of

---

[86] *Charmides* 170b–171c; *Laches* 196d, 199c; *Euthydemus* 290b–d. On this topic see also Irwin (1979, 117, 238).

[87] For this *technê* identified as true rhetoric meeting the goodness condition, see 503a–c, 504d–e, 508b–c, 517a, 527c.

[88] On the latter, see also 455b; both roles are mentioned at *Statesman* 259a.

[89] For broad contextualization of the saying (*to legomenon*) "learn pottery on the big jar," see Dodds (1959, 355).

[90] Such a stance on the part of Hippocratic doctors leads Jouanna (1999, 116) to tout their "humanism" (see also 112–15, 125). This term may be applied to the conversational praxis of Socrates, who was eager to pursue the elenchus with any takers whatsoever (*Apology* 23b, 30a; *Laches* 186b). Cf. *Meno* 71e–72c, where Socrates presses the point that *aretê* is one and the same by nature irrespective of differences in the age, sex, or sociopolitical standing of its human possessors.

[91] See more generally 515c–517c.

462c–465d, Socrates states that the care for city that he envisions is "that of striving valiantly with the Athenians to make them as good as possible (*tên tou diamachesthai Athênaiois hopôs hôs beltistoi esontai*), like a doctor"—contra toadying to them "for their gratification" (*pros charin*; 521a3–5). Likely stunning those aware of his lack of political involvement save obligatory forays, Socrates contends that "I'm one of a few Athenians—I don't say I'm the sole one ever, but I'm certainly unique among our contemporaries—to take up and practice the true political *technê* (*epicheirein têi hôs alêthôs politikêi technêi kai prattein ta politika*)" (521d6–8).[92]

Despite persisting unclarity in the *Gorgias* on the precise content of *politikê*, by the dialogue's end we know that the care and guarding of souls is lodged with legislation and judging, whose satisfaction of highly normative criteria warrants their designation as soul-occupied *technai* conjoined, in a fashion not yet specified, under politics. Even as the *Gorgias* makes clear that an integral tie exists between legislation and judging insofar as both fall under politics, which has yet to exist in its genuine form (527d, cf. 517a), the dialogue stresses the distinctness of the psychic *technai* falling under *politikê* (463a–465d, 520a–b). The precise domains of legislation and judging remain unclear in the *Gorgias*, as does, therefore, whether these are ultimately two vantage points through which one may view a single *technê*. It is thus left to the *Republic*, *Statesman*, and *Laws* to elaborate how legislation and judging figure in political expertise.[93]

The *Gorgias*' lack of detail on how its two psychic *technai* operate is coupled with even less clarity on the side of corresponding *empeiriai*, sophistry and rhetoric, alleged to correspond to legislation and judging, respectively. Officially, rhetoric's good-fostering counterpart is judging. As, however, the *Gorgias* does not differentiate the natures of rhetoric and sophistry, the *agôn* (rivalry) regarding *phusis* and *eudaimonia* here is ultimately between rhetoric/sophistry and *politikê*.[94]

---

[92] As Irwin (1979, 240) observes, strictly speaking Socrates "does not say that he *has* this craft, but that he 'undertakes' (or 'attempts,' *epicheirein*) it, looking for its principles" (italics in original; cf. 1995, 371n21). Irwin's (241) conclusion that, regarding politics, one may not properly view the *Gorgias* as "any more Platonic than Socratic" is, however, underdetermined by the evidence, which centrally includes Plato's own *technê* theory debuted there.

[93] The *Gorgias*' splitting of politics into legislation on the one side, and judging accompanied by punishment on the other, suggests that its closest fit is with the *Laws*, above all its deployment of legislative preludes; cf. Plato's mention of both "persuasion and constraint" (*peithontes kai biazomenoi*, 517b6) as means of fostering psychic improvement, the sole *ergon* of a good citizen (c1–2).

[94] Although rhetoric is the dialogue's focus by way of critique, Plato signals that its *technê* grid applies equally to another of his rivals, poetry, which is pointedly exposed as *hêdonê*-promotion dolled up in verse (501e–502d). As Sedley (2009, 70) observes, poetry is linked with rhetoric insofar as they are both "civic institutions that are disparaged in the *Gorgias*." In the *Republic*, Plato subjects poetry to its own systematic critique via the *Gorgias*' *technê* grid; for discussion see Levin (2001, chap. 5). Cf. Jaeger (1986a, 144), for whom the *Republic*'s challenge to poetry "is of the same type as his attack on sophistry and rhetoric in *Protagoras* and *Gorgias*."

Even without the *Gorgias*' cashing out *politikê*, several of its key claims together help to clarify and warrant politics' identification as supreme: (1) psychic welfare is, finally, all that counts; (2) a good psychic condition is tied crucially to order, which link makes a pleasure-centered life antithetical to the good; (3) the push for psychic remediation must be unremitting, with punishments calibrated to levels of offense and prospects of reparability; (4) the political *technê* addresses not just individual welfare but the city's goodness tout court; and (5) proceeding full force and correctly apropos of (1)–(4) requires that there exist a repository of overarching insight into *phusis* and *eudaimonia*. In the *Republic*, Plato's arguments that philosophy alone is this venue and indications of why important rivals cannot function thus unfold in tandem. One such competitor there is medicine, the dialogue's rivalry with which has yet to receive its scholarly due. Crucial work involving this rival awaits us, however, before we take up the *Republic*. While Chapter 3 concentrates on the *Symposium*, Chapter 2 illuminates the seeds of Plato's *agôn* with medicine—despite rosy appearances to the contrary—in the *Gorgias* itself.

2

Medicine in the *Gorgias*: A Collision Course with Philosophy Is Set

I. INTRODUCTION

As we have seen, the *Gorgias* debuts Plato's highly normative notion of *technê*, according to which, overall, medicine comes off well. The present chapter shows that to a significant degree, medicine appears favorably there by standards that originate in those very treatises.[1] In fact, all three of the *Gorgias'* core *technê* requirements are represented in some fashion in medical writings, down to the fact that one with insight must be able to provide accounts of causes and rationales. That said, they are not treated systematically, with identical content, or expressly united as constituting a grid of *technê* standards.

Medicine is a *technê* not only to its defenders in the Hippocratic Corpus, for the *Gorgias* assumes it to qualify as such on Plato's versions of the three conditions that together anchor his *technê* theory. Moreover, Plato concurs within limits that medicine is not merely one practice among others: not only is it, along with gymnastics, a bodily *technê*, but the two preside over all other activities that promote bodily/material welfare to ensure that the latter make only acceptable contributions vis-à-vis the goods in question (517d–518a).

[1] This study's claims about medicine are based on an investigation of the treatises comprising Loeb Classical Library, vols. 1–10 (1923–2012).

By Plato's lights, while medicine is superior to some endeavors, it is not and cannot be the *technê* par excellence as Hippocratic authors claimed. Key here is Plato's insistence that, among *agatha* (things that are good), the soul categorically surpasses all else in merit; hence, *technai* that enhance its condition are categorically superior to activities that promote inferior goods. The *Gorgias*, as we saw, locates the source of the Big Three in the soul and views those appetites as naturally insatiable (493a–494a). Wrongly indulged, they impede psychic welfare with potentially grave results. This much the dialogue makes evident. What is not brought to light there respecting medicine's limits stems from the fact that the same appetites also impact health, for which reason ancient medicine deals extensively with them. For Plato, since the Big Three and their attendant pleasure stem from the soul itself, it is inevitable that doctors' practice here will be insufficiently rigorous and ultimately misguided. In addition, this difficulty cannot be addressed from within medicine, because expertise in the relevant psychic phenomena is by definition excluded from its subject matter, falling instead, in the *Gorgias*' terms, under *politikê*.[2]

Furthermore, the *Gorgias*' account of judging, discussed in Chapter 1, suggests a need for marked revision of existing medical authority, since doctors must not treat those deemed physically incurable or psychically irremediable from the standpoint of virtue (*aretê*). While the present chapter attends particularly to appetitive indulgence and related matters from a critical perspective, it also addresses the need for adjustment of these practices' authority in a way that complements our account of punishment in Chapter 1.

2. MEDICINE'S ROLE AS AID AND SUPPORT TO THE *GORGIAS*' CASTIGATION OF RHETORIC

As we have seen, Plato deems medicine a powerful ally in the *Gorgias*' castigation of mere knacks, particularly rhetoric. Where knacks are critiqued, medicine's superior standing is regularly front and center. It is important, for instance, as a lead-up to the dramatic contrast between rhetoric and philosophy at 500b–d, with medicine corresponding to the latter in Plato's analogy. This is but one illustration of his point that medicine holds up well when judged against cookery, its shoddy bodily counterpart, and rhetoric, the dissembling knack of self-serving persuasion (see further 456a–c, 459a–460a, 464b–465e, 500e–501a, 521e–522a).[3] I concur with the reading

[2] Jaeger asserts a close tie between medicine and Plato's conceptions of reality, human nature, and the soul (1986a, 183, 321–22, 389n30, 390n48, 392n103, 393nn129, 137, 143, 394n151; 1986b, 21–27). Although Jaeger rightly calls our attention to a salutary impact of medicine on Plato's theorizing, he carries that supposed influence much too far.

[3] Cf. *Euthydemus* 289d–290a.

of Stalley (1981, 115), according to which the *Gorgias* "seems more kindly disposed towards medicine" than the *Republic*. The question is why.

The *Gorgias* offers a cornucopia of medical and health-related usage, information, concepts, and assumptions. For instance, enough is said in the *Gorgias* to ground a particularly close tie between the virtue of *sôphrosunê* (self-control) and the body (specifically, familiar sources of sensory indulgence). This view is abundantly displayed in Hippocratic writings. I submit that the stage is set there for Plato's stress on *sôphrosunê*, with its distinctive tie to the body, not only in the *Gorgias* but in subsequent dialogues, central among them the *Symposium* and *Republic*. The same applies to those writings' invocation of what becomes for Plato in the *Statesman* a core notion of *to metrion* (due measure). The existence of these parallels to medical work is fascinating in its own right and testifies to medicine's being strongly and firmly on Plato's radar screen. Evidence of his attending to it from early on is reinforced by the fact that the *Gorgias*' substantial recourse to it is accompanied by numerous references elsewhere.[4]

Medicine was lodged without privilege among ordinary crafts (e.g., shoemaking) on a widespread view dating back to Homer (Edelstein 1987b, 87; 1952, 301).[5] The Hippocratic treatise *Ancient Medicine* both notes (7) and ambitiously challenges (20) that assimilation.[6]

If people felt confident about health's preservation through routine effort but doubted that they could make their own footwear, they might view medicine as subordinate in stature even to mundane crafts like shoemaking. In fact, there is evidence in Hippocratic writings of an extreme view on which medicine does not merit placement even with ordinary crafts, instead by rights lacking *technê* standing altogether (*Ancient Medicine* 4). Showing the falsity of this view "is of great importance to the physician, for if there is really no such thing as a *technê*, then medicine is useless" (Edelstein 1987b, 101). In their own work, Hippocratic authors

---

[4] See *Euthyphro* 13d; *Crito* 47a–e; *Charmides* 155d–157c, 161e–162a, 164a–c, 165c–d, 170b–171c, 173b, 174b–175a; *Laches* 190a–b, 192e–193a, 195b–196a, 196d, 198d–e; *Lysis* 209e–210a, 215d, 217a–b, 218e–219c; *Euthydemus* 280a, 289a–290a, 291e, 299b–c; *Protagoras* 311b–c, 313a–314b, 322c–e, 334a–c, 345a–b, 352a, 353c–354b; *Ion* 531e, 537c, 538c, 539d–e.

[5] See also Dodds (1959, 208). For a contrasting view see Jaeger (1986b, 3; cf. 12), who, however, relies on Plato's depictions, which he takes to be strictly glowing; interestingly, Jaeger (15) proceeds to note that Euthydemus is "horrified" by the prospect of becoming a doctor in Xenophon's *Memorabilia* (IV.2.10).

[6] Unless otherwise noted, translations of Hippocratic treatises, with certain adjustments, are drawn from Loeb Classical Library, vols. 1–10 (1923–2012). On matters of dating, I follow Jouanna (1999, 373–416). Most writings gathered under the head "Hippocratic Corpus" were, as Jouanna points out, "contemporaneous with Hippocrates" (57) though not all written by him (56–57). As the corpus possesses a "globally coherent core that can be seen as constituting a distinctly Hippocratic style of thought" (xii), a treatise's having a later date need not be "a sign of discontinuity" (70). While the present investigation includes reference to subsequent treatises, no point central to this inquiry hinges on postclassical writings.

either argue for the claim or assume that medicine ranks as a *technê*. As to defenses of the position, according to *Ancient Medicine* (1), one may infer medicine's necessary standing as a *technê* from the very fact that medical practitioners differ vastly in caliber. While this variation undoubtedly existed, it does not obviously suffice to show that better operators possess a *technê*. From that standpoint, *Regimen in Acute Diseases* is superior, for it moves beyond comparisons (8) to argue directly for medicine's claim to *technê* standing via factors having counterparts in the *Gorgias*' formalized requirements.[7]

Plato's handling of medicine is in keeping with the *Charmides*' observation (161c) that the merit of ideas, not their source, counts for purposes of their assessment.[8] On some key issues medicine is simply mistaken. On others, Plato either concurs with medical notions or offers transmuted versions of positions whose medical framing he views as flawed. The following section of this chapter concentrates on salient points of divergence. Here, I address similarities in views and concerns.

In the *Gorgias*, Plato accepts—indeed, relies on—the claim of medicine to be a *technê*. Its standing as such was also assumed in earlier dialogues, referenced in Chapter 1, that provide a backdrop for the *Gorgias*' account. Given the controversy over medicine's standing evinced by Hippocratic writings, Plato's confidence on this point is not trivial. The *Gorgias* also concurs, to a degree, with medicine's claims to operate in an elevated way, for the dialogue presents medicine as a prominent bodily *technê* presiding, with gymnastics, over practices like weaving, cobblery, tanning, and cooking (517d–518a).

The foundational role of the *technê-empeiria* divide means that certain familiar activities would be categorically disallowed; these include oratory and cookery (i.e., the provision of foods to indulge undiscriminating urges without heed to people's welfare). Apart from what one gleans from its allusions to "true rhetoric" as politics or its tool (503a–c, 504d–e, 508b–c, 517a, 527c), the *Gorgias* does not consider whether some heretofore self-standing practices will become slighter, if not disappear, because *technai* in the dialogue's sense subsume their territory rightly approached.

Hippocratic work, however, does present medicine as seeking absorption of what falls in the spheres of physical training/exertion and cooking. Authors do not merely funnel their reflections on other domains through what they view as medicine's comprehensive vision. Though their move here goes further epistemologically, it is

---

[7] One also finds defenses of medicine's *technê* standing in *Law* (1) and *The Art* (9). Displaying a measure of hubris, the author of the latter asserts that he could also defend the *technê* standing of other crafts but declines to do so there.

[8] Cf. *Euthyphro* 9e.

not unlike what occurs in the *Gorgias*, where cooks, like shoemakers, are to operate under doctors' and trainers' supervision. Physical training—coequal with medicine, even superior to it, on the *Gorgias*' account—is subordinated expressly to medicine (*Regimen* I 24).[9] Further, medicine absorbs its knowledge and duties by declaring the fitting forms, amounts, and intensities of exertion in sickness and health.[10] Instances of silent appropriation are numerous (*Regimen in Health* 7; *Regimen* I 2; *Regimen* II 62, 64; *Regimen* III 69, 71–72, 81). The border between express and silent appropriation is sometimes blurred, as in *Regimen* III (67), whose author claims for medicine what the *Gorgias* places under physical training, namely prevention. He proceeds to assert—as his discovery no less—that the secret to maximal enjoyment of health is maximal preventive care.[11] Reinforcing this subordination, preventive activity is itself dubbed treatment (*all' ou chrê proïesthai es touto, all' ektherapeuesthai proteron hôde*, *Regimen* III 83), which strongly suggests annexation, and which would be a smart linguistic move for one aiming at this.[12]

Hippocratic doctors also place dietary guidance and food preparation under the head of medicine insofar as it alone knows what substances benefit and harm the body, including particulars like circumstances and amounts. If medicine does not supplant cooking outright here, it juts rather far into its terrain.[13] Though food and drink possess their own *phuseis* (natures) and *dunameis* (capacities), the *technê* of medicine can impact their expression (*Regimen* II 39, 56). Medicine is the true repository of wisdom here: ignorant handlers of food (or *pharmaka*, i.e., drugs or medication) oversimplify the terrain—a familiar objection of medical authors generally when contesting rivals' handling of pertinent arenas—by assimilating from the get-go all things ostensibly one in kind (e.g., sweet, 39). Due to this powerful context dependency, the *technê* of medicine, unlike skill in writing, cannot be rapidly acquired (*Places in Man* 41). Medicine can alter the very *dunameis* of foodstuffs

[9] While the author's critique of *paidotribê* does not include his questioning whether this praxis is a *technê* at all, its content is not unlike that of Plato's harangue against rhetoricians in the *Gorgias* and *Republic*. According to *Places in Man* (35), medicine and gymnastics are "naturally opposed" (*hupenantia pephuken*), since the latter maintains a salutary status quo while the former aids ailing ones in altering their conditions; this claim, unusual in Hippocratic writings, leaves both practices intact and may suggest equality, though it could be taken to imply that medicine, qua restorer of right conditions, requires a finer-grained expertise.

[10] On the pertinence of exercise to both modalities, see also Jouanna (1999, 166).

[11] On ancient medicine as claiming to preside over both the maintenance and the restoration of health, see also Edelstein (1952, 308–9).

[12] For a view stressing instead the ongoing independence of medicine and physical training, with physicians' submission "in some matters . . . [to] the authority of the trainer as final," see Jaeger (1986b, 31).

[13] This is so all the more when emphasis is laid not only on regimen's salience in combating illness but also on its being one and the same diet that preserves people when well. Even where authors contend that one's conduct when ill should redress imbalance, hence be opposed to one's usual custom, knowing right norms is requisite for proper counterbalancing.

(*Regimen* II 42, 45), whose preparation falls to doctors. Similarly, in *Affections* (47) doctors are instructed to "prepare and give to patients cereals and entrees" as per the medical author's own instructions (see also *Internal Affections* 23).[14] The more complex the food preparation guided by medicine, the closer to superfluity does cookery as an independent praxis become. One might, of course, employ watered-down practitioners, what we might call cooks versus chefs, who prepared suitable concoctions strictly in line with doctors' vision; in that case, medicine's subsuming the subject matter of bodily crafts like cookery would be not unlike doctors' common practice of using assistants, who were valued for their performance of manual labor (e.g., holding patients' limbs in place during procedures).

Medicine's annexations regarding physical training/exertion and cooking are significant as evidence of medicine's agonistic self-presentation. Medicine's competitive positioning of itself vis-à-vis other domains is evident as well when Hippocratic authors depict it as lying atop the sphere of *technai*. While this claim for medicine's preeminence is made expressly, it is regularly assumed by authors' macrocosmic visions (i.e., broad cosmological theorizing) applied to the human sphere. Figuring centrally here are *Ancient Medicine*, *Airs Waters Places*, and *Regimen* I, which are discussed further in Chapter 3.

Though such contentions on their own do not prove medicine to be a *technê*, medical writings often contrast real doctors with those who falsely claim to practice this *technê* and whose lack of insight may be dangerously cloaked by alluring facades. While consummate practitioners represent the best that *iatrikê* (i.e., the *technê* of medicine) has to offer, poor ones do not undertake a *technê*, neither medicine nor any other (*On Fractures* 30–31). The latter fail to practice *iatrikê* by standards that emerge as the *Gorgias*' core conditions involving subject matter, understanding, and goodness. These evaluative reference points are featured both when authors are keen to demarcate genuine medical experts from charlatans—as in *Regimen in Acute Diseases*, which makes use of all three Platonic requirements—and when writers tackle challenges to medicine's very *technê* standing, as in *The Art*.

First, let us consider medical writings' attention to the ontological plane, which becomes the *Gorgias*' subject-matter requirement on genuine *technai*. Hippocratic

[14] *Ancient Medicine* (3–4) takes the extreme position that cookery never truly was an independent practice; this is what one might call a genetic subsumption of cooking that preempts the emergence of a truly independent practice of cookery. Jaeger (1986b, 35) comments on "the astonishing richness and variety of diet which the civilized Greeks commanded" as evidenced by medical writings. In addition to such evidence of a clearly elaborate knowledge of foodstuffs, there is support (e.g., in *Ulcers*, *Nature of Women*, *Superfetation*) for wide-ranging attention by some to notable properties of plants and natural, inanimate substances such as arsenic, lead, sulfur, wool, and wax; while this twofold apprehension bears on physicians' handling of *pharmaka*, knowledge of plants is useful as well from the standpoint of regimen.

authors' occupation with medicine's subject matter, construed quite broadly, is ubiquitous. As one might expect, "the body's nature is the launching-point of medical reasoning" (*phusis de tou sômatos, archê tou en iêtrikêi logou*, *Places in Man* 2). Fostering bodily well-being necessitates, however, that medicine's purview include physical activity, dietetics, and *pharmaka*, as well as invasive procedures like surgery and cautery. Dietetics and the use of drugs (*pharmaka*), taken together, cover the properties of food, drink, plants, and natural inanimate entities (liquids, solids, and powders) used in medications, along with entities' combinatory features. As noted above, exertion too falls under medicine, since sound condition (not to be confused, e.g., with excess muscularity) aids the prevention of illness, and right handling of physical activity helps recovery. Proper deployment of surgery and cautery, in turn, requires both technical skill and a grasp of what was known of anatomy, itself required also for proper bandaging of fractures and dislocations.[15] Perhaps in part due to a recognition that medicine includes so much, *The Art* (3) specifies the practice's subject matter (*ho nomizô iêtrikên einai*) through an articulation of its end.[16] Casting the net more widely still, medical writings abound with cosmological commitments, as when authors posit particular material substances (e.g., air) as comprising all that is and tie illness and recovery to seasonal factors (e.g., atypical wetness or dryness), winds, particular locales, and astronomical phenomena such as equinoxes (see further Chapter 3).

Though the corpus ranges broadly in terms of medicine's subject matter, it does not suggest that doctors are somehow expert in everything. Importantly, treatises offer reasons for medicine's diversified occupation with the microcosm (e.g., the selection and preparation of foodstuffs impact bodily humors). The same occurs when authors lodge overarching cosmic principles under medicine's umbrella, the rationale here resting on Greek convictions, extending from epic poetry to pre-Socratic philosophy, that there exist deep macrocosmic-microcosmic correspondences. Compared with Hippocratic writings, the *Gorgias* substantially narrows medicine's *peri ti* (subject matter), as evidenced by 501a, which concentrates on medicine's mastering the nature of *sôma* and its sound condition.

---

[15] *On Fractures*, essentially a how-to guide for those dealing with these conditions, castigates defective practice versus that of a *technê*. See also the treatises *Anatomy*, *The Heart*, and *Nature of Bones*, which are Hellenistic or later (Jouanna 1999, 375, 394, 398). As Jouanna (308) points out, anatomical knowledge premised on human dissection did not exist in classical times but arose "as an aspect of medical practice at Alexandria during the Hellenistic era."

[16] In addition to this wide-ranging occupation with bodily states, treatises' reflections on *phusis* and health often include organic psychic concomitants (e.g., delirium, coma, madness) and broader ties between soul and body; not surprisingly, *sôma*, not *psuchê*, is typically in the driver's seat.

When praising medicine simpliciter and contrasting legitimate with sham practice, authors stress doctors' acting from insight into health and its restoration (*Regimen in Acute Diseases* 6, 40, 43, 67; *On the Sacred Disease* 2). According to *The Art* (1), only one knowing nothing of medicine's core mission to use and expand understanding (*sunesis*) and wisdom (*sophiê*) for patients' sake could deny its *technê* standing. Ignorant practice has grave liabilities, including mistaken diagnoses (e.g., *Internal Affections* 14). One finds also a version of the *Gorgias*' epistemological contrast (454c–d): intellectual conditions are two, "knowledge and belief" (*epistêmê te kai doxa*), which differ sharply in nature and efficacy (*Law* 4). Belief, hinging on sense-perception alone (*The Art* 11), cannot be trusted. In contrast, doctors' grasp of "ailments' causes" (*to eidenai tôn nousôn ta aitia*) holds the key to fitting treatment (*to therapeuein autas epistasthai*, 11). In fact, the view that physicians must know the causes of ailments for care to benefit patients reliably is ubiquitous in medical writings (e.g., *Breaths* 1–2; *Diseases* I 1; *Epidemics* II 1.7, 4.5; *Places in Man* 1).

Further, understanding must be confirmed via *logoi* (here, "explanations") that illuminate the how and why of conclusions and recommendations. *Regimen in Acute Diseases* addresses at length the cause of barley-based gruel's preferability to other cereals for acute diseases (10, 15–17), with the author consciously aware that he is providing a requisite account (*Dia tautas oun tas prophasias kai heteras toiautas*, 17).[17] In addition, since those practicing *iatrikê* must understand medications' natures and effects, which knowledge they can voice at will, an inability to explain the impact of *pharmaka* (drugs) demonstrates ignorance (*Places in Man* 46, cf. 45).

Reliable prognostication—necessarily expressed in *logoi*—is a crucial sign of doctors' insight into the subject matter of medicine (*The Art* 6–7); this understanding allows doctors not only to predict diseases' prospects of relenting but also to foretell their advent (*Regimen* I 2). Concerted investigation of medical writings thus shows the falsity of Levy's (2005) claim that ancient physicians were unable to meet the requirement (200n29) that they "be able to explain in general terms why a particular treatment cures a particular illness, not just that, in this case, such a treatment cured this patient's illness" (200). Further, the assertion of Franklin (2005, 247n36), "Physicians of Plato's day were more interested in prognosis than diagnosis," reflects an oversimplification of what one gleans from the Hippocratic Corpus, where one and the same knowledge of natures, causes, and potentialities (e.g., of core bodily

---

[17] Explanatory *logoi* are foregrounded elsewhere in the treatise (28, 35, 41).

elements and *pharmaka*) is key to (1) identifying patients' ailments, (2) treatment selection, and (3) anticipating outcomes involving (1) and (2).[18]

As *The Art* (1) observes, insight drives medicine's provision of benefit. As for direct Hippocratic formulations of what becomes the *Gorgias*' goodness requirement on *technai*, *Regimen in Acute Diseases* (43) asserts that calibrating patients' treatment based on insight into their constitutions and inclinations means the difference between life and death (*sôtêriên ê thanaton pherei ginôskomena kai agnoeumena ta toiade*).[19] Conversely, as in the *Gorgias*, ignorance of the pertinent terrain leads to harm; thus, *On Fractures* (2) condemns agents who, ignorant of anatomy and conjuring up archery instead, bind arms in unnatural positions with deleterious results.[20] Rather than take responsibility for their ignorance and pursue its remediation, they compound their shortcomings by blaming the disease, the patient, and even chance *(tina atuchiên, On Fractures* 25).[21]

Despite differences on specifics, Hippocratic treatises concur that *tuchê* (chance) either lacks merit altogether or is categorically inferior to the steady reliability that *technê* allows. According to *Ancient Medicine*, ancient discoveries involving diet, to which the author traces the advent of *iatrikê* (the *technê* of medicine), stemmed not "from chance" (*apo tuchês*) but rather from "inquiry well and correctly conducted" *(kalôs kai orthôs exeurêtai*, 12; cf. 14). In fact, one with insight relies so little on good fortune that he is able to benefit patients irrespective of whether luck is on his side (*Places in Man* 46). Even where *tuchê* is pertinent to measures' success (or failure), healing itself occurs through the agency of *technê* (*The Art* 4–5).[22] Where possessors of *iatrikê* tackle dangerous conditions, good fortune plays a role in their success (*Places in Man* 24), while its opposite leaves the patient no worse than he was before treatment.[23] Unlike those with medical knowledge, when ignorant practitioners

[18] The overall preeminence given the future-directedness of ancient medicine by Jouanna (1999, 102) must be contextualized within his recognition of prognosis' complexity (101): "For a modern physician, prognosis—clearly distinguished from diagnosis—consists in forecasting the development and outcome of a disease. For an ancient physician, prognosis had a much wider definition and assumed greater importance"; like the work of the soothsayer, "the prognosis of the ancient physician . . . bore upon the past, the present, and the future alike."

[19] See also chaps. 29, 31, 33, 66. Understanding is tethered to benefit versus harm in *Humors* 5; *Affections* 13, 45.

[20] In contrast, though they cannot formulate beneficial praxis, the manual work of assistants overseen by knowledgeable doctors redounds to patients' aid. While intellectual grasp and its guiding of praxis are far superior to mere facility in manual work, one deficient in the former but possessed of manual expertise may, e.g., at any rate, "apply dressings well and in a way that will do no harm" (*On Fractures* 28).

[21] On the divide between insightful and ignorant practice, see further *On Wounds in the Head* 21.

[22] Cf. *Diseases* I (1), where only *technê*-based activity is accomplished *akribôs*.

[23] Of course, finding a qualified physician may itself involve luck; for instance, while gout in the elderly is incurable, a young patient's recovery hinges on his own careful regimen and whether he "chances on a physician who possesses understanding" (*iêtrou gnômên echontos epituchôn*; *Prorrhetic* II 8).

fail to promote healing, they castigate chance straightaway (*On Fractures* 25), which serves merely to broadcast their deficiency in experts' eyes. On the other side, when faux doctors succeed, that result truly is the product of *tuchê* alone (*On Joints* 77).[24]

According to Hippocratic writings, a reliance on chance, which indicates ignorance, is not the sole flaw in those falsely dubbing themselves physicians. Also defective is the motivation of operators driven more by repute and greed than by a concern for patients' welfare.[25] In fact, lack of an unshakable commitment to the benefit of those who ail suffices to disprove one's legitimacy as a *technê* practitioner—a stance with which, as we have seen, the *Gorgias* heartily concurs. Rather than guessing unilaterally at how to proceed out of a selfish concern for one's reputation (*Precepts* 7), sound practitioners will not hesitate to consult other experts for the patient's sake in difficult cases (8). *On the Sacred Disease* stresses that charlatans do anything to avoid assuming responsibility for poor outcomes (2): while they eagerly claim credit for recoveries, failures are laid at divinities' feet (ibid.).[26]

A further source of unsalutary practice involves insight's not being adequately accompanied by healing action, where *empeiria* (here, "experience") is important (*Precepts* 1);[27] in fact, given its salience, laypeople may themselves hit accidentally on salutary measures (2). According to *The Art*, and contra Polus in the *Gorgias*, *empeiria* and *technê* in some way coexist in the ailing layperson's use of trial and error (5) despite his not being a knowledgeable practitioner of the medical art.[28] Elsewhere, stress is placed on the notion that abstract understanding (evinced via *logoi*) is worthless if not translated into effective practice, or deeds (*erga*, *The Art* 14; *Law* 4). On the pithy formulation of *On Joints*, "it is not enough to know the art in theory only (*ouk arkei mounon logôi eidenai tên technên tautên*); much practice

[24] The same point is stressed in *Regimen* IV (87), which critiques dream-interpreters who randomly succeed and fail in their constructions of bodily symptoms presaged by soul, ever ignorant of the cause in either case. In *Affections*, though laypeople and experts may light equally upon useful *pharmaka* by chance, what requires *gnômê* can be gleaned solely through *iatrikê* (45). According to Jaeger (1986b, 11), a lay-professional distinction, which later became quite influential, first surfaced in medical writings.

[25] On malice, virtually never mentioned as a motive, see *On Joints* 47.

[26] Cf. *On Joints* (14), which speaks of a tacit conspiring by doctor and patient toward an unsalutary result: patients are careful just at the start, while doctors "gradually withdraw and are not displeased by patients' carelessness" once they see that restoration of patients' earlier appearance is impossible. Even if malice is not a direct motivator, practitioners may be indifferent to patients' welfare (e.g., they do not involve themselves adequately to ensure that the proper regimen is followed, being concerned only to avoid negative judgments by others that might harm their reputations).

[27] The author contrasts *tribê* (experience) with patients' being harmed needlessly *têi tou iêtrou apeiriêi*.

[28] Perhaps unintentionally, *The Art* (5) blurs somewhat the boundary between the sharpest laypeople and medical professionals by suggesting that the former may go at least some way toward meeting the goodness condition; but see chap. 7, which stresses deficiencies in patients' discipline and comprehension.

is also needed" (10). Experience in the handling of congenital dislocations, for instance, deepens doctors' attunement to relevant contextual factors (*Instruments of Reduction* 40), and it has much to teach them about fevers' duration (*Affections* 18).[29]

In the clinical setting, authors demarcate doctors from their assistants, not themselves *technê* practitioners, whose duties include physically restraining patients while doctors tend to fractures and dislocations, handing over surgical implements, providing salutary baths of water or vapor, and applying herbal concoctions.[30] Hippocratic writings depict reliable assistants as effective in such elements of treatment without suggesting that they grasp the nature of health or more about anatomy than a savvy layperson might be expected to know. On these accounts, experts' good assistants are superior to bad "physicians," since at least the former operate under the command of real *iatroi* (doctors).[31] Further, even where patients' abilities are viewed with some appreciation, physicians distinguish themselves foundationally from them and other laypeople, including but not limited to patients' family members.[32] The foregoing suffices to make clear that within medical writings, as they depict and defend their views of medical insight and practice, authors are often at the same time agonistically engaged.

---

[29] On this topic see further *Regimen in Acute Diseases* 44; *On Fractures* 1.

[30] *Breaths* 9; *In the Surgery* 2, 5; *On Fractures* 8, 13, 15, 19, 39; *On Joints* 2–3, 5, 16, 26, 30, 43, 47, 70–71, 74–76, 78; *Instruments of Reduction* 5, 38; *Diseases* II 47; III 16; *Internal Affections* 53; *Regimen in Acute Diseases*, Appendix 57; *Hemorrhoids* 2. According to *Instruments of Reduction* (38), assistants differ in their own levels of instruction. See also *On Joints* (47), where manual activity may be performed by the physician or "an assistant who is strong and not untrained." Even higher-caliber assistants are limited to labor of a manual variety. While bad "doctors" are frequently viewed as ignorant of their own limits, this is not singled out as a problem with assistants.

[31] Jouanna (1999, 89–91) distinguishes "aides" from "assistants," reserving the latter term for auxiliaries of comparatively refined abilities. For the claim that most operating as doctors are no better than laypeople due to their ignorance of *ta aitia*, see *Ancient Medicine* 21; it is this knowledge that leads to praxis that is steadily correct (23). For the same unflattering conflation, see the opening of *Regimen in Acute Diseases*, whose ensuing account stresses true doctors' knowledge of signs and reasons with regard to conditions and remedies.

[32] This is so even in *Affections*, where marked appreciation of patients' abilities early on is followed by the author's demarcation (45) of what comes to light by chance, equally discoverable by expert and lay, from discoveries necessitating *gnômê*, which stem solely from *iatrikê*. Private practice in antiquity was not what we think of as such: according to Jouanna (1999, 75), "whether he received patients in his office or made the rounds of his patients in their homes, the physician was never alone with the patient. The patient's entourage of family and friends, together with other curious onlookers, made up a public before which the physician was obliged to perform." As to affiliations, medicine draws abundantly on pre-Socratic accounts *peri phuseôs*, though it may do so as their opponent. In addition, some medical treatises show a particular reliance on rhetorical techniques, while others disdain physicians' oratorical displays even as their authors deploy such techniques for their own ends; in Plato, medicine is tied to oratory via Hippias (see further Chapter 3). The *Gorgias* seems keen to sever medicine from rhetoric: while Gorgias' boast about his persuasive success when visiting patients with his physician-brother (456b–c) is telling vis-à-vis oratory, one also suspects that for Plato, Herodicus' allowing Gorgias' accompaniment reflects poorly on him qua doctor.

3. TAKING STOCK OF THE *GORGIAS*' PARALLELS AND DEBTS TO MEDICAL WRITINGS

Before turning to the roots of what becomes Plato's own *agôn* with medicine, let us address how Hippocratic presentations compare thus far with medicine in the *Gorgias.* One sees from the foregoing that medical authors are committed to the existence of a strong appearance-reality gap. Writers also attend to this point on a metalevel. According to *Ancient Medicine*, though doctors should take the readily evident as their launching point (18), they must be able to glean *ou phanera* (literally, "things that are not apparent," 14; cf. *The Art* 9, 13). If they cannot, they will wreak harm by mechanically applying opposites (e.g., hot and cold) to heal on the false assumption that an ailment's source is always clear straightaway (*Ancient Medicine* 13). More generally, they will be unable to glean whether patients are improving (*Internal Affections* 23) or will assume that patients fare well when key signs point to imminent death (*Coan Prenotions* 481). *Regimen* III (69), in turn, observes a gap between what seems to obtain and what truly is regarding a person's overall health, while *Regimen* I (10–11) foregrounds this divide from a grand cosmological standpoint giving pride of place to fire. Also operating cosmologically, *Airs Waters Places* claims that doctors must recognize *ta sêmeia* (signs) associated with seasons so that they can anticipate (*proeideiê*) how far diseases will manifest during that particular annum (10–11).[33]

The *Gorgias* too emphasizes a visible-imperceptible gap, stating that while doctors can look beneath the surface of bodily appearances to glean whether bodies' condition is sound (464a), charlatans skim the uppermost layers alone, with damage the likely result (517e–518a). Because they can penetrate beyond surface appearances in areas such as regimen, doctors can ascertain how much food and

[33] Further, *Breaths* (3) notes the impact of air as unavailable to sense-perception, requiring instead special insight to unmask. On visible versus invisible contusions and fractures, see *On Wounds in the Head* 5, 9–11, 13–14, 18. Appearance and reality may clash regarding the severity of fractures and dislocations: *On Fractures* 46; *On Joints* 14, 46, 51. In *Coan Prenotions*, a pronounced appearance-reality gap exists when patients' strong pain, coughing up pus, or becoming blind is, under relevant conditions, a sign of recovery (288); conversely, pains' vanishing may be a negative sign (364, 459). Unveiling consumption that usually stays "undetected" and gleaning post-ailment internal suppuration necessitate expertise in discerning the imperceptible through the sensible (*Places in Man* 10, 14). Moreover, where the presence of consumption is known, even good doctors may be unable to penetrate to its invisible causation (*Glands* 14). According to *Superfetation*, certain changes to women's eyes are signs of pregnancy prior to that state's being observable directly (16), and relative sizes of breasts and eyes indicate which side the fetus is on (19). On the apparent-imperceptible distinction involving procreation, see also *Nature of the Child* 17, 19; *Nature of Women* 2. As to regimen, sound practice involves one's inferring from foods' "evident" *dunameis* what their less evident capacities are (*Affections* 47); this is particularly important since the best foods for health and strength are not identical (ibid.).

drink should be offered at a given juncture with a view toward the optimal health and strength not only of each based on his size and condition but also of the human aggregate (490b–c, 504e–505a).[34] In addition to food and drink, doctors prescribe medication (*pharmaka*) with a view toward restoring the bodily balance that is health (467c), and resort when fitting to surgery (*temnein*) and cautery (*kaein*; 480c, cf. 476c–d).

On the *Gorgias*' account, to the extent it succeeds, medical practice provides "order and organization to the body" (504a3–4), ridding it of disease (477e8–478b1), in which undertaking *technê*, not chance, is decisive (506d6–7). These claims accord clearly with Hippocratic accounts. Medicine's self-conception involving its subject matter and practitioners' understanding is succinctly voiced at 501a, where it is said to investigate both (a) the nature of what it treats (*toutou hou therapeuei . . . tên phusin*) and (b) the cause of what it does (*tên aitian hôn prattei*), being able to provide an account (*logon dounai*) of each. In keeping with the *Gorgias*' insistence that *technai*, including medicine, benefit their objects, Plato stresses (500b) that they—unlike pleasure-obsessed knacks (*empeiriai*; described as charlatans and pretenders, 464c–465a)—"recognize (*gignôskousai*) what's good and bad" for the objects of their concern. If one brackets the *technai-empeiriai* split as cleaving activities systematically into two, with express conditions for *technê* standing, which are Plato's innovations, one finds the same point about experts' apprehending "what's good and bad" time and again in Hippocratic sources.

As we have seen, the *Gorgias*' *technê* criteria are strongly indebted to medical writings. In Plato's hands, however, discrete Hippocratic testaments come together in a systematic account, whose crux is a core divide between worthy and unworthy human undertakings, *technai* and *empeiriai* respectively. Moreover, Plato revamps those conditions in keeping with his own emerging views of *phusis* and *eudaimonia*. Medicine meets both its own conditions for authenticity, as I have assembled them from a range of sources, and—as far as we learn expressly there—the *Gorgias*' ontological, epistemological, and goodness requirements on *technai*. On this basis, Plato concurs to a degree (517d–518a) with medicine's self-elevation beyond other practices.

One should not, however, conclude that the *Gorgias*' praise of medicine is unqualified. The following section shows how, even as the *Gorgias* lauds medicine by comparison with rhetoric and other knacks, the dialogue's handling of desire and pleasure grounds a rivalry between it and philosophy. Plato's line of thought here not only warrants a rejection of medicine's preeminence but also threatens its very self-sufficiency.

---

[34] At 490b–c, as in Hippocratic material, Plato stresses context-dependent rightness and proportionality.

4. THE ROOTS OF WHAT WILL BECOME PLATO'S HEAD-ON RIVALRY WITH MEDICINE

4.1 Medicine on the Highest Good and the Big Three Epithumiai

In the corpus generally, Plato's rivalries with other approaches to *phusis* and *eudaimonia*, and the unfolding of his own positions, go hand in hand. In the *Gorgias*, his *agôn* with rhetoric is strongly evident and that with poetry apparent (see 501e–502d). In addition to its highly positive, albeit circumscribed, role in Plato's enunciation of the *technê* grid, medicine is a competitor with him for primacy on questions of *phusis* and *eudaimonia*—one necessarily falling short insofar as its views are premised on health's being the greatest good.[35] Though this rivalry does not become overt until the *Symposium*, with further subordination due to philosophy's preeminence in the *Republic*, key grounds of this soon-to-be unveiled *agôn* are evident in the *Gorgias*. Plato's disputes with poetry and rhetoric/sophistry have received much scholarly attention. In contrast, the very fact that there is a rivalry with medicine in Plato, let alone the significance of that dispute, has not yet received its due through concerted investigation.[36]

---

[35] According to *Affections* (1), intelligent people discern health's standing as the highest good and act accordingly. Cf. Jouanna (1999, 125) on the tie between "happiness" and health, where the latter is taken to be "the supreme good."

[36] On Plato's opposition to Hippocratic *phusis*, see also Heyd (1995, 376–77, 384–85). Carrick (2001) observes that ancient "physicians and philosophers often competed for the public's ear. . . . Both dispensed advice on the important moral issue of how citizens *ought* to live in order to attain well-being" (2; italics in original); further, "mindful of this potential competition for influence between physicians and philosophers on matters of personal conduct, philosophers from Plato and Aristotle on sought to reassert the supremacy of their discipline as the only proper authority on the ultimate questions of human value" (22). While Carrick rightly notes an *agôn* here, Plato is not "reassert[ing]" philosophy's role as arbiter but rather aiming to vigorously stake out such for the first time. Carrick contends, further, that doctors are "entitled to *describe* how one might . . . regain or preserve one's health," while philosophers "*prescribe* whether one ought to try to recover or preserve one's health at any cost" (ibid.; italics in original). From Plato's standpoint, Carrick asserts here a conceptual distinction that is unsustainable in practice. Edelstein (1952, 300) also notes that ancient philosophy chastised medicine's prescriptions on how to live. Regarding Plato (308–10), Edelstein concentrates on the suggestion of medical accounts, rejected in the *Republic* and *Laws* (the *Gorgias* is unmentioned), that "a healthy person had to watch himself continuously" (308). On the positive side, philosophers gleaned from *iatrikê* "a simile [later called an 'analogy'] of their own endeavor" (300). This account overlooks the depth of Plato's engagement with medicine as well as the interweaving of his critical and constructive endeavors. Wehrli (1951) argues that Plato takes "Hippocratic-sophistic thinking" (177) on individual pedagogical ties as his launching point, then makes those notions his own. Wehrli reads the *Gorgias* through the *Laws* such that in the former alone is it evident that Plato takes *iatrikê* as a model (*Bild*) for philosophical pedagogy centered on individuals' cultivation (181–82). Though Wehrli rightly grants salience to the *Gorgias* in Plato's handling of medicine, he overplays the extent of commonality by zeroing in on one, allegedly key, point of common ground, itself rendered questionable by his approaching the *Gorgias* through the *Laws*. Unless otherwise evident from the Bibliography, translations of French and German sources are my own.

Soul's superiority to body, foregrounded in the *Gorgias*, means that its condition is incalculably more precious and worthy of note. Medical writings convey what is for Plato the supremely wrongheaded view that "a wise man knows that health is the greatest of human goods (*toisin anthrôpoisi pleistou axion estin hê hugieiê*)" (*Regimen in Health* 9). Certain of the medical notions that impact Plato (e.g., well-being as a function of order) come to be applied by him to medicine at its own expense. This, combined with Plato's divergence from medicine on the global topics of *phusis* and *eudaimonia*, results in its being critiqued and progressively demoted compared with endeavors that directly optimize the welfare of the highest good, namely soul.

The *Gorgias*' placement of psychic above bodily welfare means that even the most competent and reliable practitioner of medicine or physical training lacks the ability to assess how people fare from a higher standpoint. As we saw in Chapter 1, these evaluations fall instead under the head of *politikê*, which comprises legislation for prevention and judging to handle transgressors. The soul's optimal condition is the crux of thriving, with supreme attention to deficiencies, once gleaned, in hopes of psychic improvement. As the *Gorgias* makes clear, the lives of those who are irremediably unjust should not continue. This means, among other things, that unjust people who are ill should not receive medical treatment; indeed, providing it under these conditions is itself unjust. While Plato's making this explicit must await the *Republic*, the *Gorgias* figures importantly on his path thereto. I hence only touch on this issue here, reserving its further treatment for Chapter 4.

Though soul is clearly preeminent, a key question that remains at the *Gorgias*' close is how its account of appetite (lodged expressly within *psuchê*, 493a–d), pleasure, and self-control (not to mention its opposite) relates to medicine's own positions. How does medicine handle the Big Three from the standpoint of health, and how does this compare with the *Gorgias*' account of the relevant phenomena? Though this dialogue does not address the foregoing queries, juxtaposing it against Hippocratic writings will show where medicine comes up short. Moreover, as I argue in Chapters 3–4, these objections form the crux of Plato's arguments involving medicine in the *Symposium* and *Republic*.

Medicine gives prominence to harmony in one's bodily condition (notably, among humors or other material substances). While Plato does not reject the idea that bodily health involves harmony, his concern is order and harmony apropos of the soul. As we saw in Chapter 1, the *Gorgias* closely links order with self-control (i.e., the virtue of *sôphrosunê*) and self-control with the good. Orderly ones (*kosmioi*) just *are* those who are self-controlled and just (493d, 504d). For Plato, self-control—at whose core is proper regulation of the Big Three—is in the *Gorgias* and remains the virtue most closely tied to the body. Obviously, Plato favors psychic harmony over that of the body if one must choose. More pressing is the fact that while the Big

Three *epithumiai* (appetites or desires) are lodged within the soul, doctors handle and impact them. As it falls outside doctors' purview as bodily experts to grasp the nature of psychic phenomena, they continually and inescapably risk prescribing in a fashion that is deleterious to patients' souls. The issue is not whether indulgence might in certain cases aid the restoration of bodily health, at least in the near term. Plato would still insist that, being bad for the soul, indulgence should not occur.

Hippocratic comments involving the Big Three, which are extensive, span two phases of medicine's grappling with health, namely lifestyle, including what causes disease, and ailments' remediation. Regarding the former, authors' stances on indulgence may be neutral, positive, or negative; as we will see, where indulgence is involved in diseases' causation, its badness is lodged on that very ground. Concerning treatment, authors tend to recommend either for or against, with crucial heed being paid to context.

Let us turn first to lifestyle and ailments' causation. Some Hippocratic material appears neutral or nonjudgmental where the Big Three *epithumiai* are concerned. According to *Airs Waters Places*, doctors must grasp not only a region's typifying features (e.g., the character of its winds) but also the patterns of consumption that please its people (*kai tên diaitan tôn anthrôpôn, hokoiêi hêdontai*, 1). The author later stipulates that individuals should not be both large-scale drinkers and large-scale eaters (4), which implies that doctors would tolerate a person's being one or the other. *Aphorisms* (7.7) notes that delirium post-intoxication, rather than drunkenness itself, is bad.[37] *Ancient Medicine* (10), in turn, references dietary habits, sparked by pleasure (*di' hêdonên*), of folks dwelling in the absence of *iatrikê*. This comment occurs nonjudgmentally as part of the author's defense of medicine's lineage reaching back to ancient dietetics. Attending to preemption, *Regimen in Acute Diseases* (Appendix 45) matter-of-factly suggests garlic consumption to minimize unwanted effects "if one is about to go drinking or is already drunk."

On the positive side, *Regimen* III recommends proper amounts of sexual activity by season, treating sex as a salutary element of people's health-preserving regimen like any other, for example, vomiting (68). Recurring to the issue, the author asserts that the staving off of illness necessitates sexual activity (*chrê de kai aphrodisiasai ti*) alongside other measures involving unguents and sleep (80, cf. 73). In chap. 85, the author stipulates both sex and drunkenness to defuse in a timely fashion preailment scenarios where exercise is disproportionate in relation to food.[38]

---

[37] In *Superfetation*, while women's inebriation may facilitate conception (29), men should stay sober (26). To foster conception, males are elsewhere instructed to consume "very potent unmixed wine" (*Superfetation* 30; *Barrenness* 6).

[38] For sex as preemptive, see also *Barrenness* 35.

Medical writings link indulgence to disease. Obesity may predispose one to sudden death (*Aphorisms* 2.44). *Ancient Medicine* (14) notes excess consumption of "highly seasoned delicacies" as fostering disease. According to *Epidemics* VI, a lifestyle of "healthy discipline" (*askêsis hugiês*) excludes gluttony and laziness (4.18). In *Internal Affections,* drunkenness and excess intake of food are identified as causes of illness (6); the dietary culprits are gray mullets and eels, which are said to "contain a fat most harmful to the human constitution." Elsewhere, weight loss is said to improve intelligence. Obesity and drunkenness are said to cause madness (*Regimen* I 35).[39]

Epidemics I (case 2) reports that one Silenus became feverish following "overexertion, drinking, and exercises at the wrong time (*akairôn*)," from which condition he perished (cf. case 12). In *Diseases* I (26), excessive alcohol gives rise to pleurisy;[40] in such cases, the author implies, people wrongly single out a chill as the cause, ignoring the role of their own conduct. Thus drunkenness, including single bouts thereof, fosters illness, sometimes fatal.[41] Further, it both causes madness and negatively impacts intelligence (*Breaths* 14).[42]

Regarding sexual indulgence, the final member of the Big Three, in *Epidemics* III, "venery and drunkenness" led to fever, from which the patient recovered (case 10 of 16). For another patient, long-standing drunkenness and sexual indulgence caused delirium, insanity, and death (case 16). *Internal Affections* (13) identifies venery as drying out marrow, which negatively impacts health. All three *epithumiai* are linked in *Affections* (1), aimed centrally at laypeople, where unfitting consumption of food or drink and venery are listed as causes of imbalance leading bile or phlegm to become excessively dry, moist, hot, or cold.

Authors also note poor lifestyles' giving rise to ailments, as when defective regimen causes scattered fevers (*Breaths* 6). In *Epidemics* VII, a man's illness culminating in death is traced to "an utterly heedless mode of existence" (*panta hêmartêkôs*, 17).[43] According to *Epidemics* III, a patient's "careless living" leading to "violent rigor and acute fever" contributed importantly to his death (case 3 of 16); in a subsequent

[39] That said, people (here, women) can be fat or thin *para phusin* (*Nature of Women* 19–20; *Barrenness* 17, 25).

[40] Cf. chap. 18, where *akrasia* is one cause of lungs' excessive dryness leading to erysipelas.

[41] *Internal Affections* (36) cites drunkenness as a cause of jaundice. For further examples, see *Diseases* II 22, 55; III 8; *Internal Affections* 28, 40; *Epidemics* V 88; VII 109. In *Epidemics* V (86), a young man passed out drunk, but not ailing, succumbs to a snakebite.

[42] On drunkenness and madness, see further *Epidemics* IV 15; V 2; VII 92. *Regimen* I (24) is noteworthy in Hippocratic writings for its suggestion that indulgence of *epithumiai*—here, that for drink—leads to others' harm through deception and violence, because, contra Plato, passages favoring restraint or nonindulgence concerning the Big Three virtually always do so strictly on grounds of health.

[43] My translation.

instance, "a thoroughly bad regimen" contributed much to the person's suffering, with death the result (case 13).[44] Even after becoming ill, some still operate "just as they please, and neither forgo nor restrict the satisfaction of their desires" (*pros hêdonên, kai out' an aposchointo oudenos hôn epithumeousin outh' huposteilainto an*, *Ancient Medicine* 5).

While Hippocratic writings contain much evidence that doctors appreciated the Big Three's role as cause or co-cause of ailments, they evince no consensus on the topic. As for the Big Three and medical treatment, Hippocratic authors' judgments oscillate between negative and positive, with indulgence of the Big Three forbidden or allowed on contextual grounds, that is, based on authors' determination of whether it aids recovery. *Internal Affections* (3) formulates the point with elegant succinctness: patients are to "refrain from venery and from drinking to intoxication, except where the latter is appropriate to [treatment of] the disease (*ên mê têi nousôi prosphoron êi*)."

Regarding indulgence as a liability, in *Internal Affections* (17), venery not only causes illness but is something to avoid during treatment. *Prorrhetic* II goes a step further: having identified sexual indulgence and intoxication as impeding recovery, the author offers practical tips to physicians on how to spot excessive pursuit of food, alcohol, and sex by patients who are diverging from doctors' instructions (4). Elsewhere, combining proscription with perhaps a note of resignation, an author advises that while the patient should "abstain from drunkenness and venery . . . if he does engage in venery, let him take a vapor-bath while fasting" (*Diseases* II 73).

Medical writings stress the centrality of *kairos*—the right or favorable moment, where opportuneness varies by setting—to determinations of whether indulgence is allowed. In keeping with the stress of *Internal Affections* (3) on context dependency respecting drunkenness and venery, these are ruled out, not categorically, but in connection with particular treatment regimens (e.g., *Diseases* II 50, 66). In one context, the author stipulates expressly that patients refrain from both just for a period of one year (51); he proceeds similarly with drunkenness and gluttony (53).[45] Elsewhere, drunkenness, with venery, is not to be shunned unconditionally but merely "at an inopportune time" (*para kairon*)—this despite the fact that the former is a cause of the very liver ailment for which the patient is being treated (*Internal Affections* 28).

---

[44] See also *Epidemics* I 19; VII 53.

[45] Cf. *Regimen in Acute Diseases* (Appendix 52), which deems *enkrateia* requisite, not tout court, but for recovery from the type of dropsy that is not always terminal.

Under medical supervision, drunkenness is at times not merely condoned but commended, as in *Diseases* II, whose author states that while drunkenness may cause illness, even death (16, 22), the imbibing of "strong unmixed wine" may also be beneficial as a facet of treatment (27; see also *Nature of Women* 32.46).[46] In *Internal Affections* (18), practitioners attending a patient are charged with making him so drunk initially that he bleeds through the nose. Notably, in *Epidemics* II (6.30), the prescribed "remedy" for hangovers is actually further consumption of alcohol. Alcohol's use in the treatment setting is recommended on many other occasions, too.[47]

Hippocratic authors may also encourage pronounced indulgence of food, again heeding context dependency. In *Internal Affections*, fattening the patient is an element of his treatment for a liver ailment (28), and the program for recovery from typhus, which usually spans two years, includes a patient's eating "whatever foods he prefers and in the largest possible amounts" (43). *Aphorisms* (1.16), in turn, prescribes a careless diet as helpful with fevers not only in children but also in adults whose dietary sloppiness is habitual.

Though authors tend to recommend against venery during treatment, it too may constitute an element thereof. In *Epidemics* VI (5.15), for instance, unhindered indulgence is said to aid recovery from diseases whose cause is phlegm. According to *Epidemics* VII, venery is the treatment of choice for dysentery (122), likely due to the drying effect of sexual activity (69; Smith 1994, 413).

Also reflecting indirect, context-dependent attention to matters bearing on *epithumiai* (desires) is medical writings' sometime allowance of what authors view as mild concessions to patients' desires; these stem, for instance, from doctors' surmising that they will aid patients' morale,[48] as distinct from what doctors commend based strictly on medical insight. Thus, doctors make modest accommodation involving food for what pleases patients at a juncture in treatment when the item is prohibited (*plên ei ti smikron hêdonês heineka*, *Regimen* III 68) and for patients' pre-ailment preferences (*tou kamnontos chroniên epithumiên*, *Precepts* 14). According to *Aphorisms* II (38), "food or drink that is a little inferior but more pleasant is to be chosen over items that are better for the patient yet less pleasing (*to smikrôi cheiron kai poma kai sition, hêdion de, tôn beltionôn men, aêdesterôn de, mallon haireteon*)."[49]

---

[46] When encountering the term "unmixed" (*akrêtesteron*), one must bear in mind that the alcohol content of Greek wines was around 18% (Jouanna 1999, 165). Davidson (1997, 40) puts the alcohol content at 15%–16%, which, as he points out, still surpasses the usual figure today.

[47] See *Diseases* II 70–71; III 6, 14, 16; *Internal Affections* 4 (give wine that is *hôs hêdistos*), 6, 21, 30, 35, 52.

[48] On this topic see also Jouanna (1999, 133–34).

[49] My translation. Cf. *Regimen* I (18), which ties cookery to pleasure-production as an illustration of human concurrence in the broader setting of macrocosmic accord. Pleasure is also the focal point of measures

Consistent with health's being the paramount good, what is preeminently virtue-, or ethics-, based terminology in Plato (*agathon-kakon*, *kalon-aischron*) regularly has health as its focal point in medical writings.[50] Thus, when the author of *Fleshes* announces at the outset that he shall handle "the good and bad in man" (*ho ti to en anthrôpôi kakon kai agathon*),[51] he means that he addresses what holds the promise of benefit or the specter of harm respecting symptoms and medical treatment. The same applies generally to ailments, their progressions, and all facets of medical praxis: hence, one who will knowledgeably frame and answer queries about healing "must consider . . . what in the body . . . is noble or base . . . what evil, succeeding another one, brings something good, and what evil follows inevitably upon some other evil" (*enthumeisthai chrê . . . tou sômatos . . . ho ti kalôs ê aischrôs . . . kai ho ti kakon epi kakôi genomenon agathon poieei, kai ho ti kakon epi kakôi anankê genesthai, Diseases* I 1).[52]

involving heat and cold (*Use of Liquids* 1–2). Further, dreams of heavenly bodies' aimless wandering are alleged to signify anxiety, for whose addressing *Regimen* IV prescribes "the contemplation of comic things if possible"; otherwise, the patient should focus on "such other things as will bring the most visual pleasure" (*allas tinas has ho ti malista hêsthêsetai theêsamenos*, 89). Medical writings sometimes attend to elements of doctors' self-presentation that, by fostering *hêdonê*, will aid their acquiring of patients. According to *Precepts*, while doctors must not cultivate lavish appearances, they may, within calculated limits, adjust such (10). *In the Surgery* includes a mélange of practical and self-promotional tips on operators' position, fingernails, and hands (3–4); even where such praxis aiming to please and comfort is distinguished from "dexterity" (*eucheiriê*), it is not deemed irrelevant (*Diseases* I 10). *Physician* suggests that patients give weight to appearances beyond what truly indicates doctors' caliber. Far from discouraging physicians' catering to that inclination, the author recommends that doctors exploit it, e.g., by self-application of "sweet-smelling unguents" in order to please the ailing (1). The text and translation of *Physician* (1) are those of Potter (1995), not Jones (1923). The author's commendation of pandering, out of a concern with favorable repute (*doxan agatha*), is direct and unabashed (ibid., cf. 8).

50 The ensuing illustrations include the aforementioned adjectives, along with comparative and adverbial forms. I do not wish to suggest that the present discussion exhausts Hippocratic attention to ethical matters, which appears elsewhere, most famously in the Hippocratic Oath, still taken in some form today by many graduates of medical schools; rather, I concentrate on what bears most directly on the present inquiry.

51 My translation.

52 Cf. *On Fractures* (30), where it is *aischron gar kai atechnon* "to make a machine and get no mechanical effect." Further illustrations of the point abound: *Coan Prenotions* 2, 35–36, 51, 278, 308–9, 320, 332, 337, 340, 363, 371, 384, 386–87, 399, 432–34, 438, 449, 454, 459, 462, 471, 482, 487, 496–97, 512, 546–47, 551, 554, 557–58, 590–91, 593, 595, 599; *Crises* 1, 3, 8, 13, 23, 29, 60; *Glands* 8; *Prorrhetic* II 19–25, 32; *Diseases* I 4, 7; III 10; *Regimen in Acute Diseases*, Appendix 23, 29; *Epidemics* V 54; *Critical Days* 1; *Superfetation* 29. The term *kakoêthês*, which has a strong moral sense (e.g., "malicious") when applied to states of character or soul, means "malignant" when used of disease-conditions (Liddell and Scott 1996): see *Epidemics* VII 82; *Prorrhetic* I 74, 126, 128; *Coan Prenotions* 31–34, 141, 278, 316, 336, 524, 603, 613. In *Girls* (1), when females do not marry and become pregnant at the usual time, due to the bad condition of their blood (*hupo de tês kakiês tou haimatos*), their spirit lures them toward what is bad (*ho thumos kakon ephelketai*): if hallucinations are present, the girls view suicide (e.g., through hanging) as better (*ameinona*) than continuing to live; when visions are absent, a pathological pleasure deludes them into coveting death as a good (*erai tou thanatou hôsper tinos agathou*). The relevant terminology here has no moral cast, the issue being unnatural psychic states due solely

In Hippocratic discussions of desire, pleasure, and indulgence, one finds only occasional attention, itself indirect, to issues of character. According to *Ancient Medicine* (5), even now *barbaroi* (foreigners, i.e., non-Greeks) and certain Greeks decline to restrict their pursuit of desires (*diaiteontai pros hêdonên, kai out' an aposchointo oudenos hôn epithumeousin outh' huposteilainto an*). Like the *Gorgias*, though without elaboration, the author negatively esteems those content with the unchecked pursuit of their desires. In addition, *Regimen* I likens the milieu of physical training to that of the marketplace, where entrants, "drinking and raving," mislead and do violence to others (24), which strongly implies that intoxication is a source of immoral conduct.

To sum up, even where authors speak negatively of indulgence as an *archê* of disease, the harm is its causing or co-causing of illness. Hippocratic writings do not suggest that free appetitive indulgence reflects an intrinsically mistaken pattern of valuation.[53] In writers' estimation, right and wrong quantities of food, drink, and sex in medical treatment are context-dependent matters, hence the prominence of terms like *kairos* (favorable moment) and *akairos* (untimely) in such discussions. From Plato's standpoint, given the natural bent of *epithumiai* toward insatiability (*Gorgias* 493a–494a), it is dangerously self-deceptive to allow selective indulgence of the Big Three, for once one opens this door, setting limits to desire and pleasure may become impossible. From the *Gorgias*' standpoint, Hippocratic prescriptions for indulgence are ill-advised at best, stemming as they do from ignorance of what human nature and thriving truly comprise.

Since the Big Three *epithumiai* are naturally insatiable, the so-called small Hippocratic concessions to what pleases patients are quite risky precisely because they appear so trifling. Further, such concessions—like outright medical prescriptions for drunkenness, gluttony, or venery as aiding recovery—occur invariably under doctors' "expert" guidance and supervision, which lends them a pronounced, reassuring air of legitimacy.

The ground of an applicable reservation is voiced in *Places in Man*, according to which "if someone wishing to harm the body should take away some part, even the smallest, the body will experience the hurt, of whatever sort it be, because the smallest part has everything that the greatest part has. . . . For this reason, a person

to physiological disturbance. "It is quite disgraceful (*panu d' estin aischrôs*) not to achieve with an operation what you wish to" in chap. 6 of *Physician*, a late work, could have a moral tinge depending on whether it is read as pertaining to doctors' reputations or to *technê*-governed criteria for what is best; either way, the context remains squarely that of medicine and health. From Plato's standpoint, the issue, ultimately, is not whether the application of such terminology (*agathon-kakon, kalon-aischron*) to the bodily domain is allowed or banned but what referents of the terms are viewed as foundational.

[53] Cf. Holmes (2010, 199–200).

experiences both pain and pleasure from the smallest members of his body, since all parts are present in the smallest, and these smallest parts pass on their experience to each of their own, and inform them of everything" (1, cf. 9). On this line of thought, small bodily pleasures and pains will not stay localized.

While *Places in Man* (1) contains a promising thought, it operates just on the plane of *sôma*. From Plato's standpoint, since doctors are anything but psychic experts, their concessions involving desire and pleasure are problematic above all for their potentially devastating impact on the soul. Some might accuse Plato of being unreasonable here: surely the concessions noted by doctors are harmless enough. A provocative feature of his writings, central among them the *Gorgias*, *Symposium*, and *Republic*, is their insight that human existence is not truly breakable into compartments such that relaxations of stringency involving desire and pleasure in, say, the medical arena implicate exclusively the person's actions in that specific time and place. The *Gorgias*' depictions of the harm to Athenian citizens wrought by earlier politicians show the insidious nature of the lead-up to full-blown injustice, whose foundations were laid by ostensibly innocuous measures serving indulgence. Thus Plato would object strenuously to the claim that doctors' flexibility is an asset, with "harmful consequences... [being] either reversible or minimal" (Jouanna 1999, 134).

By Plato's lights, medicine ventures toward a precipice regarding pleasure and desire. If, as per the *Gorgias*, overindulgence of bad desires correlates with psychic corruption, then, while doctors may deal with physical effects and precautions, their vision is limited, for they lack insight into which pleasures reflect and promote the soul's good and which are deleterious (for this distinction as key, see 499b). This understanding, however, falls under the head of a *technê* (500a–b) that is not—and can never be—their own. By allowing, even commending, indulgence and its attendant pleasure, medical practice contributes to the very corruption that, if it becomes irremediable, renders an existence no longer worth continuing.

4.2 Pain

In the *Gorgias*, body's subordination to soul means that the *technê* of judging, which handles psychic remediation, takes precedence over medicine. The result is that health is not to be pursued, even where doctors' efforts may bear fruit, if this would either clash with punishment needed to remedy psychic corruption or effectively countermand determinations that this corruption could not be removed.[54]

---

[54] The door is thus opened to the possibility that doctors and Platonic judges/philosophers may interpret differently what is needful in a given case, with the latter automatically trumping the former's determination of pressing *kaka* and *aischra* (see further the *Republic* and Chapter 4).

While poverty and disease—the negative conditions associated with financial gain and bodily welfare—surpass psychic corruption in pain, this last well outpaces them in harm (477b–e). Since psychic corruption gravely damages what is most valuable in us, it follows that "injustice, lack of discipline, and all other kinds of psychic corruption are the very worst thing of all" (e4–6). Though pain is not an infallible measure of whether and how far one is ailing, medical writings show time and again that doctors use pain, with patients' input on strength and location, as a salient measure of how far advanced conditions are and of patients' responses to attempted remedies (including type, timing, and amount). As Hippocratic treatises make clear, doctors focus extensively on the alleviation of pain not only where medical care will likely foster healing but—usually as part of a broader treatment plan—even where prospects for recovery are dim to nil.

Though pain is regularly taken as a sign of illness (including particular ailments, *Epidemics* II 1.11), it is not invariably a core indicator thereof, as people can of course be sick without it. In addition, pain's intensity may not correlate strictly with an ailment's severity (*Diseases* III 16). In *Epidemics* V (95), pain's early, temporary relenting is wrongly taken straightaway as a sign of improvement (*ham' hêmerêi de edokei . . . tôi iêtrôi . . . beltion echein*).[55] In *Coan Prenotions*, pain's vanishing is a negative sign (364, 459). Elsewhere, patients' experiencing strong pain is a sign of impending recovery (*Coan Prenotions* 288). Still others "do not recover unless severe pains invade their lower limbs" (*Crises* 55).

Although it is not a direct or reliable indicator of harm where it matters most, Plato does not deem pain meaningless. Pain associated with poverty centrally involves physical discomfort from deficiencies in food and shelter (e.g., weakness from hunger, shivering from exposure to the cold). Poverty also involves psychic distress via shame. Poverty's inclusion with disease at *Gorgias* 477b–d thus suggests that, while the pain that Plato subordinates to harm is above all physical, the psychic plane is relevant too. The Hippocratic Corpus views illness, doctors' own prime concern, as causing or correlating with psychic strains like *melancholia* (melancholy) and *mania* (madness).[56] Although Plato seems to acknowledge psychic strain alongside physical discomfort, he distinguishes crucially between such pain or discomfort and the rending of soul that occurs at its furthest remove from good condition (i.e., self-indulgence and injustice).

[55] Cf. *Prognostic* (18), where a symptom can disappear without the ailment itself remitting.

[56] Conversely, though far less often, affects are said to impact the body (*On the Sacred Disease* 13). On *melancholia* see further Jones (1923a, lviii).

People often put off going to doctors due to a fear of pain (479a6–b1).[57] In fact, the *Gorgias* suggests that people tend to fear bodily pain more than the psychic harms of self-indulgence and injustice to the extent that they are even aware of the latter. Medicine's own occupation with pain if anything reinforces that notion. As the *Gorgias* makes clear, from doctors' standpoint, the best course with serious ailments is for them to be consulted straightaway. This assumption—on regular display in Hippocratic writings—is undercut in the dialogue by the ultimate precedence of the *technê* of judging over medicine, hence of psychic optimization over physical reinstatement. As we will see, the same assumption about doctors' consulting is repudiated more pointedly in the *Republic*.

4.3 Soul

Though its focus is the body, medical writings also attend to the soul beyond organic, physiologically grounded phenomena like coma and delirium.[58] As we shall see, far from being an asset, these discussions strengthen Plato's case that medicine is in over its head when it comes to *phusis* and *eudaimonia*.

In the Hippocratic Corpus, psychic phenomena stem from the body in various ways. In *On the Sacred Disease*, the brain, a bodily organ (20), is the source of "our pleasures, joys, laughter and jests, as well as our sorrows, pains, cares, and tears. Through it . . . we think, see, hear, and distinguish the ugly from the beautiful, the bad from the good, the pleasant from the unpleasant. . . . It is the same thing that makes us mad or delirious, inspires us with dread and fear . . . brings . . . inopportune mistakes . . . and acts that are contrary to habit" (17).[59] In *Diseases* II, a tear in a bronchial tube causes irrational conduct (54), and phrenitis accounts for affects including disgust and fear (72). Similarly, a liver ailment causes rage and aggression

---

[57] As Hippocratic descriptions make clear, requisite treatments may be taxing for patients: see, e.g., *Diseases* II 27, 30, 33, 35; *Internal Affections* 13, 21–23; *Regimen in Acute Diseases*, Appendix 61; *Epidemics* V 7, 49; VII 2; *Places in Man* 25. While Hippocratic writings evince more confidence overall than Plato regarding patients' exposure to pain and consulting doctors of their own accord, mention is made of patients' delaying treatment or sidestepping doctors' recommendations (e.g., *Prorrhetic* II 3–4).

[58] On coma see, e.g., *Epidemics* II 3.1; III, cases 2 and 13 of 16; VII 11; *Prorrhetic* I 1, 74; *Coan Prenotions* 7, 36, 102, 161, 176–82, 206, 217, 600, 623, 631. Delirium is frequently mentioned: e.g., *Airs Waters Places* 7; *Epidemics* I, cases 3–4, 8–12; II 3.1; III, cases 2–3, 5–6, 8, 10–12; cases 1–4, 7–9, and 13 of 16; IV 2, 15, 45; VII 10–11, 25–26; *Prognostic* 3, 5, 22; *Regimen in Acute Diseases* 17, 42; *Places in Man* 32–33, 39; *Prorrhetic* I 8, 26, 34, 73, 97, 132; *Coan Prenotions* 80, 83, 88, 102, 129, 180, 197, 269, 456, 514, 595; *Crises* 48. As we will see in Chapter 6, the *Laws* is the sole place where Plato allows doctors' involvement with *psuchê*, and that involvement is quite limited in scope.

[59] Deviant conduct occurs when the brain is unhealthy due to extreme heat, cold, wetness, dryness, or some other "unnatural affection to which it was not accustomed" (17). For madness organically explained, see also *On the Sacred Disease* 18; *Glands* 12. For physical signs of impending madness, see *Prognostic* 3, 7.

(*Internal Affections* 29, 48), jaundice generates grief (35), and swelling associated with dropsy causes anger (26). In all these cases, causal trajectories move from the body to psychic phenomena.

In *Diseases* I (30) and *Breaths* (14), blood is the paramount contributor to intelligence.[60] What is more, "when the blood has increased in quantity, the soul and the thoughts in the soul change; the ills of the present are forgotten, but there is confidence that the future will be happy" (*Breaths* 14). According to *Regimen* IV, or *Dreams* (86), "when the body is awake, the soul serves it. Directing nothing of its own accord, the soul divides its attention among many things, assigning a part of it to each faculty of the body—to hearing, sight, touch, and walking, as well as to acts of the whole body. The mind never enjoys independence."[61]

Again, medicine impinges on terrain that, by Plato's lights, *iatrikê* is categorically unequipped to handle. Medicine's materialism doubtless contributes to its assumption that a direct occupation with soul, hence with the soul-body tie, rightly falls under its *peri ti* (subject matter). For Plato, however, medicine necessarily lacks insight, hence authority, in this sphere.

---

[60] Though Heraclitus ties cognitive efficacy instead to fire (B117–18, cf. 36), the reasoning of *Breaths* (14) is broadly similar to his, and both accounts reference drunkenness. Citations of pre-Socratic fragments are from the German edition of Diels-Kranz (1992). In keeping with this blood-based view of intelligence, blood's abnormal motion causes derangement (*Diseases* I 30). Elsewhere the heart is identified as the source of *gnômê*, which is nourished (*trephetai*) not by "visible blood" but instead by a "distillate" thereof (*Heart* 10–11).

[61] It is unusual for authors to note soul-body intertwining or suggest the soul's precedence. Having asserted the soul's subservience to the body when people are awake (*Regimen* II 60), the author contends (61) that the soul is the locus of sense-perception (it is what sees, and the audible "strikes the soul"); moreover, thoughts warm and dry it. While *Regimen* II (see also 64) stresses soul and body's interconnection, no clear account is offered, and what is said is not obviously consistent. In *Affections* (46), the greatest benefit from food and drink is asserted to stem from decisions paying heed to both body and soul. *Epidemics* VI (8.10) claims separate conscious awareness, particularly regarding affects: "Even the mind's consciousness, itself by itself, distinct from the organs and events, feels misery and joy, is fearful and optimistic, feels hope and despair." *Humors* (9) hints at a tie, though unspecified, between the soul and excess intake of food and drink, and suggests that the soul is in charge insofar as the body responds to psychic states, e.g., "with sweats and heart palpitations." For unexplained stress on psychic states' bodily impact, see also *Epidemics* VI 5.2, 5. While *Regimen* IV (86) has the body directing the soul during people's waking hours, "when the body is at rest, the soul, being set in motion and awake, is in charge, and of itself performs all the acts of the body. For the body when asleep does not perceive (*ouk aisthanetai*), but the soul . . . sees what is visible, hears what is audible, walks, touches, feels pain, ponders. In a word, all the functions of body and of soul are performed by the soul during sleep." Since one's efforts while awake are what directly impact thriving, the then-dominant body outpaces the soul in merit. The soul is not irrelevant, however, as dreams' signs of impending illness render it "beneficial to change the regimen of a healthy dreamer" (90). Though such passages suggest some awareness that the soul-body relation is more complex than meets the eye, overall they are marginal. From Plato's vantage point, what is key is that they stem from a categorically flawed approach to nature (centrally materialist) and values (i.e., health's being at the pinnacle).

Where authors recognize soul-body complexity, they are occupied more with body's impact on soul than with the reverse. From Plato's perspective, while health is and should be doctors' ultimate concern, it is not the highest good, hence health is not the right overarching standpoint. Doctors make a mess of things when they turn to the soul because they approach it through the lens of health and overarching physical/material substances and processes. Related to this, they lack knowledge of the soul itself. If doctors possessed such knowledge, they would never, for instance, treat courage (see *Airs Waters Places* 12) as "an innate quality, the product of climate, favored by law" (Jouanna 1999, 231). Nor would they endorse the triggering of affects as key to treatment, as in the claim of *Epidemics* II (4.4) that "it is appropriate to induce anger for the sake of restoring color and humors [i.e., as key to a treatment regimen], also to induce . . . fear and the like" (*epitêdeuein oxuthumiên empoiein kai chrômatos analêpsios heneka kai enchumôsios . . . kai phobous kai ta toiauta*). The *Gorgias*' account of desire applied to affect is antithetical to the view that purposive activation of the latter, regardless of whether health is promoted, is beneficial. According to *Regimen* III (71), intake of food disproportionate to exercise (i.e., gluttony) "disturbs the soul," by which is meant that "sleep is no longer pleasant, but the patient is necessarily disturbed and thinks that he is struggling." Though this impact does not involve soul qua *aretê* (virtue), it shows the author's recognition that unhealthful bodily activity can harm the soul. Plato could not agree more. If one privileges soul as the highest good—Plato's own, not medicine's view—only one who truly understands the soul can speak with assurance on bodily conduct motivated by the soul, above all pleasure and the Big Three.

4.4 Microcosmic Hubris

These objections would represent far less of a problem if medicine correctly assessed its own limitations. For all its positive talk about medicine, the *Gorgias* hints at what I call medicine's "microcosmic hubris." While it shows up well when compared with rhetoric and cookery, the *Gorgias* suggests that acknowledging its own limits may be difficult for medicine. In this way, the *Gorgias* sets the stage for Eryximachus' speech in the *Symposium*. To subordinate medicine is of course not to deny its merit altogether. Thus, *Gorgias* 511d–512d makes clear that medicine's contributions, kept within their proper limits, though inferior to those of judging, are not in doubt.

Gorgias 504e–505a on lives' prolongation connects importantly to 511d–512d, where Plato deems it critical that experts in each *technê* be aware not only of the reach of its own domain but also of what it does not properly encompass. He thus incorporates here the *Apology*'s view that while craftsmen preside expertly over circumscribed areas of human concern, they err by not seeing that their *technai* equip them only within limits to pronounce on human affairs (22c9–e1). While the *Apology* leaves intact craftsmen's limited expertise, the *Gorgias* suggests that one is not a proper expert if one fails to see this: this limitation—with experts' awareness thereof—is built into the *technê* theory itself at 511d–512d. The incorporation of this limit in the *peri ti* and understanding conditions ties it as well to the goodness criterion since *technê*-practitioners may truly and reliably benefit others just so far as their cognitive mastery extends.

Interestingly, while talk of medicine is abundant elsewhere in the dialogue, at 511d–512d Plato's prime example of professional humility is the helmsman. The doctor appears only at the discussion's close (512d5).[62] Helmsmen's modus operandi—contrasted expressly here with that of rhetoricians—is unpretentious and orderly (*prosestalmenê . . . kai kosmia*, 511d3–4; cf. 512b).[63] Their grasp of the limits attending their practice makes them consciously aware that, qua pilots, they cannot assess whether they have aided or harmed those whom they convey from shore to shore. Thus, on each occasion the helmsman, having accomplished his feat of conveyance,

> disembarks . . . with a modest air (*en metriôi schêmati*). For he's enough of an expert to conclude that it isn't clear which of his fellow voyagers he has benefited by not letting them drown at sea, and which ones he has harmed, knowing that they were no better in either body or soul when he set them ashore than they were when they embarked (*logizesthai gar oimai epistatai hoti adêlon estin houstinas te ôphelêken tôn sumpleontôn ouk easas katapontôthênai kai houstinas eblapsen, eidôs hoti ouden autous beltious exebibasen ê hoioi enebêsan, oute ta sômata oute tas psuchas*). . . . He knows that for a corrupt person, it's better not to be alive, for he necessarily lives badly (*oiden hoti ouk ameinon estin zên tôi mochthêrôi anthrôpôi; kakôs gar anankê estin zên*). (511e5–512b2)[64]

"He's enough of an expert to conclude" suggests that if the pilot fails to grasp these limitations—above all, the fact that satisfying the goodness condition for his own specialized endeavor does not include determining whether his clients are aided or harmed in body or soul through his conveyance of them—he is not truly an expert at all.

---

[62] For Hippocratic linkage of medicine and piloting, see the claim of *Ancient Medicine* (9) that most doctors are like poor helmsmen.

[63] On *prosestalmenê*, see Dodds (1959, ad loc.), who notes its "appl[ying] properly to one who compresses himself into the smallest possible space." The use of *kosmia* (orderly) here is significant given the interchangeability of *kosmioi* and *sôphrones* elsewhere in the dialogue.

[64] Note that this passage, like *Republic* 409e–410a, makes a stronger claim about the psychically irremediable than it does regarding those who are physically so.

The passage continues: "And yet if he wanted to say what you [clever speakers] do, exalting his occupation, he would bombard you with speeches, telling you urgently that people should become engineers because nothing else amounts to anything" (*kaitoi ei bouloito legein . . . haper humeis, semnunôn to pragma, katachôseien an humas tois logois, legôn kai parakalôn epi to dein gignesthai mêchanopoious, hôs ouden talla estin*, 512b8–c3). These speeches (*logoi*) would be accurate, hence defensible, if the continuation of bare existence were itself a good—which, however, it is not (512d–e). This point is later reaffirmed, with precedence given to one's psychic condition (522d–e, 526d–e). The properly self-aware helmsman knows (1) that merely existing is not inherently good and (2) that his own expertise does not permit him to glean what is apparent only to experts in justice and thriving, namely, where his passengers stand in terms of psychic well-being. Yet only these determinations permit one to know whether genuine benefit has occurred.

Key to the present investigation is Plato's linking helmsmen and doctors as practitioners of *technai* that are "devised to preserve (*sôizein*) us" (512d6). Doctors are often aware of having benefited patients on the bodily plane. If we make the relevant substitutions, we see that Plato's notion at 511e6–512a2—"It isn't clear which of his [patients the doctor] has benefited by not letting them [die], and which ones he has harmed, knowing that they were no better in either body or soul when he [finished their treatment than when he began]"—applies more to pilots than to doctors. Crucially, however, the passage's close, "He knows that for a corrupt person, it's better not to be alive" (512b1–2), concentrates wholly on people's psychic states and as such applies equally to piloting and medicine.

Helmsmen and doctors provide boons intrinsic to their own specialties. While health contributes to thriving more than geographical transposition, marked limits remain on the goods that doctors and pilots may bestow as practitioners of their respective disciplines.[65] Unlike piloting, medical practice is governed directly by the specialty's own views of *phusis* and *eudaimonia*—topics at the core of human existence, felt mastery of which by a praxis is sure to stoke its impression of supremacy. For this reason, it will likely be harder for doctors to accept firm restrictions on medicine's purview. Precisely because its action is guided by such views, however, it is all the more pressing that the true limits of medicine be revealed and the field properly lodged among human endeavors. Though on other points medicine and rhetoric are firmly opposed, respecting a failure to properly acknowledge limits on one's authority, the *Gorgias* leaves the door wide open for medicine's linkage with *rhêtorikê*. In fact, as will emerge in Chapter 3, a

[65] This point is key vis-à-vis contemporary debates about the ultimate source of values governing medical practice, on which see Chapter 7.

hubristic grasping at wholesale mastery—embedded in grand macrocosmic proclamations—is what Eryximachus instantiates in the *Symposium*, to his grave detriment as a representative of *iatrikê*.

For Plato, medicine falls short in its handling both of the microcosm (i.e., the human sphere) and of the macrocosm (i.e., in its broad cosmological theorizing), hence also in its presentation of parallels between them. Apropos of the *Gorgias*, our focus has been on flaws in medicine's handling of the microcosm. As we will see in Chapters 3 and 4, Plato's expected response to medicine based on this dialogue is itself clearly present in the *Symposium* and *Republic*. In Chapter 3, we investigate not only the *Symposium*'s microcosmic focus on medicine but also its critique of medicine's handling of the cosmos writ large. Because its supposed authority in both areas grounds claims that it is the *technê* par excellence, Plato's dual-pronged critique of medicine constitutes an argument against its preeminence.

5. LOOKING AHEAD

The *Gorgias' agôn* with rhetoric is at the same time a castigation of Athens' existing sociopolitical priorities. For cities, as with individuals, the good is tied to order and balance, the bad to imbalance and disarray. In the dialogue's critique of Athens' democratic grid and history—no distinction is made between current politicians and earlier ones—rhetoric figures importantly. In fact, the *Gorgias* blurs the distinction between one's being a political leader who is a good orator and one's being a rhetorician adept at political persuasion. This blurring is what allows Plato to treat key politicians past and present *as* orators (455d–e; cf. 515c–517c, 519a–b). Notably in this regard, Themistocles, Pericles, and Cimon are mentioned as having gorged the city on building projects and tribute payments "in the wholesale absence of self-control and justice" (*aneu gar sôphrosunês kai dikaiosunês*, 519a1–2).[66] This stress on politicians' self-indulgence and injustice even as they purport to be agents of enhancement ties them closely to rhetoricians.

Given how closely rhetoric and politics were intertwined in Plato's day, his reservations about the prevailing model of Athenian politics are significantly disclosed through the dialogue's critique of rhetoric. One gleans far less about the true political art, except by pointers filtered through the three core *technê* conditions. This is no accident. So long as rhetoric and politics are intermingled, an occupation with one's own advancement—even if cloaked in an alleged concern for the broader

---

[66] My translation.

good—will always be decisive, and at odds with what is best except haphazardly. As Plato notes at the *Gorgias*' close (527d), one cannot move straightaway from a wrongheaded pursuit of communal thriving, grounded in psychic distortion, to detailed conception and enaction of the political art. This would be premature, as one could not but transfer prevailing misconceptions to the "new" sociopolitical domain.

The *Gorgias*' castigation of prevailing competitive models is incontrovertible (e.g., 457d–458b), and 466b launches Plato's redefining of power qua competitive mastery through the goodness condition on *technai*. The *Gorgias*' take on the notion of *agôn* is multifaceted. In my view, Plato inaugurates here a balancing act that typifies relevant dialogues from this point forth. On the one side, it is essential that he dissolve the competitive paradigm long established in literary and athletic strivings, and increasingly dominant in the political sphere via rhetorical/sophistic practice.[67]

On the other, though Socrates stresses at 515b–c the nonagonistic quality of their enterprise, the *Gorgias* ends with a strong charge by Socrates issued in agonistic terms: "I call on all others as far as I am able . . . to this way of life, this contest, that I hold to surpass all other contests in this life" (*Parakalô . . . tous allous pantas anthrôpous, kath' hoson dunamai . . . epi touton ton bion kai ton agôna touton, hon egô phêmi anti pantôn tôn enthade agônôn einai*, 526e1–4). Plato, however, has reframed the competitive field through the dialogue's occupation with self-mastery, which culminates at 526e. As Irwin (1979, 248) observes, Socrates' *agôn* "is essentially different from others, since praise and success does not depend on competition with others, but entirely on the agent himself." Rather than stretching a tensive relation into an indefinite future, this *agôn*, rightly engaged, maximizes psychic order and harmony, which grounds the fitting use of all nonpsychic goods.

---

[67] Rhetoric had become central to the legal sphere as well, where trials' labeling as *agônes* underscored their deeply competitive nature (Yunis 2005, 196–97). Before the democratic reforms of Ephialtes in 462 B.C., Athenian trials were usually conducted before individual magistrates or the Areopagus, a court comprised of former magistrates (Kennedy 1963, 27). Subsequently, those bodies' purview was radically condensed; large juries of ordinary citizens came to preside over most cases and thus also to function as judges (ibid., 27–28; Yunis 2005, 194). Since laypeople now decided cases, latitude increased for involved parties to tweak legal interpretations for their own immediate ends, in which process rhetoric was an immense support (Sickinger 2007, 299; Yunis 2005; Kennedy 1963, 28)—so much so that, as the revised endeavor involved "a presentation of the case by the litigants themselves, each in a single set speech with sometimes a single opportunity for rebuttal . . . [there was] imposed on each litigant, and potentially on each Athenian citizen, a need to be an effective public speaker, to be able to organize a long speech and deliver it clearly and effectively" (Kennedy, 1963, 28; cf. Yunis 2005, 192). Sickinger (2007, 288) makes clear just how far the judicial responsibilities of ordinary Athenians surpassed those to which we are now accustomed: "As both prosecutors and defendants . . . private citizens had complete responsibility for preparing a case for trial. This entailed gathering all relevant pieces of evidence, seeking out witnesses, and finding potentially relevant laws. All these items were then woven together into a speech that litigants were expected to deliver, in person, to a court."

By pointing to the need to shift one's view of the nature of power and for a transmuted notion of the most fundamental human *agôn* (contest)—where the right change in one straightaway renders flawed constructions of the other insupportable—the *Gorgias* is precursor to the *Republic*'s sustained exploration of both themes. Meanwhile, Plato has thrown down the gauntlet, nested in the *technê* framework, that is his challenge to power seen as wedded to self-aggrandizement through honor and physical/material goods.

Though the *Gorgias* sets the stage for the *Symposium*'s handling of medicine, only the latter attends to medicine's own claims to occupy the pinnacle of *technai*, which self-positioning is prominent in medical writings. In fact, Plato's awareness that doctors do not subscribe to the self-effacing, unassuming model illustrated by the helmsman at *Gorgias* 511d–512d is abundantly clear in the *Symposium*, where Eryximachus makes unlimited claims for medicine's cognitive authority. While medicine's *technê* standing remains intact in the *Symposium*, Plato debunks its self-assertion of preeminence. However, medicine has further to fall, and fall further it does in the *Republic*. Not coincidentally, in the *Phaedo*, *Symposium*, and *Republic*, Plato articulates his own views of how the visible is like (and unlike) the invisible. Reflection on the latter, namely Forms, is the well from which his notions of *phusis* and *eudaimonia* are drawn.

While the *Gorgias*' account of *technai* benefits greatly from Hippocratic elucidations of *iatrikê*, recast as needed in keeping with Plato's own priorities, as argued in Chapter 4 on the *Republic*, medicine's own *technê* standing will be an inevitable casualty of that revamping. The assistance offered by medicine when Plato forges his notion of *technê* thus comes back to haunt it in a most unexpected and—to its proponents—doubtless horrifying way.[68]

At the close of the *Gorgias* (527e), Plato exhorts us to take the *logos* that he has provided as our guide to further reflection on what thriving consists in and the path to its cultivation. As we have seen, among the tasks of the overarching *technê* the dialogue speaks of is a deeper inquiry into pleasures and desires, including their kinds and effects.[69] Such a governing *logos* medicine cannot provide: if we follow Plato's

[68] Broadly speaking, this occurrence exhibits a similar double edge to medicine's construction of well-being in terms of order and harmony—which domain, according to Jouanna (1999, 255), in fact inaugurates "the cognitive paradigm of order and the exclusion of disorder."

[69] For stress on the *Gorgias*' pointing up a need for further Platonic inquiry into pleasures, see Irwin (1979, 205); Gosling and Taylor (1982, 82). On Gosling and Taylor's account, the *Republic* addresses the need for a comprehensive account of pleasure's nature (98), grounding it, implausibly (117), in a general application of "the physiologically inspired replenishment model of pleasure" (105; cf. 178, 184). The *Philebus*, in turn, lacks a general account of the nature of *hêdonê* (136), because Plato, having rejected the lens of "replenishment" (140), sees that the range of pleasures' types precludes an overarching delineation (163–65).

account—as presented in the *Gorgias*, and expanded in the *Symposium* and *Republic*—Eryximachus' competing *logos* in the *Symposium* is sure to lead us astray. Let us turn now to this next stage in Plato's engagement with medicine, which contains his answer to Eryximachus' grand claim—reflected in Hippocratic writings—that medicine is the *technê* par excellence, surpassing even philosophy through its penetrating vision of the nature, hence capacities, of all that exists.

3

Eryximachus' Tale: The *Symposium*'s Challenge to Medicine's Preeminence

I. INTRODUCTION

Commentators have typically dismissed Eryximachus' *logos* (here, "speech") as Plato's caricature of the self-important physician preceding distinctly more salient speeches from his philosophical standpoint. This view of Eryximachus' *logos* as unworthy of serious consideration is a great oversimplification and undervaluing of its import. Despite Edelstein's challenge in 1945, constructions of Eryximachus' speech as a parody have endured.[1] In recent decades, however, prominent scholars have contested that position,[2] which has had a salutary impact on explorations of his *logos*.

Although this is valuable as a corrective, I believe that it goes too far, as when Konstan and Young-Bruehl (1982, 44) laud what they deem an appreciable "degree of systematic exposition and intellectual rigor in the speech." In the present chapter I argue that the *Symposium* reflects a stage in Plato's engagement with medicine that is intermediate between the *Gorgias*' position and his stance in the *Republic*. There, as I argue in Chapter 4, philosophers' grasp of reality, above all the Form of the Good, and a more complex soul-body tie commit Plato

[1] See Nehamas and Woodruff (1989, xvi); Rosen (1987, 119); Dover (1980, 105).

[2] See McPherran (2006); Hunter (2004); Rowe (1999); Konstan and Young-Bruehl (1982).

to retract medicine's very standing as a *technê*—a move broadly aligning him with those critics of medicine's standing against which Hippocratic material is sometimes directed. Here in the *Symposium*, Plato shows why medicine cannot be the *technê* par excellence, thus setting the stage for the *Republic*'s withdrawal of its *technê* standing. Exploring the *Symposium*'s role in Plato's critique of medicine is thus crucial insofar as it enriches our appreciation of how deeply this opponent preoccupied him.

As we saw in Chapter 2, the *Gorgias* adumbrates critique, particularly when its account of the soul is applied to medical writings. The *Symposium* furthers Plato's criticism through Eryximachus' articulation of what he, qua medical professional, views as the nature of the cosmos itself. Eryximachus' account reveals what are for Plato grave shortcomings in medicine's orientation concerning *phusis* (nature) and *eudaimonia* (flourishing). Eryximachus, who represents physicians as a class, has not explored—and cannot uncover—what they genuinely comprise. The point is not that medical authors defend Eryximachus' specific view of *erôs* (love), which is after all a Platonic creation, but that Eryximachus' *logos* combines key strands in medical writings—ones with which Plato takes issue.

For its attention to order and balance, scholars have often claimed medicine as something of a model and complement vis-à-vis Plato's thought. From the standpoint of his rivalries, one might think medicine innocuous compared with poetry and rhetoric/sophistry, since their efforts target the soul while its work revolves around the body. Medicine's own claims are comprehensive, however, involving not only man's nature but also that of the cosmos writ large and the two planes' correspondence. Because the *Gorgias* used medicine mainly as a positive point of comparison with knacks, it focused on the microcosm (i.e., the human sphere). Heavily reliant on the earlier dialogue, the *Symposium* goes beyond it by directly criticizing medicine through the *Gorgias*' lens and by showcasing its approach to *phusis* as including the macrocosm (i.e., the cosmos writ large). Concerning the microcosm, doctors' view of *phusis* comes with a lens on flourishing by which health is the highest good. Further, medicine's context-dependent approach to conduct involving the Big Three *epithumiai* (desires)—those for food, drink, and sex—is interwoven with its handling of *phusis* and sheds partial light on what, more specifically, thriving is taken to involve.

The *Symposium* shows how an expressly framed approach to thriving might look if medicine's unquestioned confidence in its role as arbiter were taken to its natural extreme. Thus, the speech (*logos*) of Eryximachus, combined as relevant with other speeches and elements of the dialogue, illustrates the bad result when a physician's allegedly comprehensive grasp of reality is combined with a deeply flawed approach to the Big Three and the soul tout court. Although medicine need not adopt

Eryximachus' own particular stance, from Plato's standpoint it cannot forestall the emergence of this position or one much like it.

The *Symposium* does not dispute the *technê* status of true medical expertise so long as its applications are kept within proper bounds, as when Eryximachus cures the hiccups of Aristophanes (185d–e with 189a). But Eryximachus' *logos* purports to offer a comprehensive account of nature and thriving. For Plato, the error of this can be shown only by a vantage point on *phusis* and *eudaimonia* other than medicine's own. What is more, Plato must challenge medicine's ability to handle these matters as he defends philosophy's preeminence. Thus, in the *Symposium* we see Plato's critical engagement with medicine—for the first time in the dialogues overtly a rival—unfolding in tandem with his attempts to fortify philosophy's role as arbiter on the all-important topics of *phusis* and *eudaimonia*.

As is evident from our account of the *Gorgias*, interpretive claims about medicine in Plato must reflect a broad-based investigation of Hippocratic writings. Our handling of the *Symposium* also reserves an important place for this background. For Konstan and Young-Bruehl (1982, 44), "Plato's purpose in composing [Eryximachus'] speech [is] inclusiveness—the desire to represent fairly an important thesis on *eros*—rather than . . . a polemical intention to set off to advantage the position advanced by Socrates." Focusing on both the *Gorgias* and medical writings, the present account shows that this construction is far from the truth.

2. ERYXIMACHUS AS EMCEE?

A supposed presiding role granted to Eryximachus at the evening's celebration has been cited as clear evidence of his import qua physician in the *Symposium*. According to Edelstein (1987c, 164), Eryximachus is the "peer [of his fellow symposiasts], nay, in some respects, their superior. For he exercises a certain authority over them. Within the framework of the dialogue, he is indeed more important than anybody else."[3] While Edelstein rightly notes that Eryximachus is a player on what I will call here the "metalevel," this depiction of the doctor's guiding function is too strong. Moreover, it goes awry in maintaining that his role is unequivocally a point in Eryximachus' favor.

Eryximachus assumes that, qua practitioner of *iatrikê* (the *technê* of medicine), he is the one most properly equipped to oversee a gathering that includes prominent poets and a highly esteemed philosopher—and to do so in connection with a

[3] Cf. his reference to "the [physician's] exceptional rôle" (164) and to the "introductory scene . . . [as] dominated by Eryximachus," whose "outstanding part" continues (163).

topic, namely, *erôs*, that by tradition has far more to do with these other domains.[4] If Eryximachus' guiding role were overarching, it would be reasonable to view that fact as buttressing the claim of his own encomium that *iatrikê* is preeminent. Here, however, as in the content of his own *logos*, the physician's pretensions exceed his authority, for Eryximachus' efforts on the metalevel do not obviously stand above all others in import. In addition, they are far from rigorous and uncompromising regarding virtue qua *sôphrosunê* (self-control)—arguably the key *aretê* both here and in the *Gorgias*.

On the matter of drinking as discussed at the outset, instead of condemning it straightaway qua doctor on the ground that excess consumption fosters illness, Eryximachus takes his cue from others. It is Pausanias, supported by Aristophanes, who proposes a significant reduction in the usual heavy alcohol consumption at symposia,[5] as those present are hung over from last evening's celebration of Agathon's dramatic victory (176a–b). Eryximachus then consults Agathon's wishes—which happen to coincide with those of his fellow symposiasts—before declaring this suggestion a stroke of good fortune (*hermaion*, c1).[6] Further, it is Phaedrus' putting his seal of approval (d5–7) on Eryximachus' urging against heavy drinking, particularly among those "suffering the effects of a previous night's excesses" (d4), that clinches the company's decision to eschew the standard mandatory drunkenness.[7] On Eryximachus' formulation—which echoes the group's resolution to let people drink as per their pleasure (*pros hêdonên*, e2–3)—each person may drink as much as he likes (*hoson . . . boulêtai*, e5). Eryximachus vests authority here with each individual (*hekastos*, e5). Hence, far from strictly tempering their conduct from the standpoint of health, Eryximachus allows them as much scope for indulgence as they might wish.

According to Rowe (1998, ad loc.), Eryximachus' claim about heavy drinking as the fruit of insight gained from medicine (d1–3) is something that "everyone . . . knows perfectly well."[8] Whether this general awareness obtained, what is key is that

---

[4] In the case of poetry, see, e.g., Hesiod's *Theogony*. Empedocles is most central among philosophers. While *erôs* figures in Parmenides' account in the "Way of Seeming," his demonstrable philosophical investment lies solely in the preceding "Way of Truth." On these three figures as precursors here, cf. Jaeger (1986a, 182). Ancient Greek script did not distinguish between uppercase and lowercase, so demarcating the deity *Erôs* from *erôs* as an impersonal macrocosmic force or the human quality falls on the shoulders of interpreters.

[5] The very term *sumposion* literally means "drinking together."

[6] Deferential appeal to Agathon qua victor and host might well be expected, but this takes nothing away from the fact that Eryximachus' "scientific" formulation is heavily nested in remarks by all of the original symposiasts besides Socrates.

[7] Translations of the *Symposium* are either drawn from Nehamas and Woodruff (1989), with certain adjustments, or are my own.

[8] Hence, "Phaedrus' reply . . . and everyone else's ready agreement that they should listen to the expert (e1–3) . . . are then easily taken as mock-serious."

the idea of restraint was produced and affirmed by medical laypeople before Eryximachus weighed in. Hence, it arose not from medical strictures but simply because those present felt depleted from the previous evening. Given the broader context in which the decision is set, Edelstein's (1987c, 162) claim that the physician is "responsible for the decision that the symposium be not devoted to excessive drinking" is far too strong.

In fact, Eryximachus' conduct already opens him to criticisms that emerged in the *Gorgias*' critique of pleasure's handling by *empeiriai* (knacks, e.g., rhetoric, cookery), in particular that such permissiveness is not innocuous but likely instead to push people's *epithumiai* further toward insatiability. Moreover, we are primed to suspect that the doctor is not the expert (*technikos*) on this topic for which the *Gorgias* called (500a). Notably, by the end of his speech, Eryximachus' laxity about self-control—like Hippocratic discussions of regimen—has come to clearly include food, drink, and sex (i.e., all of the Big Three). These early signs of Eryximachus' looseness on the matter of drinking are thus suggestive for the anticipatory light they cast on the notion of *sôphrosunê* that guides his own encomium of *erôs*.

Eryximachus proceeds to suggest dismissal of the flute-girl, a staple source of entertainment at symposia, in favor of verbal exchanges. The doctor, who has just received support from his paramour Phaedrus on the matter of drinking, returns the favor, drawing Phaedrus into the spotlight by proposing a topic, *erôs* (love), that he claims to originate with the latter (177a). Eryximachus and Phaedrus concur, at length, on this choice of topic (177a–d). Phaedrus' vested interest is soon evident, as his own encomium, offered first, largely defends an existing kind of bond in aristocratic circles between an older and a younger male, the *erastês* (lover) and *erômenos* (beloved) respectively.[9] Among those present, Socrates has clearly the greatest cachet, as evidenced by the latitude he receives for what would otherwise be viewed as a rude, ill-timed arrival (175c–d). It is thus Socrates' throwing his weight behind the proposal (177d–e) that seals the company's approval of it (177e7–178a1).[10] Again, placed in a broader context, Eryximachus' role is far less dominant than Edelstein's account suggests.

Phaedrus and Eryximachus were linked together at the outset through their reciprocal support. In what follows, the role of authority is not lodged squarely in the latter's hands but well-nigh evenly divided between the two. While Aristophanes' hiccups—treated as a narrowly circumscribed bodily matter—are addressed by Eryximachus (185d–e), Phaedrus keeps the company on track prior to Agathon's

---

[9] For a magisterial inquiry into Greek homosexuality, see Dover (1989).

[10] Socrates' distinctive status as someone for whom such conduct is habitual and accepted is reprised at 220c; cf. Bury (1932, xix).

speech (194d–e). Moreover, Socrates turns to Phaedrus for permission both to depart in his own *logos* from the traditional form of encomia and to question Agathon before so doing (199b–c). Coming full circle, Socrates addresses Phaedrus, treating the latter as overseer, at its close (212b–c).

As at the dialogue's start, when alcohol consumption for the evening was discussed, Eryximachus' final appearance in the *Symposium* shows him once more prepared to defer to others where action bearing on *sôphrosunê* is involved. The physician is willing to tolerate the heavy drinking that Alcibiades had initiated upon his arrival (214a) as long as it is accompanied by either talk or song. Given this fact, Alcibiades' pointed lauding of Eryximachus' father, but not the son, as "most self-controlled" (b4) is partially ironic—but not merely so, as *Symposium* 214a–b involving Eryximachus tacitly supports the *Gorgias'* claim that the absence of firm limits on indulgence lowers the bar to future yielding.[11] Having acceded to Alcibiades on this point of procedure—a marked departure from the less immoderate course that he had supported early on—Eryximachus urges Alcibiades to praise Socrates instead of *erôs* (214d) in what the doctor cannot know will be a *logos* that meshes with the lauding of restraint in Socrates' own speech. Having been pivotal when the choice of *erôs* as topic was confirmed (177d–e), Socrates, not Eryximachus, now grants his acceptance to this course (214e).[12] That the lovers depart together (223b) reinforces the collaborative nature of Eryximachus and Phaedrus' earlier role.[13]

Hence, I must diverge from Edelstein (1987c, 164n38), who claims that Phaedrus' and Eryximachus' being the sole individuals mentioned by name at 223b is "a feature that stresses their moderation." Additionally, there is a telling disconnect here in Plato's underscoring the limits of Eryximachus' role on the metalevel even as the physician views his role as dominant. This discrepancy illumines—well before his own encomium—the doctor's failure to grasp the limits of his own understanding, which awareness was deemed crucial to expert praxis in the *Gorgias* (511d–512d). Further, this notable disconnect between what occurs and the doctor's impression sets the stage for and reinforces Plato's stress on the unbridled extravagance of Eryximachus' claim to cognitive authority in his subsequent lauding of *erôs*.

---

[11] Eryximachus had been identified at the outset as the "son of Acumenus" (176b5). For a different interpretation of the reference to Eryximachus' father at 214b4, see Rowe (1998, ad loc.); Bury (1932, ad loc.).

[12] As to why Socrates assents, might we have reason to think that, knowing what has—and has not—transpired between himself and Alcibiades, Socrates realizes that less of a shift than met the eye would take place? Prior (2006) offers such a justification: having glimpsed the "private face" of Socrates (160–61), Alcibiades sees that his voicing "erotic attachment to youths" qua sexual yearning is ironic (158), and Alcibiades' encomium "affirms" Socrates' completion of the ascent (164).

[13] Cf. Edelstein (1987c, 164n38).

3. MACROCOSMIC OCCUPATIONS: THE *LOGOS* OF ERYXIMACHUS AND ITS HIPPOCRATIC BACKDROP

According to Edelstein (1987c, 159), Eryximachus' speech "is not a caricature but rather an historically correct picture of a medical man of that time. It cannot have been Plato's intention to deride Eryximachus as a pedant, a system-monger, unduly fond of medicine." Though Edelstein rightly shuns the received position that the speech is a parody, I find untenable his claim that Eryximachus is not "unduly fond" of his art. Defending this position necessitates reference to pertinent medical writings.

Having argued for the ancient pedigree of medicine qua dietetics (*Ancient Medicine* 3–5), and vigorously rejecting a foundational role for philosophy in medical theorizing (20),[14] the Hippocratic author observes (ibid.) that

> certain physicians and philosophers assert that no one can know medicine who lacks understanding of what man is. . . . But the question they raise is one for philosophy. . . . My view is that . . . clear knowledge about nature can be acquired from medicine and from no other source (*oudamothen allothen . . . ê ex iêtrikês*), and that one can attain this knowledge when medicine itself has been properly comprehended, but until then it is quite impossible—I mean to possess this information, what man is, by what causes he is made, and similar points accurately.

That philosophical theorizing is useless to the topic at hand is strongly suggested by the author's comment that what philosophers "have said or written on nature no more pertains to medicine than to painting (*hêsson nomizô têi iêtrikêi technêi prosêkein ê têi graphikêi*)" (20). Philosophers like Empedocles offer accounts "on nature (*phusis*)" including man, whose broad sweep bases everything on the same *archai* (explanatory factors).[15] The Hippocratic author's perspective grounded in medicine leads him to claim, against philosophy, that there is no single human nature but rather varying constitutions (*hai phusies*, 20; cf. 12). Moreover, the salience of hot and cold—which figure heavily as opposites in philosophical theories—is discounted as the cause of health and disease (15–19).

Having inverted the direction of inquiry so that medicine's investigation of *phusis* takes precedence over philosophy's, the author makes no attempt to offer the equally

---

[14] On this function see Longrigg (1993); Jouanna (1998).

[15] *Ancient Medicine* (20) itself includes polemical engagement with Empedocles.

comprehensive account grounded in medicine that a full reversal of authority from philosophy to it requires. The more modest scope of *Ancient Medicine* (20) is suggested when the author contents himself with stating that doctors must, at any rate (*epei touto ge*), know "regarding nature" (*peri phusios*) "what man is in relation to foods and drinks"—the illustration being different reactions to cheese across constitutions—and to his lifestyle more generally.[16]

What *Ancient Medicine* provides is starkly inadequate as a *logos* grounding the all-embracing epistemological priority of medicine. Even if one concurs with Longrigg (1993) that this work construes *phusis* narrowly (84 with 239n2), Hippocratic medicine relied on placing man in his broader environment—a view inherited from philosophy, as Longrigg (99) observes. In *Airs Waters Places*, "the greatest triumphs" of the medical *technê* (2, cf. 1) depend on physicians' apprehending wider phenomena falling in the domain of astronomy. Bringing medical expertise to bear in particular geographical settings necessitates doctors' "knowing the changes of the seasons, and the risings and settings of the stars, with the circumstances of each of these phenomena" (2). As we will see, the stance of *Airs Waters Places* is far from idiosyncratic, since medical writings regularly deploy macrocosmic insights as key to health and treatment.

Like the author of *Ancient Medicine*, Eryximachus begins by stressing that all his knowledge was gained through medicine (*ek tês iatrikês*, 186a7). McPherran (2006, 79) draws on *Ancient Medicine* (20) to support the contention that "given his grand theorizing and his citation of Heraclitus, Eryximachus seems very much the kind of physician targeted by this Hippocratic author."[17] I maintain, in contrast, that Eryximachus takes the general stance of *Ancient Medicine* but that he makes in concentrated form an attempt of the sort ultimately required to support a claim for medicine's epistemological preeminence. Though it reflects this general approach, Eryximachus' vision is more ambitious still, since his cognitive authority allegedly encompasses not only the human and cosmological domains but also the deities (*hoi theoi*). While the theoretical orientation is that of *Ancient Medicine*, Eryximachus' methodology parallels—is in fact a version of—*Regimen* I's voluminous citing of *technai* (12–24) to support its case for the single governing nature of all. Hence,

---

[16] Cf. Jaeger (1986b, 19), who claims also (20–21) that even as the author of *Ancient Medicine* critiques the impact of philosophy, he himself engages in it and, moreover, is aware of himself as so doing.

[17] Cf. his assertion that Eryximachus is "Plato's response to all *other* physicians who would rank the craft of medicine as superior to, rather than subordinate to, the new craft of philosophy" (87; emphasis added). While McPherran notes that "Plato has no patience with medicine's overblown claims" (77n16), the aforementioned remark, combined with his assertion that Eryximachus "serves as Plato's model of a properly philosophically-oriented physician" (94n52), commits him to the view that Eryximachus does not represent the targeted group.

the *Symposium* both reflects medicine's own *agôn* with philosophy and contains a Platonic reply.

At *Symposium* 186a3–b2 the physician offers a general statement of his thesis (cf. its reiteration, 187e6–188a1). According to Eryximachus, medicine has taught him (*katheôrakenai moi dokô ek tês iatrikês, tês hêmeteras technês*) that

> love does not occur only in the human soul; it is not simply the attraction we feel toward human beauty but rather a much broader phenomenon (*alla kai pros alla polla kai en tois allois*). It certainly occurs within the animal kingdom, and even in the world of plants. In fact, it occurs everywhere in the universe (*kai hôs epos eipein en pasi tois ousi*). Love is a deity of the greatest importance: he permeates everything (*epi pan . . . teinei*), not only in the human domain, but also in that of the gods.

This opening supports the view that Eryximachus, like the author of *Ancient Medicine*, considers *iatrikê* to be the preeminent *technê*.[18] Eryximachus singles out medicine here as the source of his macrocosmic vision (*arxomai de apo tês iatrikês legôn, hina kai presbeuômen tên technên*, 186b2–3). Moreover, that encompassing vision informs Eryximachus' theoretical treatment of other endeavors whose *technê* standing the physician assumes. In principle one might claim that groups of experts may access ultimate truths from, or through, different initial vantage points, with its being shown here how one might do so via medicine. Paralleling methodologically *Regimen* I (12), Eryximachus' position is that medicine's comprehensive knowledge is unique among the pursuits he considers, most importantly philosophy. For Eryximachus, as is regularly stated or assumed in Hippocratic writings, medicine is the preeminent *technê*.

As often occurs in those treatises, Eryximachus ensconces his approach to health in a broader cosmological thesis from whose perspective bodily good, and the microcosm generally, is properly addressed. Hence, if correct, the view filtered through *erôs* that Eryximachus defends trumps both the stances of endeavors with circumscribed domains (e.g., shoemaking) and all rival comprehensive vantage points.[19] As we will soon see, philosophy's role as Eryximachus' key rival for authority on the real and good is front and center in the longest segment of his speech, that concerning

---

[18] While I concur with Robin's (1929, lii, 24n2) stress on medicine à la Eryximachus as the *technê* par excellence, we underscore different ties to the Hippocratic corpus. On medicine as the "primary" *technê* for Eryximachus, see Rosen (1987, 105). Cf. Hoffmann (1947, 11), who imbeds the point in a quite different interpretive structure.

[19] These would include, of course, proposals by other physicians, in keeping with the intraprofessionally competitive strain evident in medical writings.

mousikê (including for the Greeks both poetry and music). There, he polemically singles out Heraclitus, asserting the philosopher's utter dependence on him for appropriation in a manner that is clear and true.

Reinforcing his self-promotional framing remarks, Eryximachus takes every opportunity to underscore both the *technê* status of his own pursuit and the knowledge of its practitioners. Thus, early on there are ten occurrences of the former: we find *technê* or a cognate on four occasions (186a7–b1, b3, c5, e3), and *iatrikê* or a cognate on six (186a7, b3, c3, c5, d1, e4). The physician's superlative cognitive state is also foregrounded from the get-go: *epistêmê* (186c6), *ho diagignôskôn* (c7), *epistamenos* (d4), and *epistêtheis* (e1, in a reference to Asclepius). Further, this twofold emphasis remains as the speech unfolds.[20] This abundance of references to doctors' insight, which meshes with medical writings' stress on physicians' understanding, contrasts sharply with Eryximachus' treatment of other *technai*.

Eryximachus' position features both a macrocosmic vision and the view that one and the same force, *erôs*, governs it and the human realm (186a–b). Eryximachus' reliance on cosmology to understand humanity is shown by his noting the impact of weather and climate on health (188a–b). It is also displayed by his adopting the single *archê* (explanatory factor) of *erôs*, an agency that, if not itself material, operates in and through matter. This links Eryximachus' efforts, like those of many Hippocratic writings, to cosmologies of the broad sort adopted by pre-Socratic *phusiologoi* (philosophers of nature).[21] That Eryximachus' cosmological reliance is integral to his cementing of medicine's preeminence falsifies Robin's (1929, lin1) claim that in the physician's speech the two themes are distinct.

Before turning directly to Eryximachus' elucidation of his stance, let us briefly survey relevant features of Hippocratic discussions. To the degree that medical writers view man's *phusis*, including its explanatory factors (*aitia/aitiai*), as apprehensible only when humans are seen in their broader surroundings, authors' confidence in their microcosmic understandings stems crucially from their conviction that only doctors grasp the macrocosm.[22]

Encompassing visions, with crucial attention to microcosmic applications, regularly govern medical authors' accounts. While some of these visions are assumed,

---

[20] For pertinent remarks see 187a2 (*tôi kai smikron prosechonti ton noun*, doubtless meant in a self-congratulatory fashion); 187c2–3 (*hôsper ekei hê iatrikê*); c6–7 (*ouden chalepon ta erôtika diagignôskein*); e4 (*en têi hêmeterai technêi*); e6 (*en iatrikêi*).

[21] That this issue is in no way addressed by Eryximachus is but one more mark of its incompleteness and the doctor's inadequacy as a thinker.

[22] Medicine's subsumption of expertise traditionally tied to training/fitness and cookery, discussed in Chapter 2, is salient evidence of that confidence; interestingly from that standpoint, Eryximachus mentions both, with cookery singled out as his *logos* nears its close.

others are argued for.[23] Variables on which those visions concentrate include weather, which I use as shorthand for seasons, regional climates, temperature, and winds (*Regimen* II 37–38, 56, 63, 65; *Regimen* III 67–68, 70; *Humors* 17; *Regimen in Health* 1–3, 7; *Breaths* 3; *Diseases* IV 13, 19–21). Despite its initial opposition to grand cosmological theorizing, *Nature of Man* repudiates a single principle in favor of four equally weighted humors (2, 5).[24] Often particular astronomical phenomena (e.g., equinoxes) are cited expressly (*Airs Waters Places* 2; *Aphorisms* 4.5; *Internal Affections* 39; *Epidemics* I 18, 22).[25] Moreover, authors provide cosmologies along the lines of pre-Socratic accounts, where the sources of all may be one or many, with prominence given to material *aitiai*.[26]

From medicine's microcosmic standpoint, specific cosmological endorsements matter for their bearing on (1) the maintenance of health; (2) diagnoses; (3) treatment plans, including, as pertinent, regimen, medication, and invasive procedures; (4) prognoses for patients' recovery versus permanent impairment or death (*On the Sacred Disease* 11); (5) estimates of illnesses' duration where eventual recovery is anticipated (*Prognostic* 25 conjoins this variable with the preceding one); and (6) doctors' identifications of the palette of ailments to be expected in the coming year (*Airs Waters Places* 2).[27]

The point is not that macrocosmic factors alone are relevant, as authors consistently include microcosmic data like age, constitutional types, what are or should be

[23] The presence of an equally strong commitment to cosmological theorizing by medicine and *phusiologia* is defended by Vlastos (1955), who relies on a small number of Hippocratic passages. Leaving claims about strict equality to the side, the present account supports the view of medicine's pronounced theoretical occupation via a far greater range of textual evidence from medical writings.

[24] Cf. Vlastos (1955, 67), who also references this tension in *Nature of Man*.

[25] See further *Epidemics* II 3.1; V 73, 88–89, 94; VI 7.1; VII 1, 3, 5, 14, 23–24, 39, 41, 43–44, 92–93, 95–96, 103, 105. Cf. *Regimen* IV (89), which, mentioning sun and moon, treats astronomical dreams and the author's own astronomical observations. I parse the relevant territory involving weather, climate, and astronomy in the way that promotes the clearest formulation of the present argument. On *astronomia* for the Greeks as a genus that includes meteorology, see Dover (1980, 110), whose claim is clearly supported by *Airs Waters Places* (2): "Knowing the changes of the seasons, and the risings and settings of the stars, with the circumstances of each of these phenomena, he will know beforehand the nature of the year that is coming. Through these considerations . . . he will . . . succeed best in securing health. . . . If it be thought that all this belongs to meteorology, he will find out, on further reflection, that the contribution of astronomy to medicine is . . . a very great one indeed."

[26] For instance, a single *arché*, air, is favored in *Breaths* 3; *On the Sacred Disease* 19. *Nature of Man*, however, repudiates monism, though it appears to conflate the Eleatic variety (Melissus is mentioned by name), which does not involve cosmology, with sources of being and change that true *phusiologoi* provide. *Fleshes* addresses cosmogony as well (1–3). Plato castigates the emphasis on material explainers by *phusiologoi* in *Phaedo* 96a–99b (see especially 99b, which demarcates material preconditions from genuine explanatory factors, namely, Forms).

[27] Further relevant material is found in *Aphorisms*, *Regimen* I, *Nature of Man*, *Breaths* 3.

individuals' habitual regimens in health, sex (i.e., whether patients are male or female), and sociopolitical status (above all, whether patients are free or slave).[28] Writers are generally convinced of a deep macrocosm-microcosm fit: hence, to say that microcosmic factors are directly involved does not exclude a cosmological explanation. Thus, for instance, constitutions are delineated by reference to the *archê* or *archai* deemed most fundamental, cosmologically speaking (*Epidemics* II 3.15), and suitable regimen, including food, drink, and exertion, is defined by season (*Regimen in Health* 1, 3, 7).

4. ERYXIMACHUS' APPROPRIATION AND CRITIQUE OF HERACLITUS AND ANAXIMANDER

Eryximachus contends that

> dissimilar subjects desire and love objects that are themselves dissimilar. Therefore, the love manifested in health is fundamentally distinct from the love manifested in disease. . . . Whatever is unhealthy and unsound must be frustrated and rebuffed. . . . The doctor's task is to effect a reconciliation and establish mutual love between the most basic bodily elements . . . [which] are, of course, those most opposed to each other, as hot to cold, bitter to sweet, wet to dry, and so on. (186b–d)[29]

Having made this broad cosmological claim, Eryximachus undertakes his subordinating challenge to philosophy.[30] Empedocles' favoring of *erôs* (love), in his case

---

[28] Pertinent material includes *Diseases* I (22), which mentions sex, age, bodily differences across individuals, ailments' intensity in each, and "whether or not the disease has followed from another ailment."

[29] *Lysis* 215c–e voices (though does not endorse, 216a–b) a related stance involving opposites' mutual attraction and dependence, including a mention of medicine. The *Lysis*' account is similar to Eryximachus' in pairs of opposites named and in the mention of filling and emptying (186d–e). Moreover, both present their theses in macrocosmic terms and assume that the cosmos writ large and the human sphere operate in parallel fashion. Though Eryximachus is more focused than the *Lysis* on balance and the avoidance of extremes, these differences do not impact the present argument. The *Lysis*' position is unattributed (215c4–5); when expressly applied to medicine, it meshes with Hippocratic material, due obviously (though not merely) to its notions of filling and emptying, which are central to authors' treatment recommendations (e.g., their extensive recourse to purging). In *Breaths* (1), for instance, opposites are pointedly identified as "cures for opposites." The idea is voiced elsewhere: see *Nature of Man* 9; *Aphorisms* 2.22; 7.60; *Epidemics* VI 5.4; *Airs Waters Places* 7; *Regimen in Acute Diseases* 19; *On the Sacred Disease* 21; *Regimen in Health* 1–2; *Internal Affections* 51.

[30] The doctor's battling of philosophy fits with that in the Hippocratic corpus, most closely *Ancient Medicine* as Edelstein (1987c, 160n25) notes though on different grounds. While "filling" (*plêrôsis*) and "emptying" (*kenôsis*), mentioned by Eryximachus (186d), are not irrelevant, contra Edelstein (cf. Craik 2001, 110), these notions do not constitute the most fundamental points of common ground between *Ancient Medicine* and Eryximachus' *logos*.

with *eris* (strife), is the general backdrop here for Eryximachus' reflections. But Empedocles is not front and center in Eryximachus' account. Moreover, insofar as Empedocles figures as a backdrop for the physician's handling of *erôs* as a harmonizing motive force, the tie is not antagonistic. Eryximachus' handling of *mousikê*—following that of medicine and exceeding it in length—features a pointed, subordinating invocation of another eminent pre-Socratic philosopher, Heraclitus. In what follows I explore that engagement, whose salience and depth have yet to receive their due.

Eryximachus' *logos* relies heavily on what he deems a clarified or corrected version of Heraclitus' global vision centered on the *Logos*; that is, his overarching cosmic principle (e.g., "All things happen according to this *Logos*," B1),[31] toward whose complex, pervasive operations all worthy human thought and speech are directed (B1–2, 114). By operating thus, Eryximachus puts himself in a dialogue with a tradition going back to the Milesian philosophers, Thales, Anaximander, and Anaximenes, whose own comprehensive visions were intended to rival those of poets. It was from these, particularly Homer and Hesiod, that the Greeks derived their views of the divine (Herodotus, *Histories* 2.53), hence of what accounts for paramount macrocosmic operations. Philosophy, once off and running, impacted medicine, as it relied heavily on philosophy's naturalistic explanations, its positing of *archai* usually native to this world, and its emphasis on oppositional substances and properties. Medicine chafed under this reliance even as it could not escape it. Such a bind is a consequence of its seeking to establish itself as arbiter of *phusis* on macrocosmic and human planes. For medicine must then demonstrate its superiority to all else, including an important guide like philosophy.

Eryximachus initiates his handling of *mousikê* by stating that

> the entire *technê* of medicine is guided by *erôs*, just as is the case with (*hôsautôs de kai*) gymnastics and farming; and it is clear to anyone who gives it a moment's thought (*panti katadêlos tôi kai smikron prosechonti ton noun*) that the same is true also in the case of *mousikê*. This is perhaps what Heraclitus, too, wanted to say though it is hard to tell because he does not express himself well. The one, he says, "being at variance with itself is in agreement with itself," "like the attunement of a bow or a lyre." Naturally, it is patently absurd to claim that an attunement or a harmony is in itself discordant or that its elements are still in discord with one another. Heraclitus probably meant that an expert musician creates a harmony by resolving the prior discord between high and low notes, for surely there can be no

[31] Translations of Heraclitus and Anaximander are from McKirahan (1994), with slight modifications.

> harmony so long as high and low are still discordant. Harmony, after all, is consonance, and consonance is a species of agreement. Discordant elements, as long as they remain in discord, cannot come to an agreement, and they therefore cannot produce a harmony. Rhythm, for instance, is produced only when fast and slow, though earlier discordant, are brought into agreement with each other. Music, like medicine, creates agreement by producing concord and love between these various opposites. Music is therefore simply the science of the effects of *erôs* on rhythm and harmony. (186e4–187c5)

McPherran (2006, 77) notes that "Hippocratic physicians at the time did take a self-conscious interest in such things as music." In keeping with this inclination, Eryximachus takes it as natural that he is qualified to pronounce on this topic. His formulation here ("it is clear to anyone who gives it a moment's thought," 187a2; cf. "it is not difficult," c6) is ironic. Influential in *Nutriment* and *Regimen* I, Heraclitus was also relied upon elsewhere in medical writings (*On the Sacred Disease* 4; *Use of Liquids* 3).[32] According to Eryximachus, the esteemed philosopher Heraclitus does not succeed in expressing the cosmic truth about harmony and hence depends on the doctor's aid for the chance to be viewed as proffering an insight as opposed to an absurdity.[33] That Heraclitus is mentioned by name here is notable, as "the use of proper names in a polemical context was not a custom typical of [medical discussions in] the fifth century" (Jouanna 1998, 53). In fact, the use of adversaries' names by Hippocratic authors was so rare that there are just three such references in the entire corpus.[34] Heraclitus' express mention hence dramatically accentuates the polemical nature of Eryximachus' engagement with him, to which we now turn.

As Nehamas and Woodruff (1989, ad loc.) observe, Eryximachus gets Heraclitus completely wrong in his exegesis of 187a–c. Rowe (1999, 62) disagrees, interpreting the discussion as a "transparent" instance of "artfulness and wit in Eryximachus (things said with a nudge and a wink)."[35] The physician is here "*pretending* to put Heraclitus right, in a show of 'learning'" (italics in original). Rowe (ibid.) elaborates: "If Plato knows what Heraclitus actually meant, as he presumably did, there is no reason to suppose that Eryximachus is not supposed to know it—unless we have other grounds for thinking him (meant to be) ignorant of the field, including

[32] *On the Sacred Disease* (4) calls to mind Heraclitus B5 on purification, while *Use of Liquids* (3) recalls B61 on what sea water is suitable for.

[33] Indeed, the Hippocratic distinction between experts and laypeople—and between better and worse physicians—would lose its force if such an insight were not in fact a challenge to achieve.

[34] See Jouanna (1961, 461n68): as he observes, these are to Empedocles (mentioned above; *Ancient Medicine* 20), Melissus (*Nature of Man* 1), and Herodicus (*Epidemics* VI 3.18).

[35] Cf. Hunter (2004, 55).

cosmology, in which he is operating. But there are no such grounds (as everyone notices, he seems to know something about Empedocles)." On the contrary, we have very good reason for believing that Plato wishes to reveal the physician as ignorant here. When one contextualizes Eryximachus' efforts in the Hippocratic Corpus, it becomes clear that he is not pretending. In addition, Rowe's use of Empedocles to support Eryximachus' knowledge of Heraclitus is not compelling, since key notions of the former were far more routine and pervasive than those of the latter as a backdrop for medical theorizing in the fifth century.[36]

Unlike *Nutriment* and *Regimen* I, which silently incorporate versions of Heraclitus' ideas, Eryximachus treats him polemically to ground his lengthy discussion of *mousikê* as, like medicine, "everywhere guided by love" (186e4–187a1): "This is perhaps what Heraclitus, too, wanted to say, though it is hard to tell because he does not express himself well" (*hôsper isôs Hêrakleitos bouletai legein, epei tois ge rhêmasin ou kalôs legei*, 187a3–4). For emphasis, Eryximachus reiterates the same point about Heraclitus just a few lines later (a8). With regard to the caliber of Heraclitus' offering, the doctor envisions just two options, both unflattering: either Heraclitus, like Eryximachus, had the right idea—in which case it took Eryximachus to articulate the point clearly—or one must view Heraclitus as endorsing the absurd position (*esti de pollê alogia . . . phanai*) that harmony and discord may coexist (a6–8).

As McPherran (2006, 80n27) maintains, the speech of Eryximachus indeed shows that the physician is "no slave to Presocratic science." This fact is not, however, as McPherran contends, a point in its favor. Eryximachus proceeds to mangle the nuance in Heraclitus' position—as expressed by "the one . . . 'being at variance with itself is in agreement with itself,' 'like the attunement of a bow or a lyre'" (187a5–6)—via a heavy-handed pronouncement that harmony must arise in a sequential manner whose formulation features a sharp temporal disjunction between *proteron* (earlier) and *husteron* (later; b1).[37] Eryximachus insists that there can be no harmony as long as high and low are at odds (b2–4)—promptly repeating the contention so that it becomes more emphatic still (*homologian de ek diapheromenôn, heôs an diapherôntai, adunaton einai; diapheromenon de au kai mê homologoun adunaton harmosai*,

[36] For detailed treatment of Empedocles' distinctive status qua philosophical influence on Hippocratic medicine in this period, see Longrigg (1993, 26–81, 91–92). On the formulation of Jouanna (1961, 462), "whether imitated or critiqued, Empedocles remained a prominent figure for medicine at the close of the fifth century."

[37] Konstan and Young-Bruehl (1982, 41) note, though without exploring its implications for Eryximachus' standing in Plato's eyes, that the physician "ignores Heraclitus' concern with the tension in the bow or lyre themselves . . . (the bow seems to be irrelevant to this line of reasoning)." Dorter (1969, 226) asserts that Eryximachus is "almost, but not quite, aware" of his "failure to understand" Heraclitus, without indicating the basis of his claim.

b5–7). The physician then makes the same point about rhythm (*hôsper ge kai ho rhuthmos*, b7), again stressing temporal sequence via *proteron* and *husteron* (c1).

Dover's (1980, ad loc.) claim that Plato's interpretation of Heraclitus might not match the latter's intention, and that the construction attributed by Plato to Eryximachus might differ from either of these, is true in an abstract exegetical way. Given that Eryximachus' *logos* proffers what the doctor views as an account of reality proper, including human flourishing, at issue here is the extent to which Eryximachus' construction reflects what can be unveiled as Plato's own. Most specifically, if it can be shown that the physician's interpretation of Heraclitus is distinctly shallower than Plato's, this would support the view that, far from offering a tenable account of his own, Eryximachus cannot even grasp with any subtlety what others have said.[38] That Eryximachus goes so far astray in his take on Heraclitus is but one illustration in his speech of the great harm tied at *Gorgias* 511d–512d to experts' not resting within the natural limits of their disciplines, which point is directly illustrated there via helmsmanship but with medicine hovering about.

Plato's own construction of Heraclitus is more nuanced than would meet the eye based on a cursory reading of passages on flux in the *Cratylus* (439b–440d) and *Theaetetus* (181e–182d) that are not placed in the broader setting of pertinent remarks in Plato's corpus. Although Irwin (1977, 4) does not mention *Symposium* 187a–c, his account of Plato's Heracliteanism distinguishes helpfully between the notion of "*self-change*" ("*s*-change")—alteration of one entity through time (e.g., a shift in height)—and that of "*aspect-change*" ("*a*-change"), which involves the simultaneous coexistence of opposites in one entity from different perspectives (e.g., courage and cowardice, roughness and smoothness). Irwin (5, cf. 12) rightly interprets Plato as being aware of both kinds of flux and as acknowledging Heraclitus' engagement with both. The passages from the *Cratylus* and *Theaetetus* leave no doubt that Plato was cognizant of what Irwin calls *s*-change and associated Heraclitus with it. As Irwin (5) remarks, salient evidence of Plato's knowledge that Heraclitus also foregrounded what Irwin dubs *a*-change is found in the *Hippias Major*, where Plato cites that pre-Socratic philosopher (B82): "Don't you know that what Heraclitus said holds good—'the finest of monkeys is foul put together with

---

38 One finds a similar, though less obviously overarching, lack of care in *Regimen* I's (7) recourse to Heraclitus' view of soul. Contra Jones (1931, 241n2), this view of dual material *archai*, fire and water, as comprising *psuchê* is properly read as a correction of Heraclitus' view of soul as fiery. Though Eryximachus' correction is obtrusive and broader, the parallel to *Regimen* I is notable common ground. Loosely similar to Eryximachus' lack of care and systematicity is *Regimen* I's (10) singling out of *psuchê*, *noos*, and *phronêsis* as comprised of fire that is inaccessible to vision or touch; cf. chap. 21, where statue-makers *mimêsin sômatos poieousin plên psuchês*. As the author appears overall to be a strong materialist, it is not evident what he has in view.

another class'" (289a2–4; cf. b3–5, 293b–c).[39] As commentators have recognized, the *Sophist* buttresses the view that Plato was aware of his predecessor's construction of opposites as coexistent. According to the "Ionian muse" (Heraclitus), "in being taken apart they're brought together" (242d7–e3); Plato contrasts this stance with that of the "Sicilian muse" (Empedocles), who focuses on alternation (242e3–243a1).[40] Furthermore, as Irwin (5) rightly stresses, Plato foregrounds coexistence as an instance of flux at *Theaetetus* 152d: "If you call a thing large, it will reveal itself as small, and if you dub it heavy, it is liable to appear as light, and so on with everything, because nothing is one or anything or any kind of thing. What is really true, is this: the things of which we naturally say that they 'are,' are in process of coming to be."

Given that Plato himself (1) is aware of the two types of flux, (2) knows that Heraclitus had also identified them, and (3) like Heraclitus, ties coexistence to flux, it is significant that he presents Eryximachus as lacking all elements of this understanding. Using Irwin's terminology, one may attribute to Eryximachus the view that instantiating proper *s*-change eliminates tension—at least at the juncture in question. Plato foregrounds both the physician's ignorance and his presumption by having him say that Heraclitus either had the wrong idea or expressed himself poorly by not declaring plainly that he had temporal sequences in view. Supposing himself lucid where Heraclitus was not, Eryximachus states expressly that temporal shifts produce such harmony as exists. Yet the material Eryximachus cites—"the one . . . 'being at variance with itself is in agreement with itself,' 'like the attunement of a bow or a lyre'" (187a5–6)—which he construes as an unmistakable case of *s*-change, is in fact a salient expression of *a*-change. Hence Eryximachus allocates to Heraclitus a confusion that is in fact his own.

I believe that Plato attributes this muddle to Eryximachus to show that the physician (both this individual and the class) lacks insight and a refined capacity for reflection. I cannot agree, therefore, with the contention of Wardy (2002, 7) that "Eryximachus' reading remains an option in the *Symposium*." In my view, it simply cannot be available as an interpretation of the Heraclitean material in question here. The core issue is not that temporal sequences also figure in Heraclitus' thought and that Plato is aware of this. Rather, Eryximachus both limits himself to temporal sequences in his construction of flux and distorts Heraclitean material that clearly

[39] Regarding this type of flux in Heraclitus, one may also consult B8–9, 13, 37, 51 (on whose content Eryximachus draws), 59–61, 83, 91—the last of these being a place where, as Irwin (4n7) observes, Heraclitus "clearly associates compresence of opposites with flux."

[40] On the connection of this passage to Eryximachus' handling of Heraclitus, see also Robin (1929, livn2); Rosen (1987, 109–10).

singles out harmony through contemporaneous tension in order to force it into line with the sequential construction that he treats as exclusive.

Eryximachus' mistaking of Heraclitean *a*-change for *s*-change is succeeded by Plato's reconstituted notion of *a*-change in the dialogue's "ascent" (210a–212a) from qualifiedly beautiful particulars (e.g., statues) to the pure, transcendent nature of Beauty itself. Unlike beautiful particulars, the Form of Beauty is not "beautiful in relation to one thing and ugly in relation to another; nor is it beautiful here but ugly there, as it would be if it were beautiful for some people and ugly for others" (211a3–5, cf. d8–e4). The distinction between an existent's possessing a feature (e.g., beauty, justice) without and with limitation—which is key to Plato's metaphysics in the *Symposium*, *Phaedo*, and *Republic*—anchors this crucial passage (210a–212a). In addition, earlier in Socrates' speech Plato invokes his revised construction of *s*-change in remarks stressing the existence of incremental shifts within individuals moving through the life cycle (208a–b).[41] Hence, in the same dialogue where Eryximachus mangles Heraclitus, Plato incorporates his reconstituted versions of Heraclitus' twofold distinction, whose inclusion assumes the nuanced awareness of his predecessor that I have presented here. At one stroke, then, Plato both shows forth the doctor's intellectual limits and indicates how the salient topics of coexistence and alteration are rightly handled.

At the pinnacle of the *Symposium*'s ascent regarding the *kalon* (attractive, fine, admirable)[42] stands *auto to kalon*—literally, "the beautiful itself," namely the eternal, transcendent Form of Beauty (210e–211b).[43] This belongs to the macrocosmic plane of reality—comprising the totality of Forms, absolutes in the spheres of values and mathematics—that Plato believes himself to have discovered. Its predecessors on lower ontological tiers are entities in our world that are *kalon* in varying ways and degrees: from the bottom up these are the physically attractive, admirable institutions and practices, and branches of knowledge (210a–d).[44] Neither the *Gorgias* nor Eryximachus' *logos* provides an absolute touchstone against which all pertinent entities native to our world may be rightly assessed. This is exactly what Plato offers in the *Symposium*, *Phaedo*, and *Republic*. Plato is strongly of the mind that "the world

[41] Regarding 208a–b see Irwin (1977, 6): "Diotima shows how someone remains the same man throughout his lifetime; *s*-changes are regular and maintain a close qualitative similarity between the man at one time and at another." Wardy (2002) finds an unqualified reference to "the flux doctrine" at 207e1–208a3 (37), treating the notion voiced there as strictly Heraclitean (59–60).

[42] Cf. Dover (1980, 2).

[43] The pronoun *auto* serves as an intensifier in this standard way of referencing Forms, where the adjective varies depending on the feature (e.g., beauty, courage, justice) being singled out. In the *Republic*, the preeminent Form of the Good is referred to as *auto to agathon* (534c4).

[44] Interestingly, the *Gorgias* includes pre-*eidê* counterparts to these three levels: beautiful bodies (474d); "laws and practices, that is, the admirable ones" (474e); and "the [admirable] fields of learning" (475a).

inside of man, the microcosmos, is akin to the whole universe" (Tenkku 1956, 11), which stance, as Tenkku (ibid.) observes, ties him broadly to medicine. Philosophy alone, however, is equipped to speak decisively here—as Plato does at *Symposium* 210a–212a.

Eryximachus illustrates the *Gorgias*' point (511c–512a) about the dangers of experts not recognizing the limits of their disciplines. Two additional parallels involving his *logos* come to mind. First, it illustrates the flaw in craftspeople's vision of their understanding in the *Apology* (22c9–e1), which consists in their wrongly assuming that their adeptness in one arena of craft translates automatically into insight regarding core human values like justice.[45]

Second, Eryximachus' presumption involving Heraclitus ties him to Protagoras' view of poets in the eponymous dialogue. Noting this link, Konstan and Young-Bruehl (1982, 44) claim that, aside from the *logos* of Socrates, Eryximachus' "is the only one which rivals . . . Protagoras' great speech, in the dialogue named for that sophist, for philosophical significance and coherence." I maintain, in contrast, that comparing Eryximachus' speech with this section of the *Protagoras* illustrates once again Plato's concern to expose the presumption and danger of unbridled claims to authority vis-à-vis the macrocosmic and human spheres.[46]

Protagoras holds that an educated person must be "in command of poetry," which he construes as expertise in poetic exegesis (338e–339a). As one would expect given the deeply competitive spirit of sophistic practice, Protagoras' interpretation of the poet Simonides (339a–341e) shows his conviction that sophistry surpasses poetry, since poetry requires hermeneutical displays of sophistic virtuosity for the full attainment of its value to the soul.[47] Plato of course maintains that sophists do not practice a *technê*,[48] and hence denies that they can grasp what is and is not true, particularly regarding the good, in *anyone's* formulations. Thus, in the *Symposium* and *Protagoras*, Plato targets the presumed authority of activities whose practitioners, ignorant of reality, challenge their rivals for supremacy on matters of greatest import.[49]

The *Protagoras* also places Eryximachus, with Phaedrus, among auditors who were "asking Hippias questions on astronomy and physics, and he, from his high

---

[45] This parallel is also noted by Nichols (2009, 30–31).

[46] This similarity exists even though sophistry, unlike medicine, lacks all legitimacy as a practice.

[47] See further Levin (2008, 87–88).

[48] Further, sophistic activity here targets poetry, from which he also withholds that designation.

[49] There are of course differences between the two scenarios: unlike Protagoras regarding Simonides, it suffices for Eryximachus if Heraclitus turns out to be demonstrably unclear rather than simply wrong; further, if Heraclitus is incorrect, it is not, as with Simonides, because the philosopher contradicts himself.

seat, was answering each question point by point" (315c, cf. 318d–e).[50] This image of the sophist Hippias holding court, patiently taking questions from those wishing to receive the details of his wisdom, leads one to wonder whether Eryximachus has learned some of what he "knows" (and perhaps also how to present ideas involving *phusis* with maximal rhetorical effectiveness) from the likes of Hippias.[51] Reinforcing this picture of Hippias as a self-proclaimed authority is *Hippias Major* 281c–d, where the sophist maintains that his wisdom surpasses that of all other "wise" individuals, including philosophers from Thales through Anaxagoras. Subsequently, Socrates characterizes astronomy (with deep irony) as a domain comprising things that Hippias "know[s] most finely" (285b8–c1).

At 318e, Protagoras disparages Hippias, a fellow sophist, as a teacher of "arithmetic, astronomy, geometry, and *mousikê*," which suggests that what Hippias claimed to know and teach was unusually broad for a sophist (see also *Hippias Major* 285c–d; *Hippias Minor* 366c–369a). Thus, Hippias is singled out by Plato for being a kind of dabbler—a criticism leveled by Heraclitus himself at figures including Hesiod, Xenophanes, and Pythagoras (B40, cf. B57). The encompassing nature of Eryximachus' account renders fitting his linkage with Hippias at the *Protagoras*' gathering. For Edelstein (1987c, 160), Plato thinks that the doctor's "interest in questions of natural philosophy and astronomy," as shown in the *Protagoras*, will "have stood him in good stead." I submit, in contrast, that given Plato's vigorous challenge to the *technê* status of rhetoric/sophistry, the link to Hippias cannot but reflect badly on the physician.[52]

Although Heraclitus is front and center in Eryximachus' *agôn* with philosophy, further evidence for his criticism of philosophers regarding ultimate principles lies in what one may view as a correction of Anaximander's valuation of cyclical macrocosmic shifts. On the physician's formulation, which, like medical writings, allocates a causal role to seasons vis-à-vis health and disease,

> when . . . hot and cold, wet and dry, happen to be governed by the proper form of love toward one another, they exhibit harmony and a temperate mixture (*kai harmonian kai krasin labêi sôphrona*), they come bearing good harvest and health to human beings, other animals, and plants, and there is no injustice

---

50 Also in attendance was Andron, a member of the oligarchic Four Hundred of 411 (Nails 2002, 28–29) and among those linked with Callicles as *koinônous gegonotas sophias* at *Gorgias* 487c2–3.

51 For Hippias as impacting both the form and the content of Eryximachus' *logos*, see Rettig (1876, 16–17, 179).

52 It also reflects poorly on Phaedrus—Eryximachus' paramour and co-auditor of Hippias in the *Protagoras* (315c)—whose own encomium of male desire and romantic ties indirectly impacts Eryximachus' speech via its tie to Pausanias'.

> (*ouden êdikêsen*). But when the *erôs* powered by *hubris* controls the seasons of the year, destruction and injustice prevail (*diephtheiren te polla kai êdikêsen*). He spreads the plague and many other diseases among plants and animals; he causes frost and hail and blights. All these are the effects of the immodest and disordered kind of love (*ek pleonexias kai akosmias peri allêla tôn toioutôn gignetai erôtikôn*) on the movements of the stars and the seasons of the year, that is, on the objects studied by the science called astronomy. (188a2–b6)

Konstan and Young-Bruehl (1982, 43) make little of the passage, stating simply that the term *êdikêsen* here "underscores the anthropomorphic attribution of good and bad impulses to the cosmos." According to Kahn (1960, 179), Eryximachus' concern is much different from Anaximander's, involving only the human body. In contrast, in light of medical writings, I submit that Eryximachus has both a concern with human physicality specifically (in particular, its tie to desire) and a broader, more ambitious aim tied to his rivalry with philosophy over macrocosmic insight.

Eryximachus' lauding of smooth, undramatic shifts in domains like seasonal change and his rejection of disproportion mesh with a familiar strand in medical writings.[53] *Affections*, for instance, enjoins the shunning of imbalance involving excessive heat or cold (18). According to *Nature of Man*, the four humors (blood, phlegm, yellow bile, black bile) comprise the body's nature (4–5), the optimal state being their perfectly balanced mixture (*hotan . . . tauta . . . malista memigmena êi*, 4). Based on this cosmological model, the key to bodily soundness is proportionality (i.e., health is present *hotan metriôs echêi tauta . . . pros allêla*, with pain's being caused by excess, deficiency, or one humor's separation from the rest; ibid.). In *Airs Waters Places* (5), moderate climate is tethered to health, with an analogy drawn to the growth of plants. Most worrisome with respect to health are "the most violent changes of the seasons" (11). This point is echoed and extended in *Humors* (15), where the paramount cause of disease is "the greatest shifts, the violent alterations both in the seasons and in other things." According to *Epidemics* II (1.5), "in stable times and years that produce seasonal things at their proper times, diseases are dependable and have proper crises, while in unstable years" the reverse obtains.[54]

As in his reconstruction of Heraclitus, we find in Eryximachus' correction of Anaximander at *Symposium* 188a–b a macrocosmic preoccupation wedded to a confidence that he grasps both overarching principles and their governance of the

---

53 On Anaximander's tie to the Hippocratic Corpus, see also Jaeger (1986b, 6, 293–94n11).

54 As Jouanna (1999, 337) observes, in ancient medicine "the notion of crisis . . . did not have the pejorative sense it has for us; it was a significant moment in the evolution of the disease, for better or for worse." The crises at issue here are of the former sort, i.e., those that "signify . . . sure recovery of health" (338).

microcosm—the whole being a complex union that his vision alone reveals. On Eryximachus' account, justice prevails—emphatically put, there is not a whit of injustice (*ouden êdikêsen*, 188a6)—as long as each season is moderate in the befitting way.[55] Eryximachus diverges significantly from Anaximander, who claims in our sole extant quotation that ordinary shifts like those of the seasons comprise a state of affairs in which "the things that are perish into the things out of which they come to be, according to necessity, for they pay penalty and retribution to each other for their injustice in accord with the ordering of time (*didonai gar auta dikên kai tisin allêlois tês adikias kata tên tou chronou taxin*)" (B1).

The quotation's legal language is far from strictly metaphorical (McKirahan 1994, 45). It makes clear that on Anaximander's macrocosmic account—unlike that of Eryximachus—all fluctuations like seasonal change are properly viewed as transgressions needing recompense. Anaximander's negative valuation of alternations in opposed qualities (e.g., hot and cold, dry and wet) in his cosmology fits with the metaphysical subordination of opposition in his cosmogony. As Kirk, Raven, and Schofield (1983, 114) observe, if one member of a pair of opposites was foundational, due to fire and water's antithetical features (hot and dry versus cold and wet), no cosmos containing both substances could have emerged. Hence, Anaximander selected *to apeiron* (the indefinite) as his *archê*, presumably because it lacked all familiar qualitative features.[56]

While Anaximander's stance on opposition places him most obviously in the earliest critical dialogue among philosophers,[57] as applied to seasonal change it resonates with certain Hippocratic accounts of health and disease. *Nature of Man* (7), which features strong macrocosm-microcosm isomorphism, favors close explanatory ties between ordinary seasonal shifts and manifestations of human constitutions construed in light of humors. Illnesses typical of each season are traced here to humors' cyclical relations of dominance and recession. The very same humor-based cosmological system that explains propensities to ailments by season is also that by which "all things are constructed and nourished" (ibid.). According to *Epidemics* II (1.5), while irregular weather patterns negatively impact disease-conditions—which fits with Eryximachus' approach—under ordinary conditions the cyclical severity of

---

[55] Cf. Bury (1932, ix).

[56] Scholars disagree regarding the emergence of opposites in Anaximander's cosmogony, namely, whether opposites, e.g., the hot and the cold, emerge directly from the *apeiron* or whether instead what subsequently gives rise to them stems from that source. For discussion see McKirahan (1994, 36–38); Kirk, Raven, and Schofield (1983, 128–30). Either way, opposites' emergence depends on the *apeiron*, i.e., on an *archê* that lacks all familiar qualities.

[57] On this remarkable occurrence, see Popper (1963).

diseases is tied to seasonal and diurnal variation (1.4): "In autumn diseases are most acute and most deadly, generally similar to exacerbation in the afternoon. The year has a cycle of diseases, just as the day has of one disease." The approach of *Nature of Man* (7) and *Epidemics* II (1.4) resonates broadly with Anaximander's notion that even normalcy in seasonal or diurnal shifts is or may be a source of harm.

Anaximander's vision of opposition was subsequently "corrected" by Heraclitus (B80). Eryximachus differs from Heraclitus, according to whom "it is necessary to know that war is common, and justice strife" (*eidenai de chrê ton polemon eonta xunon, kai dikên erin*, ibid.), which does not marginalize "extreme," or "extraordinary," happenings as infelicitous. Quite the opposite, as Heraclitus stresses ultimate harmony even amid what may be fierce opposition (B51). As is evident in his handling of *mousikê*, Eryximachus' version lacks the intensity of Heraclitus' macrocosmic position. His handling of Anaximander at *Symposium* 188a–b valorizes moderate *erôs* against a disharmonious variety and actually converges with his handling of Heraclitus at 187a–c.

Heraclitus and Anaximander, then, represent two extremes between which Eryximachus locates himself as a more balanced voice. In fact, he recasts their views so that they match his own position. While the doctor's take on the cosmos writ large stresses balance, he never defines the elements of that balance or clearly depicts its nature. This leaves him much latitude when interpreting "moderation" apropos of the human sphere. On a structural plane, as Konstan and Young-Bruehl (1982) point out, Eryximachus' handling of *erôs* qua *epithumia* (desire) and *philia* (friendship, affection) on the microcosmic and macrocosmic planes, respectively, does not actually establish the tight link he claims. Not only is *erôs* differently construed on the two planes, but *erôs* qua *epithumia* "pertains only to living creatures or organic systems. Love as harmony, on the other hand, applies to any system of opposites" (42). This observation does not, however, lead Konstan and Young-Bruehl to consider that Eryximachus' motives may be self-serving. Instead, they take him to be intellectually earnest if not always clear (e.g., "The distinction between these two conceptions of love is to some degree obscured by Eryximachus' language," 41).

Since macrocosmic discussion is quite common in medical authors, it is not surprising that Eryximachus pursues it. His cosmological foray, incomplete and sketchy as it is, plays a crucial role in Eryximachus' account. His appeal to macrocosmic balance lends what he presumes is indisputable heft and legitimacy to his take on the human realm. Eryximachus' grand talk of cosmic moderation and assertion of a close microcosmic counterpart anchor his accord with Pausanias' stress on what the latter had self-servingly deemed right indulgence of sexual desire between an *erastês* and an *erômenos*—this desire being the second, after drinking, of the Big Three *epithumiai* (desires) that the doctor addresses.

The sequence of *logoi* originally set had Eryximachus succeed Aristophanes, who would thus have directly followed Phaedrus and Pausanias. By having Aristophanes delay on account of hiccups, with Eryximachus now sliding in as Pausanias' immediate successor, Plato arguably suggests that we should be on the lookout for thematic ties. The issue here is not whether medical authors defended precisely Eryximachus' tack on desire and pleasure: his *logos*, as previously stressed, is a Platonic creation. The point, rather, is that Eryximachus' account here powerfully illustrates Plato's view that nothing internal to medicine can impose the requisite limits on desire and pleasure.

According to Konstan and Young-Bruehl (1982, 42), Eryximachus "surprisingly declares" that the unfavorable *erôs* "must be applied [albeit] with caution." They continue: "Clearly, the doctor may cater to unhealthy appetites, provided he does not allow them to get out of control. Why he should do so is more difficult to answer" (ibid.). On the present account, it is not so mysterious why Eryximachus would embrace unsalutary *epithumiai* and why Plato would find fault. Relevant here is the *Gorgias*' notion that the more the Big Three are indulged, the harder it is to set limits to them, to the ultimate detriment of the soul. Also important is the *Gorgias*' recognition that experts may find it challenging to acknowledge the limits of their endeavors, particularly when they claim mastery of *phusis* and *eudaimonia*.

5. DESIRE, SELF-INDULGENCE, AND SELF-CONTROL: ERYXIMACHUS AND *ARETÊ*

Notwithstanding Hippocratic authors' wide-ranging occupation with cosmology, their motivating concern is the human sphere. This is certainly true for Eryximachus in the *Symposium*. Besides his wish to defend medicine's preeminence among *technai*, a microcosmic (i.e., human) self-interest broadly matching Pausanias' motivates the doctor's *logos*. Given the core role of *erôs* in Eryximachus' speech, for which Pausanias' sets the stage, the doctor's stance on desire (*epithumia*), self-indulgence (*akolasia*), and self-control (*sôphrosunê*), with his attendant view of the soul-body tie, is central to one's judging its worth from a microcosmic standpoint.[58] As we will see in Chapter 4, the *Republic*'s handling of the soul-body relationship devotes special concern to the tie between appetite and self-control, the virtue most closely linked to the body. As Chapter 1 made clear, the *Gorgias*' account of well-being already gives particular weight to *epithumiai*, *akolasia*, and *sôphrosunê*. In the *Gorgias* and *Republic*—along with the *Symposium* through Socrates' speech (210d, 211d)—Plato

---

[58] On Hippocratic treatments of this terrain, see Chapter 2.

squarely opposes latitude for the indulgence of desire. Eryximachus pays lip service to restraint through his positive spin on the self-serving dimension of his predecessors' speeches that sought to justify yielding, under the "right" conditions, to the sexual overtures of the *erastês* (lover). He thus offers a variant on Hippocratic context dependency involving the Big Three generally and sex specifically.

On desire and pleasure, a comparison of Eryximachus with Callicles, the *Gorgias*' overt devotee of pleasure and power, is instructive. Two things might be viewed as favoring Eryximachus: first, Callicles is brasher and more overtly antagonistic; second, the physician's seemingly erudite cosmological foray makes him look more deeply informed. Beneath the surface, however, no small part of the impetus to Eryximachus' macrocosmic inquiry is that it offers an intellectually respectable pedigree for Pausanias' self-serving contribution, whose governing picture of desire (and associated pleasure) Eryximachus appears clearly to share.

As we will see, the core message of Eryximachus' speech regarding desire, pleasure, and self-indulgence—and on the other side, self-control and justice—is unexpectedly similar to Callicles' view. Qua practitioner of medicine, the preeminent *technê*, Eryximachus claims mastery of psychic terrain including pleasure and desire, whose being the province of *technê* the *Gorgias* adamantly rejects.[59] Callicles never sheds light on the distinction he acknowledges between better and worse pleasures (499b, 503c–d). Not dissimilarly, Eryximachus never articulates the right conditions for submitting to an *erastês*.[60] The *Symposium* does not offer right guidelines for *erastês-erômenos* (lover-beloved) ties via Eryximachus. Through the *logoi* (speeches) of Socrates and Alcibiades, however, Plato begins to flesh out what the correct pursuit of *erôs* both necessitates and precludes.[61]

Let us begin by addressing Eryximachus' remarks involving the vice of *akolasia* (self-indulgence) in 186b–c and 187d–e. At 186b8–c1, Eryximachus offers an analogy involving body and soul—one that assumes Pausanias' infrastructure for appropriate physicality: "Just as, following Pausanias, it's admirable to submit to good men but shameful to gratify those who are self-indulgent, so too with the body" (*hôsper arti Pausanias elegen tois men agathois kalon charizesthai tôn anthrôpôn, tois d' akolastois aischron, houtô kai en autois tois sômasin*). Reinforcing the bond

---

[59] As we saw in Chapter 1, the *technê* at issue is instead an overarching one that allows one to demarcate good pleasures from bad (500a).

[60] There are of course differences, too. For instance, while Callicles' approach would upend existing political praxis, Eryximachus' *logos* functions importantly in defense of a traditional practice, namely, the existing model of homosexual *erôs*.

[61] In viewing the speeches as mutually reinforcing a defense of abstention from impassioned interpersonal ties, I diverge from Nussbaum (1986, 165–99), according to whom Alcibiades' *logos* poignantly captures for our serious attention what of merit is lost when such ties are relinquished during the ascent.

between the two *logoi* retrospectively is Aristophanes' use of a dual form (*eipetên*, 189c3) to convey that Eryximachus and Pausanias had adopted the same approach.[62] Aristophanes' account of *erôs*, displaced by his hiccups so that it follows Eryximachus', stresses that the optimal interpersonal tie is not grounded in sexual relations (192c–d). This pointedly corrects Eryximachus' and Pausanias' stance, which Aristophanes had previously signaled he would oppose (189c).[63] As Dover (1989, 44, 83–84, 157) observes, the verb *charizesthai* (to show or grant a favor) referred specifically to sexual activity. This term appears numerous times in Pausanias' speech (182a–d, 183d, 184a–e, 185a–b) and several times in Eryximachus' own (186b–c, 187d, 188c). In 186b–c, quoted above, *charizesthai* grounds an approving reference to Pausanias' account of when submission to an *erastês* is justified. In the perceptive view of Rettig (1876), Eryximachus grants top priority to sexual desire and its fulfillment (19), so much so that his speech and Pausanias' "to a certain degree form a single whole" (13).

Eryximachus formulates the issue concerning *akolasia* (self-indulgence) at 186b–c as precluding one's submission to those who are *akolastoi* (self-indulgent), implying that its avoidance is key to one's not becoming self-indulgent oneself. He later frames the point in terms of one's not forming the negative character trait of *akolasia*. Thus at 187d–e the physician asserts that

> the same account applies once again, namely, that the love felt by good people—and by those who though not yet good might become such—must be gratified and protected (*palin gar hêkei ho autos logos, hoti tois men kosmiois tôn anthrôpôn, kai hôs an kosmiôteroi gignointo hoi mêpô ontes, dei charizesthai kai phulattein ton toutôn erôta*). And this is the admirable (*kalos*), heavenly *erôs*, the *erôs* of the Ouranian Muse. The other, that of Polyhymnia, is boorish (*pandêmos*), and must be applied cautiously to those to whom it applies, in order that one enjoy the pleasure of it but instill no self-indulgence (*akolasia*), just as (*hôsper*) in our *technê* great effort is expended to use well the desires associated with the art of cookery in order that people take pleasure without illness (*tais peri tên opsopoiikên technên epithumiais kalôs chrêsthai, hôst' aneu nosou tên hêdonên karpôsasthai*).

On Rowe's (1999, 62) account, 187d4–7 introduces "the *possibility* of finding artfulness and wit in Eryximachus (things said with a nudge and a wink)," thereby

---

[62] Cf. Rosen (1987, 92n8).

[63] On the medical backdrop for the poet's own *logos* and its tying thus to Eryximachus', see Craik (2001, 111–13).

offering a partial "antidote to the attribution to him of mere pedantry" (italics in original). I differ from Rowe on this point, believing that Plato is dead serious in attributing these views to the physician. *Symposium* 187d–e spells out what the earlier, compact version at 186b–c amounts to given human fallibility, which Pausanias acknowledged (185a–b), in assessments of character when one determines with whom to engage. Further, the later passage, which mentions desires for sex and food, suggests that if desires are wrongly indulged, setting limits to them is hard. The later passage thus helps to bring out what about indulgence Plato finds deeply problematic.

Sôphrosunê, integral to thriving, entails strict appropriateness in kinds and objects of desire—already signaled in the *Gorgias*—with indulgence of a sexual nature precluded. Wardy (2002, 29) refers aptly here to Diotima's "systematic devaluation of the flesh" in philosophic guidance that Socrates claims (201d–e, 207a, 209e–210a) this figure to have provided.[64] That Eryximachus' view is antithetical to Plato's is manifest in the *Symposium*'s placing the sexual expression of *erôs* on the lowest tier of pre-ascent types (207d). This contrasts it with pursuing *erôs* correctly (*orthôs*; 210a6, 211b5) respecting interpersonal ties. On the ascent's own lowest plane, one's *erôs* is ultimately about ideas' creation and lodging in written works, not physical beauty, and does not target let alone revolve around physical consummation.[65] The *Symposium*'s juxtaposing two divergent orientations to physical attraction relies on the *Gorgias*' contrasting of lives and types of pleasures (499b). At the same time, it represents a significant advance in depth and specificity.

Plato's opposition to Eryximachus' model is reinforced by his contrasting of two incompatible lives (211d–212a) once he has depicted the ascent and its culmination. Socrates' resolve in the face of Alcibiades' persistent advances (217a–219d) is an exact reflection of the stance on *erôs* depicted in 211d–212a. What is more, Socrates' firmness in 217a–219d opposes two ways of life in a way loosely analogous to the *Gorgias*' foundational clash between rhetoric and philosophy as grounding modes of existence, with Socrates' conduct here reflecting his embodiment of true *sôphrosunê*.[66] Even Alcibiades musters respect for Socrates' possession of this *aretê*

[64] On the prominence of *sôphrosunê* in the *Symposium*, see also North (1966, 167), for whom it "alone among the cardinal virtues . . . has a prominent place in the dialectic of Beauty as well as in the dialectic of Reason." See Levin (1996, 29–30) on Diotima, whose supposed views are key to Socrates' encomium of *erôs*. As Dover (1980, 137) points out, "we do not know whether Diotima is real or fictitious, and it does not much matter, considering the extreme improbability . . . that even if she really existed she entertained" Plato's theory of Forms.

[65] On this key Platonic differentiation in the *Symposium*, see further Moravcsik (1971, 291).

[66] Cf. the reference of Bury (1932, 148) to Socrates' "inner" *sôphrosunê*.

(219d3–5). Plato's critical treatment of *mousikê* in *Republic* II–III also contains a strong prohibition against "excessive pleasure" (*hêdonêi huperballousêi*, 402e3), with a special focus on sexual activity's categorical disallowance (402e–403c).[67] Contra Hippocratic material discussed in Chapter 2, Plato's refusal of sexual indulgence is categorical. The context does not matter.

A harbinger of Plato's more developed stance regarding desire and self-control is evident in the *Gorgias*, which considers *epithumiai* and their relation to *akolasia*. Like Eryximachus, who singles out in closing *sôphrosunê* (self-control) and *dikaiosunê* (justice), the *Gorgias* puts special weight on these two *aretai* (478d, 493d, 504d–e, 507d–508a, 519a). There we find that one wishing to flourish must foster *sôphrosunê*, whose cultivation requires his "flee[ing] away from lack of discipline (*akolasia*) as fast as his feet will carry him" (507d2). The *Gorgias*' message is that one cannot indulge inappropriate desires without capitulating to badness within. At *Gorgias* 507e1–508a4 we are told that one seeking to be good

> should not allow his appetites to be undisciplined or undertake to fill them up (*ouk epithumias eônta akolastous einai kai tautas epicheirounta plêroun*)—a never-ending evil—and live the life of a marauder. Such a man could not be dear to another man or to a god. . . . Wise men claim that partnership and friendship, orderliness, self-control, and justice (*tên koinônian . . . kai philian kai kosmiotêta kai sôphrosunên kai dikaiotêta*) hold together heaven and earth, and gods and men, and that is why they call this universe a world order (*kosmon*), my friend, and not an undisciplined world-disorder (*ouk akosmian oude akolasian*).

Plato's point here, that desire as such must be tightly regulated, is lost on Eryximachus, just as it ultimately escapes the notice of Hippocratic authors. *Gorgias* 507e–508a is a useful contrast with Eryximachus' closing remarks on virtue and thriving, which issue from a divergent ontological and epistemological standpoint:

> Such is the power (*dunamin*) of love—so varied and great that in all cases it might be called absolute. Yet its power (*dunamin*) is greatest when love is directed, in self-control and justice, toward good things (*ho de peri tagatha meta sôphrosunês kai dikaiosunês apoteloumenos*), whether in heaven or on earth: happiness, the bonds of human society, concord with the gods above—all these

[67] Plato's exclusion of sexual activity from the highest expression of *erôs* is, moreover, central to the *Phaedrus*' account (250e, 253d–254e, 256a–b). On Plato and sexual activity, cf. Dover (1989, 163–64, 167–68).

are among its gifts (*pasan hêmin eudaimonian paraskeuazei kai allêlois dunamenous homilein kai philous einai kai tois kreittosin hêmôn thois*). (188d4–9)[68]

In these final remarks, Eryximachus' quest to show the all-encompassing cognitive reach of his *technê* is once again strikingly clear. But the comments' glancing, ad hoc reference to virtue and thriving shows that they are not integral to a *logos* that he alleges to be exhaustive (188d9–e2), indeed that he has not reflected at all on what they actually entail.

While North (1966, 167) sees a parallel between Eryximachus' *logos* here and what she calls this "cosmological" portion of the *Gorgias*, she wrongly takes the physician to represent Plato's own view.[69] Though at first blush one may see parallels here between the two dialogues, on closer inspection telling differences emerge. First, Eryximachus is at pains to stress that the power (*dunamis*) to ensure virtue and flourishing stems from *erôs* alone—the term appears twice in 188d4–9 (d4, 7), and the participle at d8. But Diotima, representing Plato, identifies the good as the arbiter of its proper role.[70] In d5, the physician speaks generically of goods (*ta agatha*), not of *the* good. The *Gorgias*, however, sharply demarcates external goods from the good of the virtuous life (e.g., 478d7–8). Second, *Gorgias* 507e–508a, like the *Republic* and *Laws*, ties excellence and well-being to order. It prefaced its observations on *aretê* with a reminder that self-control and justice are accessible only to those whose *epithumiai* are tightly controlled (507d6–e3). As we have seen, Eryximachus obtrusively declines to tie virtue to appetitive control.

Relevant here too is Plato's contention at *Gorgias* 503c–d that "a man should satisfy those of his appetites that . . . make us better human beings (*hai men tôn epithumiôn . . . beltiô poiousi ton anthrôpon, tautas men apotelein*), not those that make us worse, and . . . this is a matter of *technê*." Recurring to the point shortly thereafter, but here formulating it in terms of justice, Plato maintains that a *technê* is required to keep one from vice (509d–510a).[71]

---

[68] On the macrocosmic strain in *Gorgias* 507e–508a, see Irwin (1979, 226); while he references *Symposium* 186b–188e for purposes of comparison, Irwin omits mention of medicine, concentrating exclusively on Pythagoreanism and pre-Socratic theorizing.

[69] Cf. 168, where North treats the *logoi* of Eryximachus and Socrates as strongly complementary insofar as the doctor's speech explores "the cosmic implications" of *erôs,* while the philosopher "develops the political."

[70] *Dunamis* is a quite salient term in the Hippocratic Corpus: see, e.g., *Ancient Medicine* 3, 13–17, 19, 22, 24; *Regimen* I 2–4, 10, 35.

[71] Socrates' status as a philosopher is stressed (cf. the authority granted him as such, albeit tacitly, in the *Symposium*'s proceedings) at *Gorgias* 481d3–4 (cf. 482a2–b1, 484c5–486d1), and the excellent soul of a philosopher is said to fare well in the afterlife (526c). *Gorgias* 527d indicates that a turn to politics is appropriate only after one is secure in the practice of *aretê* (cf. "the true political *technê*," 521d7). Such passages, taken together, support the view that Plato envisions here a single *technê*, between the aspects of practitioners' role he has not yet clearly distinguished.

As we saw in Chapter 2, the *Gorgias*' lens on medical writings shows that this *technê* cannot be medicine. Plato stresses there, as in the *Republic* (406c–e, 409e–410a), that life is not worth preserving at all costs; doing so can be unjust. Life with a ruined body should not continue (*Gorgias* 505a). Plato elaborates in 511b–512e, including this crucial claim: "If a man afflicted with serious incurable physical ailments did not drown [while with the helmsman], this man is miserable for not dying and has received no benefit from him. But if a man has many incurable diseases in what is more valuable than his body, his soul, life for that man is not worth living, and he won't do him any favor if he rescues him from the sea, prison, or anywhere else" (512a2–b1). Philosophically, the way was paved in part for this conclusion by Socrates' argument that "injustice, lack of discipline (*hê adikia . . . kai hê akolasia*), and all other kinds of psychic corruption are the very worst thing of all (*megiston tôn ontôn kakon*)" (477e4–6)—far more serious than any misfortune and misery tied to disease (477e–480d). Since medicine is not the *technê* whose subject matter is justice, which flourishing requires, medicine cannot occupy the pinnacle of *technai*. Indeed, restoring an individual to health can work against justice, as when a soul is incurable (477e–478d with 512a2–b1; cf. the dialogue's closing *logos*, 525b–e). If so, it should turn out that medicine is not preeminent but also that its operations will sometimes require supervision by a practitioner of the *technê* that presides over justice. This latter point is not showcased until the *Republic*, where it will be crucial to the further shift in Plato's stance toward medicine.

As previously observed, the Big Three *epithumiai* are all promoted in some fashion by Eryximachus. We have already seen that the latitude that Eryximachus allows concerning sex fits with his lax take on drinking at the event. Eryximachus' tying of medicine to cookery rounds out his handling of this triumvirate. He states: "We must be careful to enjoy [the pleasure of Polyhymnia] without slipping into debauchery. This case, I might add, is strictly parallel to a serious issue in my own field, namely, the problem of handling well the appetite whose province is cookery (*tais peri tên opsopoiikên technên epithumiais kalôs chrêsthai*) so that one can reap the pleasure of a fine meal (*tên hêdonên karpôsasthai*) without unhealthy aftereffects" (187e2–6). As Rowe (1998, 150) observes, Eryximachus' remark involving cookery "hint[s] that medicine has a role to play in preventing 'immorality.'" Notably, the latitude he allows for indulgence of the appetite for food runs together with his tolerance for the indulgence of sexual desire.

In the *Gorgias*, however, cookery, whose *technê* status Eryximachus assumes (187e4–5), is firmly relegated, with rhetoric, to the plane of *empeiriai* (knacks). There Plato stresses, for instance, that *kolakeia* (flattery)—an umbrella term for the modus operandi of *empeiriai*—"considers not at all whatever is best. With the lure of what's most pleasant at the moment, it sniffs out folly and hoodwinks it, so that it gives the impression of being most deserving" (464d1–3; see more generally 464b–466a). In one of many disparaging remarks about cookery, Plato announces disdainfully that those adept at it are mere "servants, satisfiers of appetites" (*diakonous . . . kai epithumiôn paraskeuastas*, 518c3–4).[72] As Rettig (1876, 165, 172–73) rightly maintains, against this background Eryximachus' appeal to cookery cannot but lower medicine's standing in Plato's eyes.

At the *Gorgias*' close (527e), Plato exhorts us to take his account as our guide to flourishing and the path to its cultivation. Among the responsibilities of the *technê* referred to at 503c7–d2 is further exploration of desire and pleasure, including their types and psychic impacts. Such an account medicine cannot provide. We cannot follow both Eryximachus' *logos* and Plato's own as this is presented in the *Gorgias*, expanded in the *Symposium*, and brought to completion in the *Republic*. Embracing Plato's account necessarily disqualifies Eryximachus'.

Notwithstanding his lengthy treatment of *mousikê*, a domain in which, traditionally, *aretê* figures prominently, prior to his closing remarks the physician does not speak of virtue beyond a quick gesture in comments involving the vice, *akolasia*, corresponding to self-control.[73] Only in his wrap-up does Eryximachus turn briefly to *aretê*, in a passage, discussed above, whose juxtaposition with *Gorgias* 507e–508a and what transpires earlier in the physician's *logos* reflects badly on his account of human flourishing:

> Such is the power (*dunamin*) of love—so varied and great that in all cases it might be called absolute. Yet its power (*dunamin*) is greatest when love is directed, in self-control and justice, toward good things (*ho de peri tagatha meta sôphrosunês kai dikaiosunês apoteloumenos*), whether in heaven or on earth: happiness, the bonds of human society, concord with the gods above—all these are among its gifts (*pasan hêmin eudaimonian paraskeuazei kai allêlois dunamenous homilein kai philous einai kai tois kreittosin hêmôn theois*). (188d4–9)

As Dorter (1969, 234n10) observes, *erôs* and the good are the *Symposium*'s two overarching themes. For each speaker prior to Socrates, "love acquires the status of a *telos*, an end pursued or the terminus of an appetite, and for that reason stands as a final state of perfection, i.e., a god" (Schindler 2007, 207). In contrast to those earlier speakers, Plato holds that the good is the launching point for everything else, including the true nature and capacity of *erôs*. Plato's subjecting of *erôs* to the good

---

[72] See also 462d–e, 463b, 500b, 500e–501a, 517d–518d, 521e–522a.

[73] Thus far the sole use of pertinent terminology has come in 188a5, where *sôphrona* is employed regarding the seasons.

begins with Diotima's comment, well before the ascent, that "on my account, a lover does not seek the half or the whole, unless it turns out to be good as well" (205e1–3). The ascent, which renders *erôs* properly subordinate to virtue and the good,[74] systematizes Plato's reversal of the physician's ordering of fundamental principles. Plato pointedly excludes (210a6, 211b5, 211d–212a) all indulgence of sexual desire—which Eryximachus pointedly sought to encompass—as antithetical to one's prospects for *eudaimonia*.

Far from providing the foundation for an authoritative account of human flourishing, Eryximachus' brief comments at the end are merely tacked on as perhaps obligatory from one who wishes to encompass human *erôs* in a complete account of "what is" that allegedly privileges what is sound and balanced against extremes. Though Eryximachus mentions *sôphrosunê* (with *dikaiosunê*, 188d5–6), his *logos* makes clear that he has no idea what it is or how it is produced. For Plato, the doctor's remarks reflect a flawed construction of *phusis* that is hostile to human beings' cultivation of *eudaimonia*.

In closing, Eryximachus states that "if I omitted anything from my encomium, it wasn't intentional" (*isôs men oun kai egô ton erôta epainôn polla paraleipô, ou mentoi hekôn ge*, 188d9–e2). On Bury's (1932) plausible account, *kai egô* (I, too) in 188e1 means "I as well as Pausanias," which again shows the close tie of Eryximachus' speech to Pausanias'. Given Eryximachus' level of confidence, Dover (1980, ad loc.) rightly takes the doctor's claim at 188d9–e2 as wholly sincere.[75] That the doctor could brashly venture such a remark at closing indicates his lack of awareness of what would constitute a truly encompassing account of human nature and the cosmos at large. This view of Eryximachus gains further support from the fact that, by Plato's lights, he operates with a flawed construction of *technê*.

6. THE FIELD OF *TECHNAI*: ERYXIMACHUS' LOOSE CONSTRUCTION

As we saw in Chapter 2, medical presentations of what in the *Gorgias* become Plato's formal, highly normative *technê* requirements are unsystematized and largely discrete. Hippocratic authors sought to demarcate real *iatrikê* from efforts by those lacking a *technê*, with which *iatrikê* might be conflated. They were far more concerned with medical poseurs than with challenging other activities' claims to *technê* standing (see, e.g., *Regimen* I 12–24). Eryximachus uses *mousikê* (poetry and music) and *mantikê* (prophecy), not direct competitors with medicine, to help him debunk philosophy, which, like *Ancient Medicine*, he views as offering a rival comprehensive

[74] On the eventual supplanting of *erôs* by reason in the ascent, see Moravcsik (1971).

[75] Cf. Robin (1929, lvi), for whom Eryximachus "doubts not a whit his endeavor's success."

vision. Thus, Eryximachus' standards for activities' qualifying as *technai* at all are more generous than the *Gorgias*' criteria, according to which both *mousikê* and *mantikê* are excluded. This generosity typifies and grounds Eryximachus' approach throughout his speech. Hence, even as he elevates his own *technê* above all others, Eryximachus' liberal use of the designation grants it to endeavors whose *technê* standing Plato rejects. We have ample evidence already that Plato's stance on foundational matters is importantly at odds with that adopted by Eryximachus. That the physician speaks so confidently, yet ignorantly, on the crucial matter of what qualifies as a *technê* further undermines his insight and authority from Plato's standpoint.

Though his goal is to valorize his own profession, most of Eryximachus' *logos* addresses other *technai*. As the doctor assumes his medical competency is not in question, he does not devote his *logos* to its defense. What requires support, however, is his broader claim for the cognitive authority of *iatrikê*. The doctor's extensive discussion of other *technai* in his own praise of medicine reflects Eryximachus' assurance that he is qualified to grasp what they can offer. I thus diverge from McPherran (2006, 76–77), according to whom "we are no doubt supposed to read all this as a parodic example of high-flying medical rhetoric, but at the same time we should appreciate the extent to which Eryximachus is himself merely entering into the general light-hearted sympotic spirit of things by speaking as bombastically as he does."

Interestingly, McPherran's comments on Eryximachus' "good familiarity" (2006, 76) with the Hippocratic corpus do not mention the *Symposium*'s parallel here to the wealth of *technai* used in *Regimen* I to support the author's claim about encompassing cosmic principles. Like the speech of Eryximachus, *Regimen* I construes *technê* in the loose, unsystematic way that Plato challenges in the *Gorgias*. In chaps. 12–24 the Hippocratic author underscores what he views as fundamental common ground between the nature of man, which is grasped by medicine, and principles guiding effective practice in a wide range of other *technai*. Since the physician alone grasps human *pathêmata*, "both visible and invisible" (*kai phaneroisi kai aphanesi*, 12)—with their macrocosmic embedment (3–4, 10)—he alone is in a position to adduce this spectrum of illustrations. The assumption of *Regimen* I is clearly that medicine is preeminent in relation to this comparison group, whose practitioners are not in a position to reach overarching insight.[76] Eryximachus deploys a truncated version of precisely that methodology here, omitting discussion of artifact production such as

---

[76] While *Regimen* I (25) foregrounds analogy, the illustrations in chaps. 12–24 are supposed to show that *technai* operate with uniform materials and principles, hence share something foundational with human nature (24) in a fashion surpassing the merely analogical.

cobblery (*Regimen* I 15) and basket-making (19). To illustrate that Eryximachus' liberal application of the *technê* designation goes well beyond what the *Gorgias* allows, I shall examine his handling of *mantikê* and *mousikê*.

In the eponymous dialogue, Laches conjoins *iatrikê* (medicine) with *mantikê* (prophecy) due to their alleged standing as *technai* with expertise in prognostication (195d–196a, cf. 198d–e). Viewing this linkage through the *Gorgias*' lens, we see that Eryximachus' careless inclusion of *mantikê* among the alleged *technai* handled by his *logos* reflects his (and Laches') ignorance. His sloppiness here also fits with medical writings, which assume that prophecy has *technê* standing (*Regimen* I 12; *Regimen* IV 87). According to *Regimen* IV (87), prophecy fails to recognize its own limits. It purports to handle dreams that anticipate physical symptoms, while their interpretation is rightly the province of medical experts. Though *Regimen* IV and Eryximachus claim to know prophecy's legitimate scope, neither questions prophecy's rank as a self-standing *technê*.

What, then, is Plato's view of *mantikê*? The features he prizes above all (e.g., being eternal and unaltered) are ascribed to Forms (*Phaedo* 79d; *Symposium* 211a–b). Notably, Plato's account of Forms (i.e., reality proper) at *Phaedo* 80b includes the term *to theion* (divine). For Plato, *mantikê* à la Eryximachus is categorically precluded from taking as its purview the truly divine. In the *Symposium*, the divine is represented by the Form of Beauty (*auto to kalon*), which, as we have seen, lies at the pinnacle of the ascent. In addition to the Form of Beauty's being beautiful (*kalon*) without qualification, as a Form it possesses the eternality and changelessness that characterize what Plato views as divine.[77] Hence, the divine resides under philosophy's purview, not prophecy's. Failing the *Gorgias*' subject-matter condition on *technai*, *mantikê* perforce cannot satisfy the understanding and goodness criteria.

Eryximachus' discussion of *mousikê* is particularly significant for its inclusion of his most pointed challenge to philosophy's preeminence (see Section 4 above). But as we will see, Eryximachus' account of *mousikê*, like that of *mantikê*, rests on an insufficiently selective notion of *technê*.

Mousikê includes the language of poetry, along with rhythm and modes. Plato's critique of poetry's *technê* status unfolds in the *Ion*, *Gorgias*, and *Cratylus*, and culminates in the *Republic*; as *Republic* III makes clear, the target of his challenge is *mousikê* in its entirety. As I argue elsewhere,[78] the *Republic*'s critique of poetic content revolves around the goodness, understanding, and subject-matter conditions

---

[77] Nothing interpretive in the present study hangs on the *Phaedo* and *Symposium*'s relative chronology. What matters, and is uncontroversial, is that they were written fairly close together.

[78] See Levin (2001, chap. 5).

on *technai* enunciated in the *Gorgias*.[79] Briefly put, the goodness criterion is salient already in Book I, where Plato stresses that the exclusive aim of each *technê* is to do what is best (*to beltiston*) for its objects (347a1–3). Turning to poetry, he says repeatedly that its creators seek to please the audience without a concern for its well-being (387b, 389e–390a, 397d, 398a–b, 493c–d, 607a, d–e). In *Republic* II–III, Plato takes poets to task for treating as desirable a state of affairs in which one has a reputation for morality but is actually immoral. He bases poetry's failure to meet the goodness condition on its shortcomings involving understanding and subject matter (363e–364c, 365b–c, 493a–494a, 597e, 598d–602b). The conclusion to be drawn from the *Republic*'s critique of poetry is not that virtue fails to be the province of a *technê*. It is rather that this *technê* is philosophy, not poetry.

Though Eryximachus' treatment of *mousikê* encompasses the language of poetry,[80] his focus is on rhythm and harmony as traditionally construed.[81] This is the dimension of *mousikê* that Plato takes up in *Republic* 398d–403c, where he articulates the worries about poetry's pernicious impact on character that he had stressed earlier in Books II–III concerning its language. Plato tells us there that the key is to ensure that these dimensions of *mousikê* properly serve the words of poetic compositions (400c12–d3, cf. 399e–400a). Proper *paideia* involving *mousikê* is crucial to the cultivation and grasp of virtue. One's prospects for achieving *sôphrosunê* and the rest hinge on the right exposure thereto (402b–c). Plato underscores here that "excessive pleasure" (*hêdonê huperballousa*) is incompatible with this *aretê* or any other (402e) and singles out sexual pleasure as the worst culprit in this regard (403a–b). These comments gain added resonance from several *logoi* in the *Symposium*—those by Eryximachus, Pausanias, and Phaedrus—seeking to justify *erastês-erômenos* ties, which Socrates' *logos* condemns.[82] As the *Republic*'s discussion makes clear, all of *mousikê* as practiced to date is Plato's critical target. Hence, it is *mousikê* in its entirety that does not and cannot qualify as a *technê*. We see, here as elsewhere, that Eryximachus' pretentions to insight well outpace his discernment. Eryximachus'

[79] In the remainder of this paragraph I draw on Levin (2001, 132–35). Regarding the *Cratylus*, see chaps. 1–3.

[80] See Rowe (1998, on 187d2).

[81] According to Konstan and Young-Bruehl (1982, 42), the medical foundation for Eryximachus' doctrine of harmony is *Regimen* I, which "exhibits the closest agreement in both theory and association of topics." Yet on their interpretation of *mousikê* in Eryximachus' speech, *erôs* qua *philia*—versus *erôs* qua *epithumia* as in medicine—governs there, such that the musician "is doing what the doctor does when he rearranges the elements in the body. But there is nothing in a musical harmony or discord that corresponds to the various desires of bodies healthy or ill" (41–42). This construction undermines the tenability of their particular stress on *Regimen* I's foundational role insofar as, on their account, in contrast to that involving *mousikê* in *Regimen* I (18), the relationship between medicine and music—so crucial to Eryximachus' discussion—becomes in effect one of analogy.

[82] Plato's condemnation of indulgence via Socrates' speech continues in Alcibiades' (215e–216c, 217e–219e).

undiscriminating approach to what counts as a *technê* should intensify our suspicion that his claim for medicine's preeminence among *technai* is untenable.

7. CONCLUDING THOUGHTS: ERYXIMACHUS' AND OUR OWN

On the view of McPherran (2006, 77n17), at 194a "Plato has Socrates praise the beauty—hence, the correctness, it seems—of Eryximachus' speech." On my argument, the opposite is actually the case.[83] That Socrates' remark is accompanied by praise of Agathon's *logos*-to-be should render one suspicious of his sincerity given what follows involving the poet. According to Socrates, the doctor fears that nothing more remains to be said about *erôs* at this point (193e) "because you did beautifully in the contest, Eryximachus. But if you ever get in my position, or rather the position I'll be in after Agathon's spoken so well, then you'll really be afraid" (194a1–4). Eryximachus says later that Agathon has excelled (198a), and Socrates states that the poet's remarks were delivered "with beauty" (198b2–3, cf. 7). Yet Socrates proceeds to challenge Agathon's *logos* on various fronts, which indicates that the earlier observation was made ironically. Socrates' challenge also reflects poorly on Eryximachus' judgment—this time for having lavished praise on Agathon's contribution, which, like his own, displays faulty constructions of *aretai* (196b–197b). By the dialogue's standards for beauty—the value on which it concentrates—these *logoi* cannot possess that quality in any substantive way.

In the *Symposium*, the rivalry between medicine and philosophy for primacy on nature and thriving is clearly evident.[84] On my argument, via Eryximachus, who subordinates philosophy to his profession à la *Ancient Medicine*, medicine goes head-to-head with philosophy for the title of preeminent *technê*. In Plato's eyes, medicine loses this battle decisively. As the *Republic*'s *technê* par excellence, philosophy oversees all other endeavors due to the superlative, unique insight of its practitioners. In the *Symposium*'s ascent, which culminates in the Form, the placement of institutions and practices, with the fields of study addressing these, on pertinent but lower planes (210c–d, 211c) helps to bridge the gap between the *Gorgias*' *technê* of politics and the *Republic*'s *philosophia*.

---

[83] Cf. Rettig (1876, ad loc.).

[84] Brill (2006, 12) notes a clash, albeit limited, between the two practices but grounds it in medicine's exploitation of human fears of death, not fundamentally different approaches to nature and thriving more generally. Though Scott and Welton (2008) stress the *Symposium*'s rivaling of alternative pursuits, they single out poetry. In their view, Socrates' *logos* "synthesize[s] the rationalism of Eryximachus and the piety of Aristophanes" (152, cf. 192), and medicine's ultimate shortcoming is its "incomplete[ness]" (199), not fundamentally flawed constructions of *phusis* and *eudaimonia*. For an allusion to competition between philosophy and poetry in the *Symposium*, see Kahn (1987, 94).

In the *Republic*, Plato does not relinquish the notion that medicine holds up well compared with certain other activities (e.g., rhetoric/sophistry). That said, medicine comes in for further critique, including tight circumscription. What is more, the preeminence of *philosophia* in Kallipolis, the *Republic*'s ideal city, warrants philosophers' interference with medical decision making, which is thus no longer self-contained. In fact, the dialogue's line of argument commits Plato to withdraw medicine's *technê* standing altogether. This next stage in Plato's critique of medicine is made possible by the *Symposium*, whose central role in the *agôn* between philosophy and medicine I have sought to illuminate here. Let us now investigate this next phase in Plato's handling of medicine.

4

Justice and the Good in Kallipolis: Medicine's Ejection from the Ranks of *Technai*

1. INTRODUCTION

Having forged a *technê-empeiria* divide in the *Gorgias*, Plato devotes much of the *Republic* to developing his view of the earlier dialogue's preeminent *technê*. The paramount endeavor was called there *politikê* but tied closely to philosophy, as when Socrates maintains that "I'm one of a few Athenians—I don't say I'm the sole one ever, but I'm certainly unique among our contemporaries—to take up and practice the true political *technê*" (521d). The *Republic* defends philosophy's standing as preeminent by showing how robustly it satisfies the *Gorgias*' *technê* conditions. On the flip side, practices the *Gorgias* dubbed *empeiriai* are barred from Kallipolis, the *Republic*'s ideal city. These include not only rhetoric/sophistry and traditional poetry but also cookery (372c–373c), which is shed for its threat of harm as the so-called luxurious city (372e3) is distilled to forge Kallipolis.

As in the *Gorgias*, medicine falls between the highest and the disallowed. In the *Republic*, Plato cashes out the implications for medicine of the flaws the *Symposium* diagnosed in its views of *phusis* and *eudaimonia*. The *Republic* circumscribes the terrain of medicine such that lifestyle (i.e., regimen for health's maintenance), to which right handling of the Big Three is central, becomes instead the province of philosophy. Treatment is the sole area remaining for medical practice. As in Hippocratic writings, medication, surgery, and cautery are allowed, but unlike in those writings, doctors' treatments exclude regimen. Plato's view of *phusis* leads him to withhold care in the *Republic* from many people who would receive it from Hippocratic doctors (e.g., those suffering from chronic conditions). Further, as in the *Gorgias*, those irredeemably corrupt in soul are to receive no treatment at all. In the *Republic*, the judge (i.e., philosopher) oversees medicine to ensure that assessments are rightly made.

Here I shall argue, further, that key aspects of the *Republic*—its soul-body tie, the Principle of Specialization,[1] the Form of the Good, and philosophers' infallibility—commit Plato not merely to philosophy's standing atop the realm of *technai* but to the view that it alone is a *technê*. Between philosophy and the *Gorgias*' *empeiriai*, which remain forbidden in Kallipolis, there are many endeavors that make legitimate contributions to communal thriving, though the ontological merits and sociopolitical roles of their aid vary. The point to be stressed is not that Plato expressly adopts this view but rather that the aforementioned factors commit him to it. Within this broad intermediate category, our focus is naturally medicine, which is not merely one pursuit among many there. As we will see, Plato's critical response to medicine's presumed scope figures importantly in the *Republic*'s defense of his positions on *phusis* and *eudaimonia* as they come together, for the first time, in his construction of an ideal city.

2. THE HIPPOCRATIC BACKDROP

Beginning with a sketch of relevant variables in medical texts will help us appreciate how Plato streamlines medical practice. These factors include the handling of treatments, which fall into the broad categories of (1) regimen, (2) *pharmaka* (drugs, or medication), and (3) *temnein* (surgery) and *kaein* (cautery); these last two are grouped together in keeping with their frequent conjoining in the Hippocratic Corpus. Next I will turn to the diagnostic and prognostic assignment of conditions themselves to classes: chronic (i.e., long-lasting) and remediable; chronic and incurable (or at least not cured); and fatal.[2] Lastly, I touch on nondisease impairments. My discussion is not exhaustive, aiming instead to highlight what bears directly on the topic at hand.

2.1 *Treatments*

Regimen is broadly construed in medical writings to encompass people's lifestyles, particularly their conduct regarding food, drink, exercise, and sex. Unlike drugs,

---

[1] This term is drawn from Annas (1981, 73).

[2] I shall not separately address "acute" conditions.

surgery, and cautery, regimen is "something new in the medicine of the late fifth century" (Jouanna 1999, 162). Regimen caught on quickly, as it offered abundant opportunity for medicine to expand its purview. In fact, by Plato's time regimen appears to have become central to medical practice under the heading both of lifestyle and of treatment. Regimen also takes in medical authors' attempts to subsume under *iatrikê* (the *technê* of medicine) the terrain of physical activity and food preparation. Since medicine's substantial occupation with regimen was documented in Chapter 2, I refer the interested reader to that earlier discussion.

As to *pharmaka*, patients consume living materials (e.g., hellebore) and natural, nonliving substances (e.g., white lead), often in combination, to cause evacuation from "above" or "below." The goal is to help patients recover by purging direct contributors to their condition or whatever else impedes health's restoration. Expertise and caution in using *pharmaka* (drugs) are requisite because, as with so much in ancient medicine, right practice is a matter of circumstance (i.e., of the *pros ti*, or "toward what"; *Nutriment* 19). According to *Epidemics* II (3.2), medical experts "know the features of *pharmaka*, from what ones come what kinds of things. Not all are equally good, but different characteristics are good in different circumstances."[3] Such conditions include how they are prepared; the season; and a patient's disease, age, and regimen (ibid.).[4] Doctors must know not merely when to provide *pharmaka* but also when to refrain (*Affections* 14; *Airs Waters Places* 11; *Epidemics* VII 60; *Diseases* IV 16). Finally, references to surgery and cautery abound, with the two procedures often mentioned together.[5]

2.2 Conditions

Conditions that are chronic, in the sense of long-lasting (the term used may be *chronios/chronon* or *makros*, literally "long"), may be remediable,[6] so intractable as to be incurable, or fatal. Where on this list a case falls is often not a function

---

[3] Prizing automatic recall, *Decorum* (9) insists that doctors memorize all there is to know regarding *pharmaka*.

[4] On context dependency involving medication, see also *Affections* 14; *Nature of Man* 9; *Regimen* IV 89; *Aphorisms* 1.23, 4.4–7; *Places in Man* 45. Taking themselves to be experts, authors criticize others' missteps, as when *Epidemics* V (15) observes that an excessively strong *pharmakon* made one Scamandrus perish earlier than he would otherwise have done. A too-powerful purgative caused the unnecessary death of Antimachus' wife (18), who would have survived if she had just consumed water and vomited straightaway.

[5] Concerning surgery, see, e.g., *Diseases* II 24, 30, 38, 47, 61; III 10; *Internal Affections* 14–15, 17, 23, 28, 36; *Places in Man* 25, 32; *Regimen* I 15; *Physician* 2. Regarding cautery, pertinent sources include *Diseases* II 32, 34, 37, 53, 62; III 10; *Internal Affections* 18, 24–25, 30; *Hemorrhoids* 2. For the two referenced jointly, see *Aphorisms* 7.44–45; *Affections* 2, 4; *Diseases* I 10, 15; II 31, 36, 57, 60; III 16; *Internal Affections* 9; *Epidemics* V 15; *Places in Man* 40; *Prorrhetic* II 15.

[6] For *makrê* as "long" in the sense of "chronic," see, e.g., *Affections* 31; *Prorrhetic* II 7.

of the disease alone but also of contextual factors ranging from a patient's age and constitution to whether he receives treatment from the onset of his condition.[7] Medical writings virtually always call for immediate treatment as key to patients' prospects of averting a long-standing illness (*Internal Affections* 30, 36, 43), one that is serious (30, 36), an ailment's recurrence (33), an incurable though not fatal condition (47; *Affections* 18; *Diseases* II 72), or death itself (*Internal Affections* 26, 41; *Affections* 17).

That long-lasting ailments can be cured does not ensure their actual remediation. While *Precepts* (14) assumes a possible recovery from chronic ailments, an actual recovery is fostered by the lodging of regimen in experts' hands (see also *Aphorisms* VI 12).[8] The odds of a cure are greatly affected by how quickly treatment begins. If unaddressed from the get-go, a tertian fever typically shifts into a quartan and becomes chronic (*poluchronios*; *Affections* 18). When quartans hit, again, doctors must address the fevers straightaway (ibid.); these usually last awhile, though sometimes not (*lambeinei de houtos ho puretos tous men pleistous polun chronon, tous de kai oligon*). In *Affections* (19) we learn that if doctors attend to them straightaway, phlegmatic folk with phlegm-caused ailments may recover "from chronic fevers" (*ek puretôn poluchroniôn*). Otherwise, the ailment becomes dropsy, which can be fatal (ibid.). Though immediate treatment does not always lead to a patient's recovery (*Diseases* I 12), one hopes that "the disease grows old in his body" (*Diseases* II 73, see also 74) versus its remaining with him until death.

While the distinction is not always smooth, authors differentiate long-lasting, remediable conditions from those that are incurable (or at least uncured). Thus, "livid disease . . . usually continues until the patient's death" (*Diseases* II 68). In *On the Sacred Disease*, according to which epilepsy is no more supernatural in origin than any other medical condition, "once the disease has become chronic, it proves irremediable" (14). Age may impact a prognosis of incurability, as when "such complaints as become chronic in old men generally last until the end" (*hosa d' an autoisi chronia nosêmata genêtai, ta polla sunapothnêiskei*, *Aphorisms* 2.39). In certain contexts, younger men usually expire quickly, while elderly ones ail until death (*Diseases* I 22).

---

[7] Such factors impact too whether a condition attains chronicity at all (e.g., *On Joints* 50). "Chronic" in the sense of long-lasting is also used of diseases' concomitants, e.g., pains and fevers: *Diseases* I 20; *Prorrhetic* II 29–30; *Epidemics* VII 72; *Coan Prenotions* 370, 414, 500, 519; *Critical Days* 11; *Use of Liquids* 5. Cf. *Regimen in Acute Diseases* (Appendix 19), where shifts in urine are a sign of the ailment's chronicity (*chronon te sêmainei*).

[8] A necessary condition for recovery may, of course, fall outside experts' control (*Epidemics* II 6.5).

The effect of interventions' timing is often front and center. Thus, if erysipelas of the lung is not addressed via cautery straightaway, "the disease continues and rarely goes away, tending in most cases to remain into old age; often it even clings to the patient until his death" (*Internal Affections* 6, cf. 26). Further, the prognosis for a chronic ailment may depend on how responsibly patients heed doctors' instructions: "If the patient follows the [prescribed] regimen, as he reaches the prime of life he escapes, and the disease grows old in his body; if he does not take the appropriate care, the disease lasts until his death" (*Diseases* II 73). Moreover, a disease may be incurable, for though it remits, it recurs, as in *Internal Affections* (19), where the ailment returns in the twelfth year.[9]

Medical writings clearly differentiate incurable, nonfatal illness from mortal conditions. Some originally chronic ailments become fatal (*Coan Prenotions* 253). Fatal conditions, like nonfatal ones, can stem from illness but also from injuries sustained during war, work, or athletic pursuits.[10] Where injuries are the cause, death may occur either straightaway or after the passage of time. *Internal Affections* (10) instructs physicians to do their best even though the ailment in question "is usually mortal and few escape it."[11] *Diseases* II (54) ends with the instruction, "Do these things; the disease tends to be mortal" (*tauta poieein; hê de nousos thanatôdês*).[12] Similarly, *Diseases* III (5) follows a grim prognosis—for a patient in this situation, "the hope of survival is very slight" (*toutôi elpis men panu bracheê perigenesthai*)—with an insistence that "nonetheless" (*homôs de*), treatment should be pursued.[13]

2.3 Nondisease Impairments

Nondisease impairments are distinguished from illnesses by *Affections* (35), which identifies phlegm-based conditions that are "disfigurements rather than diseases" (*esti de tauta aeikea mallon ê nosêmata*). Diseases may cause nondisease impairments. According to *Aphorisms* VI (60), "chronic disease of the hip-joint" may produce lameness, which can also stem from a uterine condition (*Nature of the Child* 4; *Nature of Women* 14). In another situation, disease causes a patient's hunchback (*On Joints* 41).

---

9 Regarding long-lasting, incurable (or uncured) conditions, see further *Prorrhetic* II 11.

10 For athletes' fatalities, see *Epidemics* V 61–62; VI 8.30. A work-related injury causes a shoemaker's death in *Epidemics* V 45. For injury in battle as the cause of death, see *Epidemics* V 95.

11 Cf. chaps. 11, 29, 40.

12 Cf. chap. 48, where nontreatment is recommended unless a competent practitioner has been there from the outset.

13 For further illustrations, see *Diseases* II 46; *Internal Affections* 10; *Nature of Women* 12–13, 38. The relevant terminology applies also to conditions' concomitants (e.g., "deadly stools," *Coan Prenotions* 621); cf. 251, which distinguishes a fatal sign from a chronic one.

While some hereditary or congenital conditions take the form of diseases,[14] they also include nondisease impairments like curvature of the spine (*On Joints* 41) and dislocations (28–29, 85; *Instruments of Reduction* 5, 20, 40). Other conditions depicted as congenital are ankylosis (*On Joints* 21),[15] clubfoot (62), and cockeye (*Epidemics* II 6.14).[16]

3. THE *REPUBLIC*'S ACCOUNT OF MEDICAL PRACTICE

Against this background, I turn to the *Republic*'s view of medicine, including Plato's limiting its sphere and investing philosophy with key oversight responsibilities. As he necessarily viewed medical practice from the standpoint of his own positions on *phusis* and *eudaimonia*, that vantage point will be central when we address why Plato curtails its purview, transferring some of its terrain to philosophy and appointing the latter as medicine's supervisor. As we will see, Plato would both remove the maintenance of health entirely from medicine and severely limit its treatment responsibilities as compared with Hippocratic doctors' wide-ranging involvements.

Salient to medicine's occupation with health is its maintenance and restoration through regimen, with maintenance a matter of people's lifestyle choices. In the *Republic*, regimen is a concern solely for health's preservation. Far from leaving lifestyle decisions to individual discretion, Plato replaces medicine with philosophy as the arbiter of the best way of life. *Republic* 403a–410a—crucial to the dialogue's handling of medicine—opens (403a–404e) with Plato's "prescribing" to us qua philosopher just how the Big Three together with physical training are rightly handled. The operative reference point is Plato's views of *phusis* and *eudaimonia*, to which, as is clear from the *Gorgias* and *Symposium*, right constructions of desire and pleasure are central. Here and elsewhere in the *Republic*, Plato's rationale for philosophy's serving as arbiter is that its practitioners alone have insight with an unflinching commitment to promote the good of individuals and the community. The *Republic*'s opposition to poetry, centrally including Book III (386a–402c), has received tremendous scholarly attention. The same is not true of Book III's critique of medicine. I aim here to remedy that neglect.

---

[14] On dropsy, gout, consumption, and epilepsy, see *Prorrhetic* II 5; on epilepsy, see also *On the Sacred Disease* 5.

[15] Ankylosis is "immobility and consolidation of a joint due to disease, injury, or surgical procedure" (*Dorland's Illustrated Medical Dictionary* 2012, 94). For instance, ankylosing spondylitis is "an inflammatory disease that can cause some [spinal] vertebrae . . . to fuse together" (http://www.mayoclinic.com), and ankyloglossia limits "the tongue's range of motion . . . [because] an unusually short, thick or tight band of tissue . . . tethers the bottom of the tongue's tip to the floor of the mouth" (ibid.).

[16] Cf. *Prorrhetic* II 2: "Cases of impending mental derangement are not very likely to escape one's notice if one knows in which persons this condition is hereditary."

Attending to his work of subsumption, Plato concentrates first on health's preservation (404a).[17] Turning directly to the Big Three, Plato staunchly opposes all sexual pursuits (403a–c): "The pleasures of sex must not come into" relations between people connected "for the sake of what is fine and beautiful" (b1, 6).[18] Socrates' deprecatory mention of "Corinthian girlfriends" shortly thereafter (404d) reinforces the prohibition. Drunkenness too is condemned (403e, cf. 398e). Rounding out Plato's invocation of the Big Three here is his repudiation of indiscriminate eating, including gluttony (403e–404e). Note Plato's utter lack of concern for circumstance in how far conduct involving the Big Three is allowed, whereas context dependency, as we saw in Chapter 2, figured prominently in medical writings. As for exertion, which Hippocratic writings often subsume under medicine's head, Plato prescribes "simple and decent physical training, especially the kind involved in training for war" (404b).[19]

The Big Three were previously singled out in Plato's critique of existing poetry: "Aren't these the most important aspects of self-control for the majority of people, namely, to obey the rulers and to rule the pleasures of drink, sex, and food for themselves?" (389d9–e2). He comes down hard on literary exhibitions of drunkenness (389e–390b), gluttony (390a–b), and sexual appetite (390b–c) by characters presented as admirable. Plato adds his opposition to "money-lovers" (390d–391a)—an adumbration of Book IX's close linkage of a love of gain to the Big Three "because such appetites are most readily satisfied by means of money" (580e5–581a1).[20] In sum, Plato qua philosopher should dictate how the pertinent *epithumiai* (desires) are rightly handled in everyday life.[21]

---

[17] See also 404b–e. Unless otherwise noted, translations of the *Republic* are drawn from Grube (Cooper 1997) or Shorey (Hamilton and Cairns 1963), with adjustments.

[18] In Book V, we learn that procreation itself will be carefully managed, at least for guardians (458e–460b). *Republic* 461b–c seems casual on sexual activity of those past the age of having children, but such a view clashes with Plato's otherwise uncompromising stance against non-procreative sexual activity: in addition to the *Gorgias*, *Symposium*, and *Republic*, see *Phaedrus* 250e, 253d–254e, 256a–b.

[19] When he mentions food and drink as a treatment in Homer at 405d–406a, Plato hastens to include the caveat, "though such treatment is now thought to cause inflammation." One point on which Plato and Hippocratic doctors concur is that one can overdo physical training and be excessively fit (407b–c). In medical writings, see *Regimen* III 84; *Aphorisms* I 3; *Nutriment* 34.

[20] His rationale for poetry's constraint features role-modeling (391e): since children will absorb whatever is presented as admirable, what they are exposed to in literature and life must be genuinely good (cf. *Gorgias* 512e–513c regarding *mimêsis* with bad results). Davidson's (1997) account of "the consuming passions" (xvi) in classical Athens (i.e., what this study calls the Big Three *epithumiai*) stresses the integral role of money in their gratification (190–94); cf. his observation (208) that "anxiety about expenditure is anxiety about appetite itself."

[21] See also Holmes (2010, 205–6): for Plato in *Republic* III, doctors "are simply treating the symptoms of diseases that can be traced to a breakdown in a population's mastery of its desires. The *sôma* is a casualty of this crisis. The real problem . . . lies with a soul that indulges its desires." According to Carrick (2001, 188), "many [philosophers] wondered aloud (as did Plato) whether doctors were really qualified to prescribe to the ordinary citizen intimate patterns of daily living that ideally presupposed a deep understanding of the ultimate values and ends of life."

Further evincing his intent to remove regimen from medicine's purview is Plato's insistence that, from his standpoint as a philosopher, medicine is rightly deployed only for those who are healthy both by nature and in lifestyle. Asclepius

> taught medicine for those whose bodies are healthy in their nature and habits but have some specific disease. . . . He cured them of their disease with drugs or surgery (*pharmakois te kai tomais ta nosêmata ekballonta autôn*), then ordered them to live their usual life so as not to harm their city's affairs. But for those whose bodies were riddled with disease, he didn't attempt to prescribe a regimen, drawing off a little here and pouring in a little there, in order to make life for them long and bad (*makron kai kakon bion anthrôpôi poiein*) and enable them to produce offspring in all probability like themselves. He didn't think that he should treat someone who couldn't have a normal life. (407c–e; see also 408a–b)

Unlike medicine, which uses terms like *kakon-agathon* (bad-good) and *aischron-kalon* (base-noble) for physical states of affairs, Plato uses *aischron*, with the meaning "shameful," at *Republic* 405d5 (cf. *kakon*, 407d6) to suggest that one's needing care for anything besides mild or localized conditions, that is, not being healthy in nature and lifestyle, constitutes a moral failing: "Doesn't it seem shameful to you (*ouk aischron dokei*) to need medical help, not for wounds or a seasonal illness, but because, through idleness and the lifestyle we've described, one is full of gas and phlegm like a stagnant swamp, so that sophisticated Asclepiad doctors are forced to come up with names like 'flatulence' and 'catarrh' to describe one's diseases?" (405c–d).

Plato's claim in 407c–e that medicine is exclusively "for those whose bodies are healthy in their nature and habits" (c8–9) strengthens his earlier comments on the specifics of health's maintenance. Again, it is Plato qua philosopher, not doctors, who will dictate how the pertinent *epithumiai* (desires) are rightly handled in everyday life. In addition, the passage stresses that for Asclepius, allowable medical treatments comprised just drugs and surgery (d2–3). The import of Plato's construction of the myth of Asclepius is that the treatment practices of medicine's own founder excluded regimen.[22] Further, Plato's locution "drawing off a little here and pouring

[22] Cf. Carrick (2001, 22), for whom *Republic* III "reduce[s] the authority and role of the physician by restricting medical assistance to cases of an emergency nature only." While Jouanna (1999, 161–62) rightly notes Plato's critique of "the dietary medicine of his contemporaries" (161) in *Republic* III (449n82), he does not see that Plato goes further than this to withdraw regimen from medicine's purview.

in a little there" (d5–6) pokes fun at doctors' handling of serious cases,[23] which could be extensive and painstaking (e.g., *Places in Man* 13, 27, 41–45; *Diseases* III 16; *Epidemics* VII 1–3; *Superfetation* 29). As we will see further below, on Plato's account doctors' treatments should be withheld not just when ailments are likely fatal but also in cases of serious illness, where recovery following sustained treatment might occur.

Plato reinforces his point about medical practice by asserting that Asclepius' sons too "considered their drugs sufficient for curing men who were healthy and living an orderly life before being wounded even if they happened to drink wine mixed with barley and cheese right after receiving their wounds. But they didn't consider the lives of those who were by nature sick and self-indulgent to be profitable either to themselves or to anyone else. Medicine isn't intended for such people and they shouldn't be treated, not even if they're richer than Midas" (408a–b). Since—again, on Plato's telling—*pharmaka* (drugs) alone do the job here, the practice of renowned earlier doctors remains essentially severed from regimen. In *Republic* III, then, Plato removes a central element of doctors' work from medicine's purview altogether. Its withdrawal here diverges from the *Gorgias*, where, as Moss (2007, 238) observes, regimen as an aspect of treatment is the most evident counterpart to cookery in the dialogue's contrast of *technai* with *empeiriai*.[24]

Epidemics VI (5.1) claims that "the body's nature is the physician in disease," referring to nonconscious bodily processes like the watering of eyes, sneezing, yawning, and excretion. While Jaeger (1986b, 28) rightly draws attention to Hippocratic confidence in the body's "natural urge to self-healing," he overstresses the extent of common ground between medicine and Plato respecting treatment. The ensuing, more specific discussion of legitimate recipients of doctors' care deepens our sense of just how far he departs from medicine in that regard.

As Plato narrows the range of medicine's tools, he restricts the diagnostic and prognostic scenarios that doctors may address. While context-dependent factors such as age, constitution, season, and locale are key for Hippocratic doctors, Plato shuns them. His attention to "context" involves the question of how ailing ones fare vis-à-vis the Principle of Specialization (370a–c). By this principle, everyone

---

[23] See also 405c–d, where Plato takes a jab at physicians who create fancy terms to cover ailments caused by the bad lifestyles of those whom, by his lights, they should not treat.

[24] *Republic* III also departs from Plato's claim in Book I, as in the *Gorgias* (456b, 464d–465d, 504e–505a, 517d–518a), that the art of medicine whose benefit is health (346a) "provides drugs, foods, and drinks to bodies" (332c9–10). One must not, therefore, draw conclusions about the *Republic*'s stance regarding medicine based only on Plato's stage-setting in Book I—i.e., prior to the main argument—any more than one would portray the dialogue's conception of justice based solely on Socrates' exchanges with Cephalus, Polemarchus, and Thrasymachus.

is naturally equipped to perform one sociopolitical role and in Kallipolis must perform that function alone. This notion is strongly operative in the *Republic* generally and in Plato's discussion of medicine specifically (406c–e, 407c–408b, 409e–410a).

The Principle of Specialization is central to the *Republic*'s handling of *phusis* and *eudaimonia*. On Plato's construction, human nature comes in three types, which are ranked hierarchically based on the resident strength and directive ability of souls' rational dimension. The notion of natural types may owe something to Hippocratic constitutions, particularly those grounded in humors, where constitutional types are dubbed, for example, bilious or phlegmatic. In addition, Plato's view that the most talented are the most dangerous if poorly educated (491d–e) is not unlike the Hippocratic claim (*Nature of Man* 10) that the fiercest ailments' source is in the body's strongest part (*Hosa de tôn nosêmatôn ginetai apo tou sômatos tôn meleôn tou ischurotatou, tauta de deinotata estin*). That said, the *Republic* is distinctive for focusing on the *phusis* of *psuchê* (soul), which is responsible for people's intellectual ability and ethical caliber. Plato's view of *phusis* anchors the dialogue's account of *eudaimonia*, which is gauged by the absolute measures of (1) what caliber of soul a person has and (2) how fully she realizes the psychic capacity and sociopolitical role made available by her native endowment.

Plato's discussion of the ailing carpenter (406c–d), which references drugs, surgery, and cautery (406d), illustrates how treatment decisions should be approached: "If anyone prescribed a lengthy course of treatment (*ean de tis autôi makran diaitan prostattêi*) for the carpenter, telling him that he should rest with his head bandaged and so on, he'd reply without hesitation that he had no leisure to be ill. . . . After that he'd bid his doctor good-bye." Plato's comment that this is the fitting way of seeing medical care in a context of this sort (406e5–6) is a pointed injection of his own view. The same obtains at 407e, where Socrates is told, "your Asclepius was quite a statesman (*politikon*)." In these comments, Plato is the present voice of Asclepius (cf. 407c) and then of Asclepius' sons (408b).

Not coincidentally, following these comments Plato invokes "the good judge" (*ton agathon dikastên*, 409b4–5; see also d6–7) as arbiter in the weightiest cases. As I argue in Section 5, the "good judge" of Book III, who makes judgments needing insight beyond doctors' medical awareness, is the philosopher. In the meantime, it is worth noting that through its use of the terms *politikos* (statesman) and *dikastês* (judge), the *Republic* harks back to the *Gorgias*' overarching psychic *technê* of politics and its restorative counterpart to medicine, namely judging. What a comedown Plato orchestrates here for medicine, which is wont to exaggerate its own importance: "Don't medicine and law give themselves solemn airs when even large numbers of free men take them quite seriously?" (405a). This claim is apt when one recalls Eryximachus' *logos* in the *Symposium* and considers Hippocratic writings like *Ancient Medicine*.

Let us look again at medical writings to see how far the treatment approach illustrated by the carpenter (406c–d) diverges from them on who warrants treatment. Hippocratic authors often assume and regularly maintain that enduring diseases warrant treatment even when they are prolonged, as when *Diseases* II (49) speaks of consumption that "lasts seven or nine years; if the patient is treated from the start, he recovers."[25] Protracted care may be provided even when the outcome is always death (*Glands* 14). Treatment is also given for ailments whose level of seriousness becomes evident only with time (*On Joints* 58). As a wait-and-see attitude is virtually always deleterious,[26] treatment should begin straightaway to minimize the chances of serious illness (*Internal Affections* 36), an ailment's recurrence (33), its incurability (26),[27] or the patient's death (*Affections* 17). Plato's handling of the carpenter, in contrast, shows that he rejects treatment for serious illness and even lengthy care that may be needed for doctors to learn the seriousness of an ailment.[28]

The *Republic*'s Principle of Specialization closely aligns people's human worth with the successful performance of their naturally befitting societal roles. On this basis, the life of one not able to perform her function is no longer worth continuing. Taking further Plato's departure from medicine, one may note that lives that the *Republic* would view as deeply marred are not valueless according to Hippocratic doctors, who attend to amputations and gangrene (*Instruments of Reduction* 34; *On Joints* 68–69). While medicine views congenital clubfoot as typically curable and addresses it (*On Joints* 62), progeny with such traits in Kallipolis would not see the light of day (460c).[29]

In the *Gorgias*, Plato stressed the need for the physically ill to get to doctors straightaway, enduring pain if need be for healing's sake. As we have already seen, the *Republic* heavily qualifies this broad recommendation. Plato follows up his account of the carpenter (406c–d) by claiming expressly that patients' pursuit and doctors' provision of more than circumscribed care is pathological:

---

[25] See also *Internal Affections* 43.

[26] While medical writers disagree on whether measures should be taken in cases known to be incurable, they do not indicate that an incurable person's life is worthless.

[27] See also chap. 47.

[28] Plato's limitation of cases treated includes *makros* (long; 406d3, 407d6), a term used for "chronic" in medical writings, where such cases are handled as a matter of course.

[29] When medical writings recommend against treatment or make it optional, the reason is worry for doctors' reputations and/or a genuine concern to avoid dispensing what will not aid and may do harm (e.g., by causing needless pain).

> Excessive care of the body, over and above physical training, is pretty well the biggest obstacle of all [to one's conduct of a virtuous life]. It's troublesome in managing a household, in military service, and even in a sedentary public office. Most of all, it makes any kind of learning, thought, or private reflection difficult, for it's always imagining some headaches or dizziness and accusing philosophy of causing them. Hence, wherever this kind of virtue is practiced and examined, excessive care of the body hinders it, for it makes a person think he's ill and be all the time concerned about his body. (407b–c, cf. 405c–d)

Apart from the damage wrought by unsalutary lifestyles, marked occupation with the body both leads to excessive bodily care and distracts one from what should be a paramount focus on soul.

Drawing *Republic* III's handling of medicine to a close, Plato grants good judges authority over medical decision makers, with *phusis* and *eudaimonia* as guiding concerns: "Then won't you legislate in our city for the kind of medicine we mentioned and for this kind of judging so that together they'll look after those who are naturally well endowed in body and soul? But as for the ones who are naturally unhealthy or whose souls are incurably evil, won't they let the former die of their own accord and put the latter to death?" (409e4–410a4). This course is endorsed as "best both for the ones to whom these things happen and for the city" (410a5–6).[30] The *Republic*'s prescription that the irremediably unjust be killed is more concrete and extreme than the *Gorgias*' claim that no benefit accrues from their lives' continuing. Among psychic defects, *akolasia* (self-indulgence) is central, as it is the contrary of *sôphrosunê* (self-control), the virtue tying soul most closely to body. It should come as no surprise that non-medical judges who are expert in psychic phenomena are solely qualified to make these evaluations. While medical writings do not focus on character, either virtue or vice, doctors likely treated many who by Plato's lights were psychically flawed in the relevant sense. Thus, Plato further limits the cases that doctors may handle, whether because they never reach physicians or because, having stopped there initially, they straightaway become the province of judges.

For Jouanna (1999, 108–9), Plato's view of treatment's scope is a comprehensive application of *The Art*'s, according to which good craftspeople attempt what is possible (*dunaton*) as befits their own *technê*. Relying on *Republic* II alone here,

---

30 Carrick's (2001, 159) claim that the *Republic*'s support for involuntary euthanasia of adults "remains an open question that [Plato] does not speak to explicitly" seems untenable in light of *autoi apoktenousin* (410a4) about the psychically incurable, who would presumably oppose philosophers' determination that they should be put to death.

Jouanna does not remark that Plato radically subordinates Hippocratic notions of the possible (*dunaton*) in Book III in holding that medicine may not always implement the medically feasible, as on the Principle of Specialization some cases ought not be treated even if doctors *can* do something. Further, the presence of unremitting psychic injustice makes wholly irrelevant the question of what if anything medical could be done.

4. PHILOSOPHERS, THE BIG THREE, AND THE SOUL-BODY TIE

As we have seen, the *Republic* severs medicine's tie to regimen and removes its handling of the Big Three. As psychic welfare is primary, and central to it is right management of the Big Three, it is crucial that real experts address these *epithumiai*. In the *Republic*, philosophers are these psychic experts. The critique of medicine in Book III is not a freestanding discussion, for as we saw with the *Symposium*, Plato's development of his own theories and engagement with rivals are deeply intertwined. A central strand in the *Republic* is its more complex account of the soul and increasingly nuanced soul-body tie. Plato's views involving the soul are integral to his presentation of philosophers as infallible and solely equipped to rule. *Sôphrosunê* has special standing as the virtue most closely linking body and soul. Given the *Republic*'s conviction that children, being most impressionable, must form right attitudes early on, waiting until problems arise before tackling appetitive challenges is a recipe for individual and sociopolitical failure. Hence, it is all the more urgent that this terrain be handled not as a medical matter but as involving one's way of life tout court. Since Plato's recognition of the soul's complexity and nuanced soul-body tie have powerful implications for the *Republic*'s account of Kallipolis, his optimal city, we must explore these matters before addressing philosophers' preeminence.

When Plato's account of the optimal city opens in Book II, we are told simply that this finest of cities will require guardians (374e). Subsequently, based on natural human aptitudes, Plato divides guardians into philosophers and auxiliaries (i.e., the city's protectors).[31] Society itself encompasses three groups, with producers (e.g., farmers, cobblers), far and away the largest, added to the former two. In Book IV, having shown how the virtues—*sophia* (wisdom), *andreia* (courage), *sôphrosunê* (self-control), and *dikaiosunê* (justice)—map onto societal groups, Plato turns to argue that the soul also has three aspects. Specifically, he shows that we learn, feel, and gravitate toward the Big Three via distinct psychic elements (436a–b).

[31] Auxiliaries' protective role covers what might jeopardize the city's security from within or without (i.e., it encompasses, broadly speaking, police and military functions).

Plato's argument here for the soul's tripartition builds on the *Gorgias*' recognition (493a–d) that the Big Three have their source in the soul, which means that the soul already consists, at minimum, of intellectual and appetitive faculties. According to what Annas (1981, 137) labels the Principle of Conflict (see 439c–d), one may illustrate this multiplicity by a case in which the rational principle (*logismos*) pushes the individual to refrain from consuming a beverage as advised on grounds of health while appetite presses hard toward indulgence. The same notion of conflict is used to differentiate feeling from appetite (439e–440a), while Plato's demarcation of feeling from reason is ontogenetic (i.e., children display the former but not yet the latter, 441a–b). By distinguishing the wellsprings of feeling and of familiar desires for "the pleasures stemming from food, drink, sex, and other things akin to these" (436b1–2), Plato reaffirms a budding commitment to the soul's complexity in the *Gorgias* (493a–b) and *Symposium*. At the same time, the *Republic*'s account of the soul is deeper and covers more ground.

Though the tripartite conception of soul is not formally introduced until Book IV, one must bear it in mind not only when considering what Plato says elsewhere in the *Republic* about intrapsychic ties but also when interpreting his guidelines for children's education, comprising *mousikê* (poetry and music) and *gumnastikê* (physical training) in Books II–III.[32] In what follows I attend to Plato's remarks on both topics as avenues through which he depicts the substantive, nuanced ties between soul and body.

Plato prefaces his discussion of gymnastics in Book III by stressing that an excellent soul renders the body as good as possible (403d). Building on the *Gorgias* and *Symposium*, the *Republic* foregrounds a distinctive tie between the body's condition and the appetitive aspect of the soul, the firm regulation of whose resident desires yields *sôphrosunê*. At 403e–404e, prospective guardians are urged to avoid drunkenness, lethargy, and the injudicious consumption of food. Following up, Socrates states that the sons of Asclepius at Troy would not offer medical care to anyone "by nature sick and self-indulgent" (*nosôdê . . . phusei te kai akolaston*), since such an individual lacks value to himself and others (408b).[33] The body's close link to appetite comes to the fore in Book IV's remarks on the special standing of self-control, compared with wisdom and courage, to which we turn later in the present section.

Both *mousikê* and *gumnastikê* are pursued by guardians-in-training for their souls' sake. At 410b Plato specifies that guardians do gymnastics to properly

[32] The two can be difficult to tease apart in practice, hence the flexibility in my ensuing categorization of passages.

[33] This soul-body tie is anticipated at 396d.

cultivate spirit, that is, the psychic aspect of feeling (*pros to thumoeides tês phuseôs blepôn*),[34] as opposed to mere athletes who pursue diet and exercise strictly for bodily enhancement. Enriching the point about integration, Plato maintains that reason and spirit should be fostered in the young "not for the soul and the body in isolation but rather for the harmonious adjustment of these two principles by the proper degree of tension and relaxation of each" (*ouk epi psuchên kai sôma, ei mê ei parergon, all' ep' ekeinô, hopôs an allêloin sunarmosthêton epiteinomenô kai aniemenô mechri tou prosêkontos*, 411e6–412a2). More generally, "the person who achieves the finest blend of music and physical training and impresses it on his soul in the most measured way (*ton kallist' ara mousikêi gumnastikên kerannunta kai metriôtata têi psuchêi prospheronta*) is the one we'd most correctly call completely harmonious and trained in music, much more so than the one who merely harmonizes the strings of his instrument" (412a4–7). As Plato's treatment of early education and optimal intrapsychic ties makes clear, such individuals can resist the pull of such pressures as fear (503a2–4) precisely to the extent that they have reached a proper collaborative relationship between body and soul.

As to soul and body's linkage vis-à-vis psychic tripartition, Plato states that those obsessed with proliferating laws to "ensure" the best sociopolitical outcome are like "the sick whose immoderation blocks them from altering their harmful regimen" (*tous kamnontas te kai ouk ethelontas hupo akolasias ekbênai ponêras diaitês*, 425e8–10).[35] Striking as regards soul-body intertwining is the case of one Leontius and the corpses (439e–440a), where Plato uses the Principle of Conflict to differentiate spirit from appetite as a distinct element of *psuchê*. Leontius,

> becoming aware of dead bodies that lay at the place of public execution, felt simultaneously a desire to see them and a repugnance and aversion (*aisthomenos nekrous para tôi dêmiôi keimenous, hama men idein epithumoi, hama de au duscherainoi kai apotrepoi heauton*). . . . For a time he resisted and veiled his head, but overpowered in the end by his desire (*kratoumenos d' oun hupo tês epithumias*), with wide staring eyes he rushed up to the corpses and cried, "There, you wretches, take your fill of the fine spectacle."

While this account is not detailed, it surpasses the *Gorgias* and *Symposium* by intertwining *aisthêsis* (sense-perception), appetite, and feeling in a single episode of human experience. This illustration captures vividly how, once perception alerts one

---

[34] For a comprehensive statement of the point about psychic impact, see 410b10–c6.

[35] My translation.

to relevant stimuli, the dominance of appetite over spirit steers the body to take the action required for entities' absorption via sight or other sensory modalities. Leontius' hankering, victorious over the attendant feeling of shame, is not really about the dead but is instead "sexual in nature, for . . . Leontius was known for his love of boys as pale as corpses" (Grube 1992, ad loc.). This clarification makes it more evident how *aisthêsis* operates at two junctures in the case of the Big Three (e.g., with sexual indulgence, visual identification followed by touch). Crucial to *eudaimonia* is what happens as soon as the operative sense (here, sight) lights on the object for the first time.

The following passages involving the tripartite soul also have implications for early education. Suggesting a fairly complex soul-body tie, Plato notes that during their physical growth to maturity, philosophers should "take right good care of their bodies, thus securing a basis and a support for the intellectual life" (498b). At 503a2–4, referenced above, Plato avers that guardians-in-training will triumph over fear and other *metabolai* (pressures) if soul and body are properly harmonized. This harmony is fostered by spirit's right cultivation so that as reason unfolds, in situations like Leontius' (439e–440a) one can succeed in keeping one's appetites (*epithumiai*) at bay. *Mousikê* and *gumnastikê* foster this alliance in the young (441e–442a). Since reason has yet to unfold, early *paideia* (education) cannot target it directly. This *paideia*, however, markedly impacts its ability to express itself rightly when it does emerge. On the best scenario, reason and spirit (i.e., feeling) are able together to keep the soul's appetitive dimension in check, this being "the largest part in each person's soul and . . . by nature most insatiable (*phusei aplêstotaton*)" (442a6–7). Plato builds here on the *Gorgias*' image of the leaky jar (493b), which represents appetite's insatiability (*tên aplêstian*, b3). If reason and spirit cannot successfully align, appetite, the soul's worst aspect, dominates (*Republic* 442a–b). For Plato (558b), no one becomes good (*agathos*) unless from childhood his play and all other activities revolve around what is admirable (*ei mê pais ôn euthus paizoi en kalois kai epitêdeuoi ta toiauta panta*). This discussion makes clear both Plato's view that education is properly a lifelong affair and his deep conviction that role modeling, particularly for the young, is crucial to how their natural abilities will unfold.

Plato sees in the *Republic* not only that soul and body are interwoven but that the impact is bidirectional. Influence moves from body to soul and vice versa.[36] As we have seen, gymnastics should target spirit's proper cultivation (410b). More generally, both *mousikê* and *gumnastikê* are undertaken for the soul's sake (410b–c,

[36] On this point cf. Heyd (1995, 380).

cf. 412a). In addition (455b–c), success in any occupation for which one is suited by nature necessitates one's having a body that adequately serves the mind (*ta tou sômatos hikanôs hupêretoi têi dianoiai*). Building on this point, Plato distinguishes between coveting bodily excellence strictly for its own sake and its pursuit to maximize self-control and virtue generally: "One will not even privilege health above all, nor ways of becoming strong, healthy, and pleasing in form, unless these activities promote self-control (*ean mê kai sôphronêsein mellêi ap' autôn*) but will instead always modulate bodily harmony for the sake of psychic accord" (591c–d).[37] To proceed aright, the handling of physicality must therefore be guided by one whose *technê* features the soul.

While Plato comments more often on what the body's caliber must be with the soul's welfare in view, he also notes the reverse, namely, that the soul by its excellence renders the body as good as possible (403d). From the vantage point of medicine's status in the *Republic*, one should observe that it is not just in one person (here, the patient) that a psychic condition affects the body. Plato also points out that physicians treat their patients' bodies via the practitioners' own *psuchai* (souls, 408e). The quality of treatment one receives, therefore, will have much to do with the caliber of doctors' souls. Bearing this in mind is important when one considers the level of cognitive attainment required to steadily promote what bears on character, hence flourishing.

At times when speaking of body and soul, Plato stresses that the two directions of impact—body on soul and vice versa—are themselves closely intertwined. *Republic* 408b, on *akolasia*, seems to envision that scenario with the virtue of *sôphrosunê*. Plato's clarification that children's education is directed not to soul and body separately but seeks their maximal harmony (411e–412a) also expresses that relation. Though the *Republic* surpasses the *Gorgias* and *Symposium* on these topics, Plato has not fully elaborated the relation of body to appetite. Reading between the lines of what he does say (439e–440a, 442a, 485d, 584c), one may infer that through sense-perception (*aisthêsis*) the body alerts the soul to the proximity of relevant objects without itself generating *epithumiai* for them. While the soul is the ultimate source of those desires (i.e., the impetus behind the person's quest for their satisfaction), the results of their gratification are shared by *psuchê* and *sôma*, negatively impacting both.[38]

---

[37] My translation.

[38] To the extent it succeeds in showing the inner workings of those whose *epithumiai* have surged toward full insatiability, Book IX's depiction of the tyrant is a viable response not only to Thrasymachus' fantastical picture in *Republic* I (pace Annas 1981, 302–5) but also to Polus' extravagant lauding of Archelaus in the *Gorgias* (470d–472d, 479d–e).

In the *Republic*, the tight link between soul and body is vividly captured by Plato's emphasis on the special status of self-control (*sôphrosunê*), as compared with wisdom (*sophia*) and courage (*andreia*, 430e; see also 431e–432a). Unlike courage and wisdom, self-control involves not only the superlative condition of the pertinent psychic element (here, appetite) but all three aspects of the soul at once. At 432a6–b1 (with reemphasis at 442c9–d2), Socrates proclaims that "we should be quite right in affirming this unanimity to be self-control, the concord of the naturally superior and inferior as to which ought to rule in both the state and the individual."[39] While 389d–e may constitute a harbinger of the twofold nature of self-control, Plato points ahead to this more directly and via analogy when he notes (425e) that those wrongly obsessed with proliferating laws to bring about the best state are like those whose *akolasia* prevents their rejecting a bad lifestyle. For Plato, *sôphrosunê* involves "concord and harmony" (*sumphôniai . . . kai harmoniai*) more than wisdom and courage (430e1–2). He characterizes it preliminarily as "some order" (*kosmos tis*) and "mastery" (*enkrateia*) apropos of pleasure and desire (e4–5). Plato builds here on the *Gorgias*' noting of an integral tie among order, self-control, and the good (507e–508a). In the *Republic*, the paramount distinction between the self-controlled and self-indulgent is that the former's soul is steered by reason, its finest element, whereas the latter's is straightjacketed by a tangled mass of *epithumiai* (431a–d). On Plato's account, one's prospects for *eudaimonia* hinge on how far appetite can and does submit to directives from the soul's rightful ruling principle.

Further evidence of the *Republic*'s interweaving of body and soul comes through a striking image, deployed to accentuate that the ideal community is a unity that far transcends the grouping of its constituents as a mereological sum. The cohesion of said polis

> is most like that of an individual human being (*engutata henos anthrôpou echei*). For example, if the finger of one of us is wounded, the entire community of bodily connections stretching to the soul for "integration" (*pasa hê koinônia hê kata to sôma pros tên psuchên tetamenê eis mian suntaxin*) with the dominant part is made aware, and all of it feels the pain as a whole, though it is a part that suffers, and that is how we come to say that a person has a pain in his finger. And for any other member of the person the same statement holds. (462c9–d4)

---

[39] For a clear formulation of the twofold pertinence of *sôphrosunê*, applied to the communal plane, see Annas (1981, 116): "There is . . . a way in which moderation is displayed by all the citizens, but also a way in which it can be thought of as peculiarly the virtue of the productive class, because it is only from them that this common agreement demands restraint in the way they behave."

This image is telling as an indication that in the *Republic*, the human being is a unity in a way that, while consistent with key strands in the *Gorgias* and *Symposium*, well surpasses their depictions.[40]

We can now see why one who handles the Big Three cannot neatly demarcate bodily from psychic strands. In the *Republic*, only philosophers have a nature and education that equip them to be arbiters of ways of life. Most specifically, they alone understand reality, above all the Good, and this insight makes them intellectually and ethically infallible. To see more fully what warrants their rule, we must therefore attend to these other matters.

5. INFALLIBLE PHILOSOPHERS AND THE GOOD

According to the Principle of Specialization, different people have native aptitudes for different jobs, and each individual should pursue the occupation for which he is suited *kata phusin* (in accordance with nature, 370a–c; see also 374b–c). For instance, based on that principle, philosophers will oversee the production of poetry but not themselves compose it (379a).[41] One's assignment to a particular group in society is based ultimately on the caliber of one's soul. A refined version of the Principle of Specialization forms the core of Plato's conception of justice in *Republic* IV (433a, cf. 443b–c).[42] Plato's greatest concern (434a–c) is to avoid shifts across basic groups in society, above all from producer to philosopher-ruler, which would spell disaster for the community.[43] Each citizen of the ideal polis must contribute to its welfare. Hence oligarchy, one form of degenerate constitution discussed in Book VIII, violates the aforementioned principle by allowing a person to abide in the city "as a pauper and a dependent" (552b1). Such a one drains the city's resources without giving anything back. Still worse, where one finds beggars, one will also discover criminals (552d–e). Individual and communal welfare coincide only if the Principle of Specialization is observed, and its following eliminates the conflict between furthering one's own and others' interests that anchored Thrasymachus' encomium of the tyrant in Book I (343e–344c).

Philosophers alone bridge that gap. That bodily and psychic conditions are mutually influential with respect to an excellent soul, and that "one with a good soul is

---

[40] This is not to say that the *Republic*'s view is univocal, as a look at Book X (especially 611b–d) against the backdrop of what precedes makes clear.

[41] For comments regarding this principle, see also 394e, 397e, 406c.

[42] On this point cf. Annas (1981, 118).

[43] The formulation of London (2000, 145) smacks excessively of Rawls: "For . . . Plato . . . politics is the discipline whose function assures that the structures of society are arranged in such a way as to allow individual citizens a fair opportunity to pursue those activities that make their lives valuable."

good" (*ho . . . echôn psuchên agathên agathos*, 409c2–3), underscores the pivotal tie between human nature and the good.[44] As we saw in Chapter 1, the *Gorgias* distinguishes time and again between seeking merely to please others via flattery and truly benefiting those toward whom one's activity is directed. The *Republic* grounds philosophers' unique capacity to promote at once their own and others' welfare in their grasp of reality, above all its highest element, the Form of the Good.[45] Before Forms are expressly introduced into the *Republic*'s discussion in Book V, Plato forcefully rejects the notion, cherished by many Athenians, that the welfare of the optimal community is necessarily based in law (4.425b–e). He lauds here in contrast a select few whose exemplary character is pivotal to civic order and harmony since their vision alone attends to the city's welfare tout court (428c–d). Only they have *sophia* (428e–429a), whose practical import Book IV stresses (428b–d). Once Forms are front and center, Plato adds that contemplative insight is forged through *dialektikê* (dialectic), namely, direct investigation of Forms' natures and interrelations. This inquiry, preceded by work in mathematics, astronomy, and musical harmony (524d–534e), culminates in philosophers' apprehending the Good itself.[46]

As nothing imperfect (*ateles*) provides a firm reference point, or "measure" (*metron*), for thought or action, only Forms, unchanging and unchangeable in their perfection, function thus (*metron tôn toioutôn apoleipon kai hotioun tou ontos ou panu metriôs gignetai; ateles gar ouden oudenos metron*, 504c). It is best for philosophers to govern the community, because only they truly understand the elements of reality, particularly values, and their interconnections. Philosophers assimilate themselves to the harmony that they glimpse among these entities (500c), which apprehension and its resulting psychic harmony enable them to foster harmony without (500d, 501b–e).

Having firmly established this causal tie between apprehending perfect objects and securing social benefit, Plato introduces the capstone of his theory, the Form

[44] Fully exploring this tie necessitates consideration not just of human nature but also of reality proper, namely Forms; the nature and possibility of knowledge; freedom; power; education; character; optimal and inferior sociopolitical frameworks and institutions. On grounds like these, Annas (1981, 13) dubs the *Republic*'s approach to justice "expansive."

[45] Here and in the following two paragraphs, I draw on Levin (2001, 138–39).

[46] Strictly speaking, philosophers "recollect" knowledge of Forms. In the *Phaedo* (72e–77a), Plato resolves via Forms the famous Learner's Paradox, stated at *Meno* 80e, according to which learning is impossible: if we know what we seek, a quest is otiose; whereas, if we are unacquainted with it at the start, we would not recognize what was sought as the object of our quest even if it were thrust upon us. In the *Phaedo*, Plato presents our grasp of concepts in the domains of values (e.g., beauty) and mathematics (e.g., equality) as innate insofar as we work to recover understanding of ultimate realities in the relevant cases that our souls previously acquired while disembodied. On the highly plausible view that recollection continues to undergird Plato's notion of learning in the *Republic*, philosophers strictly speaking recover rather than acquire knowledge of the Good and other Forms.

of the Good (*auto to agathon*, "the good itself"; 534c4),[47] which sits atop the *Republic*'s hierarchy of Forms and is the ultimate object of human aspiration (504d–509d, 517b–c, 518c–d, 534b–c). While everyone wants to promote what they view as good, particularly for themselves (505d–e, cf. 521a), only insight into the Good allows the self and community to approach perfection as closely as is possible for what is colored by mortality (505a–506b, 509b, 514a–521a). Since apprehending the Good allows philosophers to maximize the beneficial across human institutions and endeavors,[48] the attainment of best results in all fields requires philosophers' expertise and supervision.[49]

Most, far from knowing the Good, lack even stable true belief about it. The result is that nothing they do is truly a boon. Although this claim, as formulated, pertains specifically to individuals' securing of their own benefit, it cannot but apply also to one's benefiting others. That it does so apply is affirmed by Plato's later contention that one who fails to understand the Form of the Good will "know neither it nor any particular good" (*oute auto to agathon . . . eidenai . . . oute allo agathon ouden*, 534c4–5). What is more, philosophers alone, with this knowledge, can glimpse a soul in its entirety (579d–e). These remarks unpack Plato's insistence at 517c3–4 that "anyone who is to act sensibly in private or public must grasp [the Good]" (*dei tautên idein ton mellonta emphronôs praxein ê idiai ê dêmosiai*).

On the *Gorgias*' account of *technê*, the central measure of one's having knowledge, or understanding, is a capacity to articulate an activity's goal and measures' pertinence to that end. Plato's view that what is knowable must be unaltered and unalterable[50] emerges post-*Gorgias* when he identifies transcendent Forms as the objects of understanding (*Symposium* 210a–212a; *Phaedo* 72e–77a, 78b–81a, 100b–105b; *Cratylus* 439a–440d). As one would expect, philosophers, accessing Forms with cognitive directness, can provide the requisite *logoi* (534b3–6).

Through the *Republic*'s account of the Good and of philosophy's standing as preeminent, Plato shows as unfounded the worry voiced in Book I that expertise is intrinsically value-neutral (i.e., that it can be used equally for good or ill).[51] Applied to medicine, the concern is that what physicians know (e.g., about the properties of plants) makes them equally capable of promoting health or illness (332d, 333e). The

[47] Cf. 534b9–c1.

[48] Controversy surrounds the matter of whether it is in philosopher-rulers' interest to divide their time between contemplation and governance rather than devoting themselves exclusively to the former. In my view, while the issue is challenging to resolve, Kraut (1992, 328) is ultimately correct that "one's highest good is not always served by purely contemplating the Forms."

[49] On the philosopher's role as overseer, cf. Kato (1986, 23, 47, 76); Anagnostopoulos (2000, 282).

[50] Cf. Parmenides B7–8.

[51] For this view of expertise, see also *Hippias Minor* 366c–369a, 375b; the latter passage addresses medicine.

problem of error is also raised. Here, Thrasymachus claims that although practicing doctors slip up, they do not blunder qua *dêmiourgoi* (practitioners of the craft) of medicine (340d–e, cf. 341c). The way is thus paved for Socrates' two-pronged query (342a): (1) Is medicine defective due to the lack of some excellence (*aretê*) such that it needs another *technê* over it to ensure that medical practice successfully promotes the good of patients? (2) If so, will there not be an infinite regress of *technai*, since none has an ultimate supervisory role? In what follows, the *Republic* addresses both through its defense of philosophers' intellectual and ethical preeminence.

Plato's post–Book I response to (2) is that one avoids a regress problem due to the anchoring role of the Good.[52] He addresses (1) by maintaining that apart from philosophy, all endeavors are limited in scope. This is not a defect per se as long as agents (e.g., doctors) respect and remain within the bounds of their own pursuits. Oversight of each nonphilosophical domain is nonetheless required, since the Good qua unqualified order and harmony equips solely those who grasp it to ensure that non-*technai* allowed in Kallipolis actually benefit the community. Moreover, proper supervisory-subordinate relations between philosophy and all other activities eliminate value-neutrality. As regards medicine, philosophers ensure that efforts to heal and the withholding or withdrawal of care achieve what is best as contexts demand.

To put in perspective the *Republic*'s handling of the Good as compared with the *Gorgias*, let us recall Plato's claim there that our aim in everything is to promote what we view as good (468b, 499e–500a), his tying of order and harmony to goodness (503c–504a, 506e–507a), and his view that flourishing is an objective matter (470c–471a with 472c–e). One might think that benefit is assured by the fact that the *Gorgias*' *technê* framework gives a crucial role to the goodness condition. However, while the goodness criterion captures Plato's insistence that harm, whether from self-absorption or culpable ignorance, be barred from the sphere of *technai*, it does not itself explain how this exclusion is possible.[53] In the *Republic*, we learn that the good (now, the Good) is paramount by comparison even with other Forms. Further, Plato addresses its apprehension as the paramount intellectual achievement and the practical impact of that insight on *eudaimonia*, including why it is that only one grasping the Good can reliably direct the attainment of goodness in all nonphilosophical domains, including medicine.

Republic V's finger analogy (462c–d, cf. 464a), quoted above regarding the soul-body tie, vividly shows Plato's concern with unity surpassing mere aggregation. Book V contains three "waves," which are the *Republic*'s dramatic sociopolitical

---

[52] For discussion of the *Parmenides*' Third Man Argument, which would take us far afield here, see Levin (2001, chap. 4).

[53] In this and the preceding sentence, I draw from Levin (2001, 142).

innovations to foster thriving. The first two—women as by nature (*kata phusin*) potentially belonging to any of the city's three groups (453b–457a)[54] and no private property or families for guardians (457c–465e)—are entwined in a description that stresses their purpose of fostering unity (466c–d). This unity, where nothing is strictly mine as opposed to shared (462b–c), is presented as a regulative ideal: it will be sought "so far as practicable" (464d3–4). Pressing queries include: does the city to be founded embody this unity more than any other they might envision (463e)? and "in what way is [that city] possible" (466d7; cf. 471c7, e4)?

At issue sociopolitically is the "smallest change" that would produce the outcome that Plato has in view (473b). This is the third "wave," which is the uniting in rare individuals of philosophical insight and ultimate political authority (473c–d). Otherwise, "there can be no cessation of troubles for our cities or for humankind" (d5–6).[55] Plato's extensive discussion in *Republic* V–VII spans the classification of faculties and their proper objects (475d–480a); the three figures (Sun, Line, Cave) and the Good (507a–519b, 531c–534e); and an advanced curriculum culminating in dialectic (522e–534e). This account makes clear how far Plato thought that philosophers surpassed all others as "participants" (*metechontes*) in relevant Forms (i.e., as bearers of qualities like self-control and justice by entities that, unlike Forms, are native to the spatiotemporal realm).[56] Once reacclimated to this realm following protracted occupation with Forms, these few people "will know what each of the images is and what it resembles because [they have] seen the Beautiful, the Just, and the Good" (520c4–5).

Plato's likening philosophers to painters (484c–d, 501b–c) brings out that the same individuals both envision what they seek and enact what they have glimpsed. When these rare individuals have been properly educated, "would you not entrust the state exclusively to them?" (487a8). What Plato proposes is best, and difficult yet not impossible to attain (499d, 502c).

---

[54] For discussion of women's nature and role in Kallipolis, see Levin (1996). In making the case for women, Plato cites as ludicrous (454c) the idea that differences in amounts of hair, specifically baldness versus hair's abundance, reflect divergence in possessors' natures. Interestingly, there is Hippocratic evidence of a view that baldness correlates with "a wasting" (*hê analôsis*) of the brain (*Epidemics* VI 3.1) and a propensity to *mania* (II 6.14).

[55] Cf. 484b–485a, 487a–489d, 496a–497a, 499b–d, 500d–e, 501d–502b.

[56] In Plato's view, "if anything is beautiful besides the Form of Beauty (*plên auto to kalon*), the only way in which it can be beautiful is by participating in that Form" (*Phaedo* 100c4–6); this and the following translation are mine. The same applies mutatis mutandis in all other relevant cases. While the details are rather mysterious, the core idea is that whatever measure, e.g., of beauty, entities in our familiar world possess stems from their relation (dubbed participation by Plato) to the pertinent element of reality proper. Based on that ontological relation of dependence, "the other things . . . are named after" the Form (102b2–3, cf. 103b6–8); for instance, a statue is properly called "beautiful" (*kalon*) based on its participation in *auto to kalon*.

According to Plato's metaphysics, any ideal formulated for the spatiotemporal realm will necessarily be modeled on Forms and by nature only qualifiedly what the Form is without restriction; that is to say, nothing in our world can possess without limitation features like beauty and justice. Supposing one could take an ontological "snapshot" of a being unrestricted in beauty or justice, even the best entities in our world have a beginning and an end, and so do not have these qualities eternally.[57] Thus, in addition to stressing philosophers' preeminence, Plato points out that they too number among Forms' participants (500b–d).[58] This does not, however, cause him to waver in contending that the best people should have absolute political authority and that the ultimate guarantor of order and harmony is not the law but rather their character: "Can anyone show that if so born they must necessarily be corrupted?" (502a8–9).

If confronted here with the *Laws*' voluminous legal provisions (see Chapters 5 and 6), Plato would likely repeat *Republic* IV's observation that those obsessed with laws as the route to *eudaimonia* are like "the sick whose immoderation blocks them from altering their harmful regimen" (425e). In this passage's broader context (425b–e, cf. 427a), Plato notes that philosopher-rulers' discretion, not legislation, will dictate the handling of many activities, for instance, treatment of elders, commerce, and the forming of juries. Included here is much that, as Klosko (1988, 83) points out, is encompassed by the legal code of Magnesia, the *Laws*' optimal city.[59] Because the character of those in charge will lead to right practice in such domains (*Republic* 425a, d–e), the key is to ensure that those with the most promising natures receive the right upbringing and education (491d–492a, 536b).

As Vlastos (1957, 234) observes, the *Republic* rejects a common Greek view, found in Herodotus, about absolute authority and corruptibility. On Herodotus' account, the tyrant's overreaching is not due to ordinary envy, since he possesses all goods (3.80.4). Rather, if given untrammeled power, even the best man (*kai . . . ton ariston andrôn pantôn*) will be corrupted (80.3).[60] In contrast, Kallipolis' rulers have surmounted tests showing their proper mastery of pleasures, pains, and affects such as fear (503a, d–e). For Plato, these select few have actually been "struck free of the leaden weights" represented by *epithumiai* (appetites; 519a–b).[61]

---

[57] Cf. *Phaedo* 75b with 76d–e; *Symposium* 210e–211b.

[58] Cf. 490a–b, 472c1–2.

[59] Hall (2001) unjustifiably assumes that "the prescriptive standards of the forms" necessitate philosophers' subservience to established law (116), hence that philosopher-rulers' not being constrained by law is equivalent to their "rul[ing] arbitrarily" (108).

[60] Cf. Vlastos (1953, 359).

[61] The cause of the "perversion and alteration" of the philosophical nature is its residing in a sociopolitical setting antithetical to its thriving (497b), not an inherent, inevitable tendency toward intrapsychic corruption (497b–c, 485d–e).

I thus diverge from Laks' (1990, 221) reading of 571b–d (with 572b), on which "even . . . the philosophical soul [will not] be a true community."[62] At 571b6–7, Plato holds expressly that the best people can avoid disruptive appetites. *Republic* 572b might seem to retract this claim: "There exists in every one of us, even in some reputed most respectable (*hekastôi enestin, kai panu dokousin hêmôn eniois metriois einai*), a terrible, fierce, and lawless group of desires." This remark, however, connects back to 571b3–5—"Among our unnecessary pleasures and appetites, there seem to me to be some lawless ones that probably are to be found in us all"—which immediately precedes the caveat pertaining to philosophers rather than qualifying their distinctiveness. Those "reputed most respectable" in 572b4–5 are not identical with those in whom unnecessary desires have been eliminated at 571b6–7. That philosopher-rulers lack such desires is strongly suggested by 586d–587a (e.g., "When the entire soul accepts the guidance of the wisdom-loving part . . . the result for each element is that it keeps to its own task," 586e4–6).

Plato does not worry that philosophers will be beset with desires for personal gratification and self-aggrandizement once they are in charge.[63] They retain their intellectual vision and unsusceptibility to moral corruption. However, hard as it is for "a state thus constituted to be shaken and disturbed," deterioration is inevitable for it as a created thing (546a). As Vlastos (1957, 234n19) observes, rather than stemming from a defect in philosophers' insight or character, Kallipolis starts to deteriorate due to a miscalculation involving the timing of procreative activity (546a–547a). Plato's explanation of this shift is not unlike the sort of allowance that Aristotle will make for imperfect action—not due in any way to vice—even by those who are morally virtuous when discussing involuntary action in the *Nicomachean Ethics*. There Aristotle differentiates fundamentally between action due to ignorance about a specific feature of the means by which one acts (*Nicomachean Ethics* 1111a4–5), where the *telos* (goal) is right, and culpable ignorance of general truths (1110b28–33) or nonvoluntary acts stemming from a disruptor like anger (1110b25–27). While the error made by the morally virtuous person is cognitive, it pertains strictly to particular information, and that on rare occasions.

In the *Republic*, the Good is introduced with the claim that it surpasses justice and other *aretai* (504d–505a), being that "by reference to which just things and all the rest become useful and beneficial" (505a3–4).[64] For Plato, "if their relation and reference to the good itself is not known, the just and admirable will not have secured a guardian of much worth in the one thus ignorant. . . . No one will understand them

---

[62] See also Kraut (1992, 325).

[63] Cf. Bobonich (2001, 226).

[64] Cf. 508b–509b, 517b–c, 518c–d.

adequately (*hikanôs*) before he knows this" (506a4–7, cf. 505a–b). Plato frames the point most powerfully when discussing the advanced education of philosophers-to-be: "One who is unable to define in his discourse and distinguish and abstract from all other things the Form of the Good . . . knows neither it nor any particular good" (534b8–c5).[65] For this reason, no one failing to possess this knowledge can have freestanding authority in any province of activity, let alone preside over the city (534d; cf. 506a–b, 519c–d, 540a–b). This calls into question Kamtekar's (1997, 250) claim that while there is evidence in the *Republic* that philosopher-rulers can exist not merely as approximations, "this assertion is not the linchpin of [Socrates'] presentation—and indeed, it seems to be of relatively minor political significance." Instead, it is the cornerstone of the sociopolitical framework whose operations most closely approximate unqualified order and harmony.

6. MEDICINE A *TECHNÊ* NO MORE

On the *Republic*'s elaboration of the *Gorgias*' account, medicine fails to qualify as a *technê*. In the *Symposium*, though its preeminence is rejected, Eryximachus' handling of Aristophanes' hiccups fosters the impression that medicine's *technê* standing is not in doubt so long as doctors observe requisite limits on what they address. The *Gorgias*' treatment of judging and of *epithumiai* as applied to medicine already suggests, however, that since it lacks a genuine grasp of *phusis* and *eudaimonia*, medicine cannot truly be a freestanding practice. In the *Republic*, it is clear that this apprehension is needed so that care or its withholding may reliably occur to patients' benefit, particularly given soul and body's intertwining. Even if one assumes doctors' competence, medical practice is not simply a matter of their fixing on technically available means in the case at hand and applying these straightaway. Medicine's necessary lack of independence, budding already in the *Gorgias*, comes to the fore in the *Republic*'s commitment to its loss of *technê* standing.

In Kallipolis, philosophers, who alone grasp values and the Good, will impinge on medical decision making when treatment would undermine justice. On the individual plane, justice exists when each element of the soul plays its proper role (443c–444a). While this notion of psychic justice derives ultimately from the Principle of Specialization (370a–c), communal justice, which involves members of each societal group actively doing their naturally appropriate jobs (433a–d), has a direct connection thereto. For Plato in the *Republic*, if a person's capacity to execute his

[65] This is but one illustration of the *Republic*'s carrying further the *Gorgias*' efforts to redefine power as mastery that is and conveys a genuine boon.

role is seriously jeopardized, this is straightaway sufficient to render his existence objectively lacking in merit. Sometimes the just thing is not to treat even though the treatment is not medically unreasonable, as when Plato eschews care that would be needed to reach a conclusion about whether the carpenter's illness is chronic, fatal, or neither (406c–e).

Like Hippocratic doctors, Plato is concerned to weigh in on cases of what we would call debilitating, chronic illness. That he reaches a quite different conclusion, however, is evident from his account of Herodicus' existence (406a–b), such as it was given his state. Due to the "perpetual observance of his malady, which was incurable . . . by reason of his skill Herodicus won the prize of a doting old age." Plato shows here his awareness that a chronic illness whose addressing is all-encompassing or nearly so may not itself be terminal. In his view, such cases should not be treated. As Stalley (1981, 115) observes, Plato contests here the notion, illustrated by the plethora of health recommendations in Hippocratic writings, that it is acceptable "to make the care of one's health a full-time business." Plato goes further, however, for his claim that the carpenter "enters upon his customary way of life, regains his health, and lives attending to his affairs—or if his body is not equal to the strain, he dies and is freed from all his troubles" (406e) indicates a wish also to deny treatment when protracted care is needed to determine whether a serious condition is actually chronic or terminal. Since Plato's concern about health is our capacity to lead human lives as befits our natures, in such cases what medical expertise supports as practicable will, with the good in view, be ill-advised (i.e., unjust).

Plato makes clear (407b–c) that his strictures regarding serious maladies, as illustrated by the carpenter, a producer, also apply to the other two groups in Kallipolis. His thinking about auxiliaries, whose work is referenced at b6, reflects a concern with conditions and measures impeding the sustained, vigorous activity needed to protect the city courageously from such threats as may arise. Finally, the rationale behind Plato's denial of treatment for the carpenter applies when those with souls governed by reason ail insofar as illness interferes with learning and thought and prevents the effective discharge of the sedentary duties tied to rule (b7–c1).[66]

The psychically corrupt may benefit from medication, surgery, or cautery, which, given the parameters of their own specialty, doctors should provide. But if a philosopher deems irremediable the psychic injustice of a member of Kallipolis, no doctor may undertake treatment, however practicable, on that person's behalf. Instead, the

[66] That physical ailments do not invariably preclude theoretical engagement is suggested by Plato's later mention of Theages (496b6–c3), whose particular *nosotrophia* kept him from a vigorous life in politics but did not prevent his doing philosophy. Plato presents Theages' illness as functionally equivalent to Socrates' *daimonion*, which kept him from seeking political engagement in the Athens of his day.

individual will be put to death (410a). In the *Gorgias*, Plato had said that for one who is wholly corrupt, "it's better not to be alive, for he necessarily lives badly" (512b). In *Republic* III (409e–410a), verdicts in all extreme situations—letting die from physical ailments, killing when flaws are psychic—will not fall to the medical profession but instead to a judge (*dikastês*) who has a higher form of expertise. The *Gorgias* allocated soul-remediation to judging, medicine's psychic counterpart. The *Republic* builds on this by clarifying the implications for medical practice. A judge must know (i.e., be *sophos*, "wise," about) both virtue and vice (409a–e).[67] This insight renders his soul good, and "one who has a good soul is good" (c2–3). Given what is required, a person can qualify as a *dikastês* (judge) only late in life (b4–5). When this is read in light of Books V–VII, which concentrate on philosopher-rulers, it is evident that these judges are none other than they.[68]

When deliberating about whether lives should continue, one must ascertain the true condition of this human being and consider whether she can achieve or be restored to what counts as a flourishing life given the parameters of her nature. Hence Plato's insistence at 591c–d that, among bodily conditions, not even health (*oude . . . hugieian*) is worthwhile (c7) unless it conduces to *sôphrosunê* and psychic harmony more generally. How can this be ascertained if the assessor does not apprehend *phusis* and how to evaluate individuals' participation in the virtues and in the Good itself? In assessments bearing on health, then, ultimate pronouncements in the *Republic* are philosophers' as sole experts on the Good whose interventions remove doctors, qua medical decision makers, from the equation.

A doctor's judgment may be subordinated from the vantage point of philosophical insight or, less frequently, by a patient (here a carpenter, 406c–e) who, unlike the physician, happens to recognize that treatment should not occur. Though the *Gorgias* too holds that continued existence for some may be at odds with justice, this claim does not itself commit Plato to a specific way for injustice to be detected. The *Republic* opts to impinge on doctors' decision making as doctors, leaving them unable to do as a matter of course what is practicable (*ta dunata*, 360e7–361a1) to promote the good qua health. As a result of this impingement, medicine is no longer a free-standing praxis; that is to say, medicine loses its *technê* status.

In the *Republic*, then, treatment recommendations are context dependent—albeit not as Hippocratic doctors think—as they hinge on sophisticated judgments about how far a given ailment incapacitates the patient for the sociopolitical role made available by her nature. Those who are psychically corrupt are denied medical

---

[67] For Plato as differentiating physicians from judges here due to their possessing experience and knowledge respectively, see Stalley (1981, 115).

[68] On this topic see also Anagnostopoulos (2000, 277).

treatment altogether. The foregoing judgments ground determinations of whether measures that are technically *dunata* (possible) also promote individual and communal well-being, this being the only acceptable ground of decisions to treat (410a5–6).

The same *technê* criteria that elevate philosophy to preeminence in the *Republic* demote medicine from the ranks of *technai* altogether. My claim here is not that Plato expressly retracts its *technê* standing. Rather, the withdrawal of this rank from medicine follows from the *Republic*'s handling of medicine combined with its overall argument, in particular its notion of the soul and soul-body tie, the Principle of Specialization, the dialogue's position on the Good, and its commitment to philosophers' intellectual and ethical infallibility.

Medicine's loss of *technê* standing in Plato's eyes, which may surprise us, broadly aligns the *Republic* with those against whose charge of failing to qualify as such Hippocratic writings sometimes defended medicine. When one combines the *Republic*'s critique of it with the dialogue's defense of philosophy's preeminence, medicine is the most visible loser of *technê* standing there. That said, the *Republic*'s elaboration of the *Gorgias*' *technê* conditions commits Plato to withdraw the rank of *technê* from all endeavors save philosophy. Again, my point is not that Plato explicitly makes such a claim but rather that the *Republic*'s elevation of philosophy commits him to it.

While talk of "the good" will most likely call morality to mind, Plato's notion is wider. He weds the good to order and harmony (*Republic* 508d–509a)[69]—a linkage that was already evident in the *Gorgias* (493c7–d2, 506e–507c). This means that goodness is broadly operative, including the subject matter and aims of arithmetic, geometry, astronomy, and musical harmony, all of which appear in the advanced educational curriculum of *Republic* VII. Astronomy, for instance, studies the ordered movement of celestial bodies. This fosters the inner harmony of those whose natures include an aptitude for the level of abstraction—though less than complete (510b–511d)—that is involved in its pursuit.

For Sprague (1976, 92), the "first-order" *technai* "are introduced as steppingstones to the good and the good *then* descends to make them truly useful" (italics in original). According to Kahn (1996, 209), "the Good itself . . . must be the object . . . for the art of the philosopher-kings. And such knowledge will be useful precisely because, in the hands of the rulers, it will guide the right use of the workings and products" of the remaining *technai*. Such statements rightly emphasize a strict hierarchy, but a further step is needed. On the *Gorgias*' presentation of the *technê* theory, experts reliably and free-standingly provide the benefits native to their ordered, knowable domains. In the *Republic*, however, one who does not know the

[69] On these features as signs of goodness, see also Kraut (1992, 323).

Good knows no good whatsoever (534c4–5). This means that practitioners of other endeavors cannot reliably satisfy the goodness condition absent philosophers' aid. To that extent, their endeavors cannot themselves count as *technai*.

7. THE *REPUBLIC*'S HIERARCHY OF HUMAN ENDEAVORS AND MEDICINE'S DISTINCTIVENESS

Kallipolis' thriving hinges on philosophy, the sole *technê*. All other pursuits are not, however, equal in merit. Activities that the *Gorgias* dubbed *empeiriai* (knacks), including rhetoric/sophistry, cookery, and poetry, continue to be excluded from *technê* standing in the *Republic*. There remains a swath of endeavors, some of which the *Gorgias* saw as *technai*, and all of which Kallipolis allows for their ability to contribute something, however limited, to *eudaimonia*. These activities include the work of auxiliaries and producers (e.g., carpenters, farmers, and doctors). Located too in this broad group are mathematics, astronomy, and musical theory.[70]

On a widespread view, which Plato contests, not the reality but only the semblance of virtue is worthwhile, and that on external grounds for its benefits to reputation (358a). To show its radical insufficiency, Plato is not content merely to substitute his own model without arguing at length for his stances on *phusis* and *eudaimonia*. Further, showing them correct necessitates his continued dispute with rival approaches. Thus, he pinpoints how they fall short by the very *technê* criteria whose satisfaction warrants philosophy's preeminence.

So far as it belongs among non-*technai* with something to offer Kallipolis, medicine is one of many endeavors. But it is more than this. Medicine is distinctive because the *Republic* continues the *Symposium*'s handling of it as a rival of philosophy's for primacy on the crucial topics of *phusis* and *eudaimonia*. As we saw in Chapter 3, the *Symposium* denied medicine's preeminence. This chapter has argued that *Republic* III advances Plato's critique by specifying further where medicine falls short and by arguing that only philosophy can assume important duties that medicine is fundamentally unable to address.

It is unsurprising that in Kallipolis, philosophy presides over all practices directly orbiting the soul, including poetry. But it is striking that it curtails and inserts itself in decision making in medicine, which is the only important Platonic rival whose defining sphere is the body. As we have seen, Plato's central motivation was his conviction that medicine's focus on the body was a dangerous oversimplification

---

70 For comparative purposes, one may wish to revisit Chapter 1, Section 8, on the *Gorgias*' final hierarchy of human pursuits. While I recognize that the claim about mathematics in particular will be controversial, addressing the issue further falls outside my purview here.

of what doctors' activity crucially affects. For its claims to primacy on nature and thriving, Plato took medicine to be an important rival. Suitably revamped medical practice, like the poetry allowed in Kallipolis,[71] will no longer be a threat. Indeed, once Plato has severed regimen and serious illness from medicine's sphere and invested philosophy with oversight over medical decision making, medicine is highly diminished compared with its Hippocratic self.

As noted in Chapter 2 regarding the *Gorgias* (511d–512d), medical practice, unlike piloting, is governed by the specialty's own views of *phusis* and *eudaimonia*, matters lying at the core of human existence. One therefore expects that doctors would resist a marked curtailing of their purview. Because medicine, which regularly impacts body and soul, is governed by false views of human and macrocosmic reality, it is urgent that its limitations be disclosed and that it be relocated accordingly in the hierarchy of human endeavors. In the *Republic*, Plato completes this task through a further critique of medicine that is integrally tied to the dialogue's defense of philosophy's preeminence.

8. A BRIEF LOOK AHEAD

Through the *Republic*'s critique of medicine, Plato builds on the *Symposium*'s denial of its claim to preeminence. His conduct of the *agôn* with medicine and defense of philosophy's standing commit him by implication to retract medicine's *technê* standing. Chapters 5 and 6 address the *Laws*, where medicine is not a subject of critique and Plato's rivalry with it appears to have dissolved. In the *Laws*, medicine operates in a sphere unto itself in the sense that a good physician may implement straightaway what he deems medically practicable. Burkholder's (1978, 32n12) contention that "the physician himself must decide whether a patient would benefit from treatment" thus applies only to the later dialogue. In the *Laws*, unlike the *Republic*, Plato resolves the *Gorgias*' lurking tension in medicine's favor by showing it to be a self-standing *technê* in Magnesia, that dialogue's favored city.

The *Laws* makes key adjustments to Plato's view of optimal governance that stem from his recognition that human understanding and character are—by nature—fallible. Due to this recognition, Magnesia, the *Laws*' ideal city, contains no philosopher-rulers or close counterparts thereto. Far from expressing great pessimism about human nature across the board, Plato's deep acknowledgment that even the best among us are fallible promotes his greater appreciation of the intellectual and ethical capabilities of ordinary folk. By key measures, Magnesia's metics

[71] As argued elsewhere (Levin 2001, 149–50), poetic composition, optimally pursued, rises in Kallipolis to a plane comparable in value to the work of auxiliaries.

(resident aliens) come off better than Kallipolis' producers, which enhancements necessarily apply to physicians as members of that class. Further and more specifically, Plato's appreciation of good medical practice in the *Laws* is substantially greater than in the *Republic*. Magnesia's legislative and judicial infrastructure for fostering justice, along with Plato's enhanced confidence in doctors, means that no one disrupts doctors' implementation of the medically feasible on those grounds. The *Laws*' positions on human nature, governance, and medicine do not, however, first surface there fully formed but are instead crucially anticipated in the *Statesman*. Hence, before turning to the *Laws*, Chapter 5 addresses those salient developments.

5

Approaching the *Laws* by Way of the *Statesman*

I. INTRODUCTION

In recent times, scholars have strongly challenged the view that Plato moves from optimism about the best sociopolitical condition in the *Republic* to great pessimism in the *Laws* about our nature and prospects for thriving. This disjunction is indeed too simplistic, and recent scholarly emphasis on the regulative nature of the *Republic*'s ideal of unity is salutary. That said, I diverge from prominent accounts of how to interpret the ideal thus construed and the implications of its regulative status for the *Republic*'s tie to the *Laws* concerning human governance. I will argue that while unity through *aretê* (virtue) remains the guiding telos of Magnesia, the *Laws*' optimal city, the route through which it is sought diverges substantially from Kallipolis'. It therefore stretches the notion beyond reasonable limits to call the *Laws*' unity an approximation of the *Republic*'s, as has been claimed, and its infrastructure for communal maintenance—above all the nocturnal council, which comprises Magnesia's finest—the approximation of philosopher-rulers for which the earlier dialogue calls. Instead, the *Laws* relinquishes the idea that anyone, even the best, is infallible. Far from expressing great pessimism about human nature as such, this recognition fosters Plato's appreciation both of the intellectual and ethical capabilities of ordinary folk and of nonphilosophical professionals' contributions to communal thriving.

Constitutional and legislative measures for Magnesia establish many checks and balances to foster justice, with no single individual or official body the arbiter in every situation. As we saw in Chapter 4, the *Republic*'s supervisory framework is rigidly top-down, with philosophers ultimately dictating what happens in all spheres, including medicine. In Magnesia, the evaluative function always vested with Kallipolis' philosopher-rulers alone is often performed by citizen jurors who assess perpetrators' psychic standing. As it supplants Kallipolis with Magnesia, the *Laws* cashes out the *Gorgias*' claim (see Chapter 1) that *politikê* comprises legislation and judging, which have distinct, complementary roles. While legislation went unexplained in the *Gorgias* and was relatively trivial in Kallipolis, both it and judging are extensively developed and pivotal to Magnesia's constitution and operations.[1]

While his opposition to poetry and sophistry/rhetoric abides in the *Laws*, Plato no longer views medicine as a rival concerning *phusis* and *eudaimonia*. On my account, the *Laws*' developments with a bearing on medicine stem ultimately from his recognition that no one is incorruptible. By key measures, central among them the domain of virtue, metics (resident aliens) come off better in Magnesia than producers, their counterparts in Kallipolis. These enhancements necessarily apply to good physicians as members of the metic class. Further, the *Laws* singles out medicine for recognition.

Magnesia's web of oversight roles, which crisscross the legislative and judicial spheres, leaves Plato confident that psychic incurability will be brought to light outside the medical arena; hence, no one disrupts doctors' implementing the medically feasible on grounds of justice. The aforementioned shifts bearing on medicine stem ultimately from the *Laws*' position that since no one's incorruptibility is assured, no pursuit can operate as a *technê* à la *philosophia* in Kallipolis. The richer appreciation of good medical practice that ensues, combined with an array of sociopolitical mechanisms for detecting injustice, means that the health-care setting in Magnesia is not—as in Kallipolis—a crossroads where judgments of the whole person must be made. For the first time by Plato's lights, medicine may be a truly self-standing endeavor.

The *Laws*' positions on human nature and fallibility on the one side, and medicine on the other, do not first surface there fully formed. Instead, they are crucially anticipated in the *Statesman*. While it, like the other dialogues featured in this study, warrants a doctrinal interpretation, the *Statesman* has a semi-exploratory cast in keeping with its status as transitional and at least in part a testament of ambivalence.[2] Thus, the dialogue struggles with the question of

[1] The city's own legal code ingeniously fuses prevention via legislative preludes with punishment as detailed in the text of the laws themselves.

[2] For the *Statesman* as "hesitating as it were between" the *Republic*'s and *Laws*' models of governance, see Kahn (1995, 51). According to Annas and Waterfield (1995, xvi), Plato was of two minds there, finding it difficult to relinquish the *Republic*'s notion of expert governance even as he becomes more aware of its inadequacies. While I concur that the *Statesman* evinces ambivalence, I must diverge from their further claim that it exhibits "confusion" on Plato's part (xxii).

whether Kallipolian autocracy or a law-based approach—the latter foundational to Magnesia—is the best path to genuine unity, hence *eudaimonia*. Gravitation toward governance by law necessitates Plato's greater trust in ordinary people, which the *Statesman* reflects both in its more inclusive view of what occupations directly promote thriving and in its higher estimation of ordinary folk's human aptitudes. At the same time, the dialogue suggests that Plato has yet to decide precisely how to broaden horizons regarding both the expert-lay connection and the interweaving of expertises while keeping the involved parties sufficiently distinct from one another.

Annas and Waterfield (1995, x) rightly observe that the *Statesman*'s role in Plato's political thought has often been undersold.[3] Fortunately, over the last couple of decades, the dialogue's import has received greater scholarly attention. On my account in Sections 2–4 of the present chapter, the *Statesman* plays a key transitional role between the *Republic* and *Laws* regarding Plato's constructions of human capacity and expertise, gesturing forward to Magnesia more than backward to Kallipolis as is often claimed.[4] Centrally, the *Statesman* shows at once Plato's diminished confidence in those who are best and growing appreciation of ordinary folk.[5] Against this backdrop, Sections 5–7 address the *Laws*' handling of *phusis* and fallibility. The implications of these developments for medicine, including the broader sociopolitical context in which it functions in Magnesia, are the focus of Chapter 6.

2. HUMAN CAPACITY IN THE *STATESMAN* AND *REPUBLIC* COMPARED

In the *Republic*, philosophy is effectively the encompassing science of the divine (i.e., Forms, called divine at *Phaedo* 80b), by whose imitation philosophers' existence assumes an order most admirable. Though by no means erasing the boundary, presentation of the tie between philosophers' superlative character and intellect, on the one side, and the nature of their *technê*'s objects, on the other, downplays

[3] For stress on its importance, see also Cole (1991, 195).

[4] See also Samaras (1996), for whom the *Statesman*'s import lies not in its attachment to the *Republic*'s ideal, which Plato "was already in the course of abandoning, but rather in the ways it anticipates [his] final political statement in the *Laws*" (113). For Neiman (2007, 415), in contrast, Plato "move[s] away from the idea of a constitution with changeable laws because . . . given the limitations of non-philosophical citizens no one with genuine knowledge of statesmanship can be distinguished from sophists who only appear to be statesmen." Skemp (2002, 51) claims that while Plato of the *Laws* "no longer stands by the contention . . . that a philosophical ruler can rule without laws," in the *Statesman* "there is still hope—hardly less so than in the *Republic*." Cf. Vlastos (1957, 237), who has "reasonable confidence that Plato's early faith in enlightened absolutism was still intact" at the time of the *Statesman*.

[5] Often only one prong is recognized (e.g., Neiman 2007, 414–15).

at times the distance between them. The philosopher-Forms connection debuts in the *Phaedo* (72e–77a, 78b–80b, 100b–e) and is extended in the *Symposium*'s ascent (210a–212a), whose linkage of those who ascend with the divine (212a6–7) is therefore not a rhetorical flourish. Philosophers' tie to Forms reaches its apex in the *Republic*'s sociopolitical application of that idea. Thus, for instance, "the philosopher, by consorting with what is ordered and divine [namely, Forms] . . . himself becomes as divine and ordered as possible for a human being" (*theiôi dê kai kosmiôi ho ge philosophos homilôn kosmios te kai theios eis to dunaton anthrôpôi gignetai*, 500d1–2).[6]

Tellingly, the *Republic*'s handling of inferior constitutions in Book VIII applies considerations involving participants' intrinsically inferior standing to Kallipolis without attributing its shift away from glory to intellectual or ethical imperfections of those in charge. In Chapter 4, I concurred with Vlastos (1957, 234n19) that the error leading to Kallipolis' deterioration (546a–547a) is a miscalculation of the timing of procreative activity. Plato's distinction between qualities (e.g., eternality) that unite Forms and Forms' own individuation via each one's being *F* (e.g., just) unqualifiedly[7] offers a helpful perspective on an existing tension involving philosophers in the *Republic*. Philosophers' justice, for instance, looks incalculably more like that of the Form (*auto to dikaion*, the just itself) than like that of the city's misfits—as indeed it must for Kallipolis, the dialogue's ideal city, to be a live option. The same likeness and dissimilarity operate, mutatis mutandis, with self-control, courage, and so on. That from a position centered on individual Forms philosophers come off extremely well is reflected in Glaucon's comment (540c3–4) that "like a sculptor, Socrates, you've produced ruling men [and women, a6–7] who are completely fine (*pankalous . . . tous archontas*)" (540c).[8] Yet no amassing of one-to-one affinities between philosophers and specific Forms can alter the fact that when Forms as a group—whose members are necessarily incomposite, eternal, and unalterable—are set against their composite, spatiotemporal participants, philosophers belong among the latter.[9] Although

---

[6] See also 500b–e generally, along with 490a–b, 501b–d, 521c, 534b–c.

[7] Cf. Moravcsik's (1992, 69–74) threefold distinction, on which eternality falls in category one.

[8] See also 500b–c, 520c, 537b–d. On those ruled by Kallipolis' philosophers as "slaves," see Annas and Waterfield (1995, xiv); for stress on the "metaphorical" standing of the *Republic*'s (590c–d) labeling of producers as slaves, see Bobonich (1995, 327n39).

[9] This divergence helpfully contextualizes Plato's well-studied claim at *Republic* 519c–d that philosophers will be compelled to rule if a preference for uninterrupted communion with Forms makes them reluctant to leave off doing this, even temporarily. While I concur that the conflict involving philosophers' rule and their *eudaimonia* should not be minimized, Brown's (2000, 9–11) and Phillips' (2011, 117n26, 119–20) dissolutions of the tension rely excessively on law and the *Crito*'s notion of obedience thereto. On dual metaphysical perspectives, cf. Vlastos (1957, 232) regarding the *Timaeus*: "Plato's cosmological pattern is systematically ambiguous. One can look at this world thinking 'It is *only* a copy' and feeling a kind of malaise or nostalgia . . . or, with equally good warrant from the metaphysical design, one can say to oneself, 'But it is an excellent copy, such as only supreme intelligence joined with perfect goodness could produce'" (italics in original).

this tension exists in the *Republic*, Plato's arguments there regarding *phusis* and *eudaimonia* for individuals and the community fundamentally rely on a strong affinity between a select few and Forms, the unqualified divine.

From this vantage point, it is notable that the *Statesman* sets humans' mutual proximity against the divine.[10] Opposing our Age of Zeus under human control to the earlier Age of Cronus, Plato says that "the divine shepherd [of that era] is so exalted a figure that no king can be said to attain his eminence. Those who rule our states in the present era are much more like their subjects in nature, and far closer to them in training and nurture than ever a shepherd could be to his flock (*tous d' enthade nun ontas politikous tois archomenois homoious te einai mallon polu tas phuseis kai paraplêsiaiteron paideias meteilêphenai kai trophês*)" (275b–c).[11] Divine rule over humans as in the previous age comprises a grid in which ruler and ruled differ so far in their cognitive and ethical natures as to effectively occupy distinct planes. This paradigm is opposed to governance premised on all being *essentially* peers, which obtains in the Age of Zeus.[12] Readers of the *Republic* would expect divine governance—in political terms, rule of the categorically superior—to be categorically preferred. The *Statesman*, however, stakes right judgment of which era better fosters *eudaimonia* on how human beings passed their time (272b), in particular on whether and how far all were searched to see what any capable of thought might "contribute to swell the common treasure store of wisdom (*eis sunagurmon phronêseôs*)" (272c). Such remarks tell against the claim of Sprague (1976, 102; cf. 117) that "Plato by no means intends to give up the characteristics of the divine shepherd in defining the statesman."[13]

Strengthening this impression of budding movement away from an embrace of radically divergent intellectual and ethical aptitudes splitting ruler off from ruled is Plato's insistence shortly thereafter that, when investigating human governance, one must properly differentiate between voluntary and compelled "care" (*epimeleia*).

---

[10] See also Annas and Waterfield (1995, x), according to whom Plato is "moving towards a more egalitarian view of the relation of ruler to ruled" (cf. 30n31); Bobonich (1995, 325); Schofield (2003, 10).

[11] While Socrates is usually the central character in Plato's dialogues, in the *Statesman* that role is played by the Eleatic Visitor, who is the speaker here at 275b–c. Translations of the *Statesman* are from Skemp (1992), with adjustments.

[12] Cf. Owen (1953, 92), for whom the *Statesman* "can be read as arguing that the very appropriateness of the *Republic*'s institutions to a Golden Age should have removed them" from consideration for politically engaged human beings.

[13] Mishima (1995, 312) favors the Age of Zeus on pessimistic grounds, claiming that bleak political circumstances led Plato to conclude that, regrettably, the best possible community must be built around less unevenness among citizens. See also Neiman (2007), for whom the Age of Zeus represents a clearly inferior scenario vis-à-vis *eudaimonia*: unfortunately, we must settle for its model of rule "due to the limitations of human beings" (407).

The *Statesman*'s early neglect of this distinction, we now learn, led to a foolish, inaccurate conflation of the king with the tyrant (276e). Blurred boundaries, if not this same conflation, obtained in the *Republic*,[14] where philosophers' extraordinary standing warranted conduct verging on tyranny, that is, compulsion from without, with authority stemming not at all from law qua established norms. Although Plato prefers there, all things equal, that people's assent to philosophers' prescriptions be internally spurred, he is not confident that such will occur and is therefore quick to indicate that those in charge should do whatever is needed for order's sake. In the *Republic*, Plato does not distinguish—more precisely, does not see the need to differentiate—willing from compelled "care." Envisioning the possibility (415d–e) that producers may revolt against the polity of which at least technically they are citizens,[15] Plato sets no limits on allowable means by which communal harmony is preserved or restored. Against this backdrop, Plato's distinction at *Statesman* 276d–e between the king and the tyrant in the dialogue's quest to articulate the unique nature of statesmanship is notable, signaling his awareness of a need to revise the *Republic*'s approach to governance.[16]

Plato thought that Kallipolis achieved unity as fully as possible (*Republic* 464d3–4) despite the fact that it sought harmony by dissolving the nuclear family and private property for rulers and auxiliaries alone (416c–417b, 464a). Strengthening its earlier uniting of *phusis* in ruler and ruled (275b–c), the *Statesman* reveals Plato's concern to weave all (apart from those whose ignorance and vice are unremitting) into a unity maximally distant from plain aggregation (308e–309b).[17] The epistemological correlate of this scenario is that *orthê doxa* (true belief), properly instilled via *paideia* (education), is depicted (309c–d) in unprecedentedly positive terms:

[14] Cf. Neiman (2007, 412). McCabe's "benevolent despotism" (1997, 116) risks downplaying the possibility of unchecked compulsion, indeed violence, as needed to maintain order in Kallipolis.

[15] On this possibility cf. Laks (1990, 220).

[16] I thus diverge from Bobonich (1995, 321–22), who discerns marked movement away from compulsion only in the *Statesman*'s final section. See Schofield (1997) for Plato's depiction of the *Laws*' young tyrant (710d–711c) as signaling his acknowledgment that "if the ruler of the *Rep.* is to have a good chance of introducing radical change into society, he will ideally be an *absolute* despot" (235; italics in original); at this juncture, Plato sees clearly "the dangers of absolute despotism" (ibid.), hence the seasoned, self-controlled figure of Nestor is preferred (237–38).

[17] The deepening of Plato's engagement with the topic of what makes for genuine unity is evident in his late philosophy of language, which depicts the final *logos* in the *Sophist* as an interweaving of *onomata* (268c5–6, 259e4–6). Plato's repeated use of an alphabet analogy (*Theaetetus* 202e–206a; *Sophist* 253a; *Statesman* 277e–278e; *Philebus* 17a–b, 18b–d) provides further evidence of his conviction that the most revealing *logoi* are always more than mereological sums. On pertinent *logoi* as transcending their aggregated parts, see also Moravcsik (1973a, 165).

> I call divine, when it comes to be in souls, that opinion about what is fine, just, and good, and their opposites, that is really true and is guaranteed; it belongs to the class of the more than human (*Tên tôn kalôn kai dikaiôn peri kai agathôn kai tôn toutois enantiôn ontôs ousan alêthê doxan meta bebaiôseôs, hopotan en tais psuchais engignêtai, theian phêmi en daimoniôi gignesthai genei*).... It belongs to the statesman and the good legislator alone to be capable of bringing this very thing about ... in those who have had their correct share of education—the people we were speaking of just now (*touto auto empoiein tois orthôs metalabousi paideias, hous elegomen nundê*).[18]

In Kallipolis too, without *paideia*, *eudaimonia* is precluded and disaster all but assured. Key guardian-centered observations in the *Republic* (456d, cf. 466e–467a) are, however, tantamount to an admission that producers receive only vocational training. For Plato this is not, strictly speaking, *paideia* at all. It is the relatively select group of auxiliaries whose early *paideia* brings them to *orthê doxa*, of a stable kind, regarding courage (429b–c), and presumably other values by extension. Due to this broadening of access to *paideia* at *Statesman* 309c–d and its positive disposal toward the resulting *orthê doxa*, Samaras (1996, 112) thus rightly observes that the passage "brings the [*Statesman*] much closer to the *Laws* than to the *Republic*."[19]

At the *Statesman*'s close, Plato stresses that the unity at issue "enfolds all who dwell in the city, slave or free, in its firm contexture.... This polity lacks nothing that makes for happiness so far as happiness is obtainable in a state" (311c). While "free-slave" and "citizen-noncitizen" are not equivalent, as "noncitizen" covers both alien and slave, this notion of weaving all into the rich unity that is the city meshes broadly with the dialogue's earlier claim (262c10–263a1) that the familiar bifurcation of human beings into Greeks and barbarians is unnatural. The *Statesman* thus anticipates the *Laws*' elaborate provision not only for citizens' mutual relations but also for ties involving citizens, metics (resident aliens), and slaves.

The *Statesman*'s stance on governance and ability is, however, unresolved. Ambivalence is evident when one juxtaposes the material treated above against the dialogue's suggestion—though without obvious resort to the *Republic*'s metaphysical machinery[20]—of Plato's indulging expertise deployed in service of the good (e.g., 296c–297b). Additionally, the statesman's essential co-belonging to the "fabric" that is the city is veiled, if not belied, by his role as the "weaver" (309a–b, 310e–311a) of

---

[18] The translation of 309c–d is from Rowe (1997), slightly adjusted.

[19] Cf. Annas and Waterfield (1995, xx–xxi).

[20] Annas and Waterfield (1995, ix) make the stronger claim that here the metaphysical foundation "has dropped away."

its unity. Plato is clearly struggling with the question of whether it matters only that boons be conveyed or also how—in particular, whether it is salient that beneficiaries embrace measures willingly on account of seeing how they enhance the commonweal.[21] That said, the manifold presence of new thoughts regarding *technai* and human capacity in the *Statesman* suggests that it points ahead to Magnesia as much as—or, as I would claim, even more than—it clings to Kallipolis.

3. THE *STATESMAN* ON HUMAN ENDEAVORS

Together with evincing a shift in Plato's view of human nature, through its handling of (1) expert activities' mutual reliance and (2) the tie between expert and lay, the *Statesman* suggests a richer, more appreciative view than the *Republic* of what expertise involves. I address the former setting here and the latter in Section 4.

In its quest for a superlative response to the question, what is the nature of statesmanship? (*politikê*, 259c3),[22] the *Statesman* shows Plato's newfound attunement to dependency relations among the manifold pursuits that are needed for a city to thrive. Thus he accentuates, for example, a broad distinction between theoretical (*gnôstikê*) and applied (*praktikê*) forms of expertise (258e, cf. 259c–d). The former activities are classified as either (a) abstract pursuits like calculation (*logistikê*) or (b) occupations such as master building, depending on whether experts' grasp translates directly into praxis or instead guides others' work (259e–260b).[23] Within (b), statesmanship, which like master building functions directively, is marked off from endeavors like prophecy and heraldry that pass along commands from higher authorities (260c–261a).[24] And Plato is just getting started!

My focus here is the dialogue's later demarcation of statesmanship from "contributory" *technai* on the one side and from auxiliary expertises on the other. The term rendered "contributory" here is *sunaitioi* (289c9), which literally means "causing or responsible [for something] along with [something else]." Concerning this type of activity, the *Statesman* sets a path toward the *Laws*, which features the interdependence of manifold forms of direct and indirect collaboration. Notoriously,

---

[21] Regarding the latter, see 285e–286a (cf. 286e–287a).

[22] Significantly, at 259d "statesmanship" is used interchangeably with "kingship" (*basilikê*). As Cooper (1999a) observes, in this dialogue "the king is assimilated to the statesman, not the other way about" (190); he notes, further, how antithetical this collapsed distinction would have been to Plato's contemporary readers (168–69).

[23] Specifically, calculation fits under *kritikê*, while statesmanship and master building fall under *epitaktikê* (260a–c). Plato's precise reference is to the master builder (*architektôn*, 259e9), not the practice itself.

[24] See Kamtekar (1997, 246) on epitactic apprehension as for all intents and purposes already present in the *Republic*.

the *Republic*'s references to producers are meager despite their vast contributions to Kallipolis' infrastructure, through which they support communal thriving. Producers' virtual invisibility in the *Republic* itself reflects their marked devaluing.[25] Moreover, what little is said about producers is ambivalent.[26] Against that backdrop, the *Statesman* evinces Plato's striking insight into just how many types of activities are truly needed for communal thriving: "Any form of expertise that fashions any object, large or small, that ministers to the needs of a state must be classed as contributory, for without the things provided by these activities, there would be no state and hence no art of statesmanship" (*Hosai gar smikron ê mega ti dêmiourgousi kata polin organon, theteon hapasas tautas hôs ousas sunaitious. Aneu gar toutôn ouk an pote genoito polis oude politikê, toutôn d' au basilikês ergon technês ouden pou thêsomen*, 287d).

The dialogue's paramount concern is to differentiate statesmanship from these other pursuits. What one finds in 287d–289b, however, is not simply a longer list of contributory occupations than in the *Republic* but a deeper apprehension of their nature and offerings. *Statesman* 287d–289b includes a sevenfold classification of these *technai* and their interrelations. For instance, Plato demarcates storage vessels from instruments, since the former are "not made . . . with a view to the production of something but to preserve a thing once it has been produced" (287e). Elsewhere in the passage, crafts preparing materials on which others' contributions depend (e.g., that devoted to readying the wood on which carpenters rely) are cordoned off from activities like farming and hunting that directly foster bodily welfare (288d–289a). Insofar as they pitch in to serve the commonweal—as all worthwhile endeavors must, Plato insists from the *Gorgias* on—activities have genuine, distinctive merit.[27]

One might wonder how this discussion of *technai* in the *Statesman* fits with my claim that the *Republic* commits Plato to the view that philosophy alone is a *technê*. My contention, one may recall, was not that he asserts this in the *Republic* but rather that its deployment of the *Gorgias*' core *technê* conditions—subject matter, understanding, and goodness—necessitates that outcome. Not only does the *Republic* not directly embrace this stance, but it indicates Plato's belief that there exist at least some nonphilosophical *technai*, including the fields that comprise the advanced *paideia* of Book VII (e.g., geometry and astronomy). Hence, on my account, the *Republic*'s handling of the *technê* requirements has an important result that, as far as one can tell, Plato does not see.

---

[25] On this point see also Skemp (2002, 43).

[26] Positive (431c9–d2; cf. 465b, 499d–500a); derogatory (415d–e, 425c–d, 589d–590d).

[27] Cf. Skemp (2002, 43–44).

One should note that in addition to showing change in his views of human nature and activities, the *Statesman* reflects a shift in Plato's conception of philosophical method (i.e., dialectic). In several late dialogues, including the *Statesman*, the Method of Division (*diairesis*), combined with other tools, becomes important. Briefly, in dialectic thus construed one moves from a single encompassing genus (in the *Statesman* and *Sophist*, *technê*) through intermediate planes until one has accumulated as many increasingly specific points as exist where that praxis overlaps with and diverges from other endeavors.[28]

While the *Statesman* concentrates on statesmanship, the *Sophist* aims to pinpoint the nature of its slippery eponymous figure. In these dialogues, the goal of dialectic is the most revealing specification, in a *logos*, of the natures of statesmanship and sophistry, respectively. One should not conclude from this that sophistry (and thus rhetoric) suddenly qualifies as a *technê* for late Plato by the *Gorgias*' own standards, as nothing could be further from the truth. Instead, where *diairesis* is prominent, Plato retains the criteria for discerning activities' legitimacy that were front and center in that dialogue without also framing the matter via its *technê-empeiria* divide. In the *Statesman*, Plato distinguishes crucially between endeavors that are and those that are not "contributory" to *eudaimonia* (287d).[29] As before, familiar rhetoric/sophistry fails that test (*Sophist* 264d–268d), while statesmanship and other truly beneficial pursuits make the grade (*Statesman* 287d–289b). Though not front and center here, the *Gorgias*' *technê-empeiria* divide does not disappear. As I show in Chapter 6, the *Laws*' critiques of sophistry/rhetoric and poetry involve that contrast.

The *Statesman*'s greater perceptiveness about what kinds of infrastructure contributions exist and how they foster thriving contrasts with the *Republic*'s largely undifferentiated referencing of producers' infrastructure work.[30] The earlier dialogue's comment that at most minimal harm could result if producers switched functions within that class of work strongly implies that the expertise required for such duties is so undistinguished that shifts could readily enough be undertaken (434a–b). The

---

[28] *Diairesis* debuts in the *Phaedrus* (265d–266c, 277b), which postdates the *Republic* and antedates the *Sophist* and *Statesman*. "Collection," division's counterpart, involves the dialectician's synthesizing the terms (*onomata*) yielded by stepwise definition in a *logos*. Accounts of natures (*phuseis*) are identified as the goal of *diairesis* in the cases of sophistry (*Sophist* 264d–265a) and statesmanship (*Statesman* 275c). Investigation of *diairesis* itself would take us far afield here. For discussion see Levin (2008); Sayre (2006); Notomi (1999); Skemp (2002); Moravcsik (1973a; 1973b); Cornford (1957).

[29] See especially *theteon hapasas tautas hôs ousas sunaitious* (d2–3).

[30] A hint at difference is found at *Republic* 428b–c (cf. 420e–421a), and Kallipolis' third class is sometimes referenced by occupational names standing in for the whole, e.g., farmers (412c, cf. 415a) or potters (421d). This group is also singled out as the money-making class (434c, cf. 434a). While these references are notable, they fall well short of the *Statesman*'s rich differentiation of pertinent activities.

Statesman's account, which treats infrastructure contributions as genuine expertises differing appreciably in nature and function, implies a tempering, if not a retraction, of such fluidity.

Having delineated contributory *technai*, Plato turns to "the precious elements that are [most closely] akin" to statesmanship (*ta timia kai sungenê*, 303e). Auxiliaries (*epikouroi*), who had military and police functions, were the only ones identified thus for Kallipolis.[31] In contrast, the *Statesman* designates four activities—political oratory, generalship, judging, and education—as aids to *politikê* (303e–304a, 304c–305c, 308d–e).[32]

Traditional oratory was disavowed in the *Gorgias* as antithetical to thriving. Building on that dialogue's cryptic identification of true rhetoric with statesmanship, the *Phaedrus* both continues Plato's critique of existing oratory and develops the genuine kind—premised on a real grasp of *psuchê*—as a tool deployed by philosophers (270e1–271c1, 276e–277c).[33] In the *Statesman*, however, suitably revamped political oratory has expert practitioners of its own. Moreover, it "is closely allied with the kingly art because it persuades people to do what is right and hence shares in controlling what goes on in the state" (*hosê basilikêi koinônousa rhêtoreia, peithousa to dikaion, sundiakubernai tas en tais polesi praxeis*, 303e–304a).

The ancillary practices of generalship (304e–305a) and judging (305b–c) too are the province of distinct groups of practitioners. Kallipolis' philosopher-rulers emerged from the original guardian group—formed so that the budding state would have protectors—that the *Republic* later divided into rulers and auxiliaries. While police and military functions do not constitute philosopher-rulers' own naturally befitting work, their background in that area allows them to impact not just the telos but also the specifics (e.g., strategies and procedures) of auxiliaries' job performance. As Cooper (1999a, 181n25) observes, philosopher-rulers "possess all the expertises of their assistants—indeed only they possess these in the highest degree and the most perfect form. They do not practice them . . . but they are fully capable of doing so." The *Statesman*, in contrast, proposes that the city's leader defer to a separate group of military specialists on how best to wage war.

---

31 There are presumably distinct groups of experts in the fields designated in Book VII's advanced curriculum. While supporting philosophers' work, they are not philosophers' aids in the *Statesman*'s sense. When one combines Book VII's account with the Divided Line (6.510b–511d) and philosophers' exclusive grasp of the Good, it is clear that those experts could not teach without the ever-present specter of philosophers' intervention. Further, having received this advanced *paideia*, philosophers could themselves do the relevant teaching.

32 According to Sprague (1976, 111–12), "we have encountered [the first three] before, so that it is no surprise to learn that these are the arts considered by Plato to be the chief rivals of statecraft."

33 On the *Phaedrus* as continuing to embrace the *Republic*'s notion of the philosopher, see Levin (2000).

Judging has a salient Platonic history antedating the *Statesman*. As we have seen, the *Gorgias* placed judging (*dikaiosunê*), the psychic *technê* handling punishment, under *politikê*, while the judge of *Republic* III (409e–410a) is none other than the philosopher whose nature and rightful dominance occupy Plato in Books V–VII. In the *Statesman*, judging comes into its own as a distinct endeavor with its own experts. Here it is tied to statesmanship not as one activity among others that a leader himself performs but rather as a distinct locus of expertise whose practitioners collaborate closely with the statesman.

Finally, *paideia* joins political oratory, generalship, and judging as a fourth ancillary *technê* (308d–e), though we do not learn here who the teachers are and what they transmit.[34] As we have seen, Kallipolis' producers are all but sure to receive only occupational training without also participating in the early *paideia* comprising *mousikê* and *gumnastikê* discussed in *Republic* II–III. In contrast, the *Statesman* trumpets loud and clear that all citizens receive this *paideia* (308d–310a).[35]

All four expertises the *Statesman* identifies as close aids (*sungenê*) of statesmanship are activities that were previously handled by philosophers themselves (true oratory, judging) or fully performable by them though practiced by others (generalship, education). On the *Republic*'s formulation, "anyone who is to act sensibly in private or public" must have glimpsed the Good (517c). What is more, one must know the Good in order to grasp how best to implement goodness in particular domains (534c). While the four *sungenê* proceed under the statesman's supervision in the *Statesman*, each involves distinct expertise that Plato acknowledges statesmen to lack. Statesmen directly rely, therefore, on those who "possess co-working . . . expertises of their own" (Cooper 1999a, 178). These are "independent experts, knowing things that the king or statesman does not know, about how to achieve the particular outcomes the statesman knows to ask for in the formation of the characters of the general citizenry that it is their responsibility to undertake" (180).[36] The *Statesman*'s move away from strict autocracy to include something closer to genuine sociopolitical collaboration is at once a strong departure from the *Republic* and a harbinger of the *Laws*.

---

[34] For Schofield (1997), the *Statesman*'s "'top-down' strategy" (221) explains the paucity of its attention to education (222).

[35] On this point see Bobonich (1995, 322).

[36] Cf. Márquez (2007, 47): "If the statesman knew *how* to command so that his commands would be sufficiently persuasive, then rhetoric would be a part of his art; but this is not the case. . . . The classification of statesmanship as a commanding form of knowledge thus points not to the statesman's unquestioned or actual preeminence in the city, but rather to the fragility of his claim to rule, which must be mediated by the agency of other arts" (italics in original).

In sum, the *Statesman*'s account of expertise foregrounds manifold experts' mutual reliance, with Plato's clear recognition of this fact and his richer, more appreciative view of these reciprocal ties. Let us next see how—unlike Kallipolis, where producers performed their naturally fitting societal jobs even as their broader human abilities were disparaged—the *Statesman*'s more expansive handling of expertises is joined with a higher estimation of the capacities of ordinary folk.

4. MEDICINE IN THE *STATESMAN* AND ITS SOCIOPOLITICAL MILIEU

The *Statesman*'s handling of medicine is notable for its suggested enrichment of the tie between expert and lay concerning health's promotion.[37] Plato claims (295c–d) that doctors, upon returning from sojourns elsewhere, are justified in revising written instructions previously lodged with patients for observance. In addition, if a patient's health-related circumstances change while his physician is away, a patient may adjust those prescriptions based on his consideration of the best response to unexpected shifts in his condition.[38] Salutary adjustments to a doctor's written instructions can thus stem from either the physician himself or the patient. Plato's presentation suggests that in many cases the patient's (i.e., layperson's) common sense and grasp of relevant health-related and medical processes is functionally similar, if not equivalent, to physicians' apprehension.[39]

Such a notion of likeminded cooperativeness in medical practice, in which the *Statesman* anticipates the *Laws*, is absent from the *Republic*'s depiction of the doctor and carpenter (406c–d). There, the craftsman rejects his doctor's treatment recommendation because he sees clearly that as things stand he can no longer function effectively as a carpenter. Because the *Republic* limits people's value to their active ability to perform their naturally appropriate functions without interruption (or with brief stoppages to address circumscribed conditions), substantive disturbance here suffices to render their existences no longer worth conducting for them or the community. Since the carpenter gleaned treatment's inappropriateness on his own, versus philosopher-rulers' actively blocking his medical care, the passage fits with an occasionally more optimistic thread in the *Republic*'s take on producers. Even so, what the carpenter acknowledges has nothing to do with health and medicine, stemming instead from his awareness as a practitioner of his own craft.

---

37 For a different view of the dialogue's use of medicine, see Annas and Waterfield (1995, xvii).

38 Broadly speaking, this confidence in the patient even as the doctor's expertise is given its due resonates with the view of the tie between expert and layperson in chap. 1 of the Hippocratic treatise *Affections* (cf. 33, 37).

39 Alternatively, one could have an assistant of the doctor attend to the patient in his absence, but this option is not broached.

He might simply recognize, for instance, that he no longer has the energy and concentration needed for making well-functioning tables. The carpenter's acknowledgment therefore differs from the more than rough grasp of medical remediation that the *Statesman*'s patient requires in order to adjust his doctor's prescriptions. Moreover, the later dialogue moves toward cooperation serving a shared, harmony-centered goal, namely restoration within the patient, via carefully chosen measures, of the balance that is health. This development is in keeping with the *Statesman*'s broader move toward greater appreciation of human abilities, including the potential of those differing in expertise to reach together toward a rich unity far surpassing the sum of its individual contributions.[40]

Concerning the *Statesman* and medicine, one must also cite the dialogue's notion of *to metrion* (due measure, 284c1), which is key to its delineation of the statesman's expertise. *Technai* centered on *to metrion* feature judgments of appropriateness, which assessments involve "the befitting, the right moment, the needful, and all such standards . . . settled about the mean" (*to prepon kai ton kairon kai to deon kai panth' hoposa eis to meson apôikisthê tôn eschatôn*, 284e). No one is mentioned by name as the concept's inspiration: Plato offers just the vague "many of our erudite friends" (*polloi tôn kompsôn legousin*, 285a1).

Skemp (2002, ad loc.) takes Plato's target here to be Pythagoreans, who failed to see a natural divide within the art of measurement (*hê metrêtikê*) between comparisons with fixed reference points, as in arithmetic and geometry, and those resting on contextual discernment of what is fitting (285a, cf. 283e).[41] Even if one accepted this speculative claim about Plato's target, the question remains, what inspired Plato to deploy the notion of due measure (*to metrion*) in the *Statesman*, and to do so in such a foundational way?[42] According to Schofield (1997, 229), the concept originates with Plato's own Academy, stemming from either an unknown individual or the school's general milieu. I suggest instead that the concept's most likely source

[40] The patient himself will of course usually have his own area of expertise, which is not (except coincidentally) medicine.

[41] Cf. Annas and Waterfield (1995, 44n41), who treat the reference to Pythagoreans as possible but not certain.

[42] Though the *Statesman*'s notion of due measure is a substantial advance over Plato's earlier attention to proportionality and context dependence, it has antecedents in earlier dialogues (e.g., *Euthydemus* 299a9–c1, which stresses proportionality apropos of medicine and health). At *Protagoras* 357d, we find that "those erring with regard to the choice of pleasure and pain, that is to say, regarding good and bad, go astray due to a lack of knowledge, and not merely a lack of knowledge but a lack of the knowledge that was agreed to be measurement." This art of measurement is sharply opposed to "the power of appearance," which "often makes us wander all over the place in confusion" (356d; cf. *Regimen* I 12). While the art of measurement (*metrêtikê*) sketched in the *Protagoras* has been much attended to apropos of pleasure, which is the impetus to Plato's handling of measurement in 356c–357e, the notion also has a pertinent tie to medical writings.

is Hippocratic medicine, in which it and closely related notions, above all that of *kairos* (the "right moment"), figure prominently.[43]

Nature of Man (4) announces that proportionality (among the humors: blood, phlegm, yellow bile, and black bile) is the key to health (*Hugiainei men oun malista, hotan metriôs echêi tauta*). As proportionality is its crux, "all diseases arise from bile and phlegm, [which] produce ailments when [things such as food, physical exertion, heat, and cold] are applied to the body at the wrong time, against custom, in too large an amount and too strong, or in too small a quantity and too weak" (*Affections* 1).[44] Further, "all sudden changes departing widely from the mean" (*panta exapinês mezon pollôi tou metriou metaballomena*) must be avoided (*Regimen in Acute Diseases* 46). Since "everything is good or bad contextually" (*Nutriment* 44),[45] doctors can err even with items that usually aid if these "are employed at an inopportune time (*mê en tôi kairôi*) or in an excessive amount" (*Affections* 50). Honey and wine, for instance, are "the best things for human beings as long as they are administered at the right time and in fitting amounts (*sun kairôi kai metriotêti prospheromena*)" (61).[46]

Surgical incisions too must be made at the right moment (*Diseases* II 61), and the pace of surgery once begun hinges on circumstance (*Physician* 5).[47] Where drugs' use is warranted,[48] their distinctive features must be tied rightly to the setting

[43] According to Kahn (2010), the *Statesman*'s concept of *to metrion* figures importantly (75–76) in the late dialogues' expansion of "[Plato's] own philosophy to occupy the field of natural phenomena studied by the Presocratics" (77). Even if one granted a tie along these lines between the *Statesman*'s handling of *to metrion* and the pre-Socratics, this leaves unaddressed the question of what most directly inspired the notion. Eskin (2002) rightly stresses the frequency and salience of Hippocratic references to *kairos*; however, while she asserts that medical usage strongly impacted Aristotle (108–9), with Plato she notes a similarity but no causality (105). For the *kairos* of rhetoric in the *Phaedrus* as having "interesting connotations in Hippocratic literature," see Heidel (1941, 12). According to Solbakk (2014), the *Phaedrus* grants "epistemic validity . . . to Hippocratic medicine" (46-47) and lauds medicine as having "managed to introduce the dialectic ideals of collection . . . and division . . . into its own procedure" (41). Though the *Phaedrus* falls outside the scope of the present inquiry, this study does not support Solbakk's account of Plato's extraordinary esteem for medicine.

[44] Cf. *Physician* (3) on the need for quantities' selection to be "well-timed (*eukairos*)." Further, "both sleep and its lack, surpassing due measure, constitute disease (*amphotera mallon tou metriou ginomena, nousos*)" (*Aphorisms* 7.72).

[45] My translation.

[46] In *Affections* (12), doctors must provide helpful items at the right time (i.e., before bile and phlegm attack a bodily part) lest patients contract pneumonia, pleurisy, or phrenitis. Moreover, context dependency obtains in the provision of light versus taxing foods; for example, what is salutary for athletes and manual laborers would overwhelm both the ailing and ordinary healthy individuals (52). On context dependency in this treatise, see further chaps. 3, 14–15, 27, 44, 46.

[47] On context dependency and surgery, see also *Affections* 2. Regarding cautery, see *Epidemics* V 7, 29–30. Concerning phlebotomy, one may consult *Epidemics* VI 3.24; *Ulcers* 25.

[48] *Affections* 14; *Nutriment* 19.

(*Epidemics* II 3.2). Further, once *pharmaka* are chosen, doses must be calibrated to patients' levels of strength (*On Wounds in the Head* 20). "The whole point" in bandaging, in turn, "is to know the correct method and due measure (*metriôs*)" (*On Fractures* 27).[49]

In short, what befits a given context is *kata phusin* (according to nature), hence salutary, while its opposite is, perforce, *para phusin* (counter to nature) and deleterious (*Places in Man* 44). Thus, "if you minister to patients in accordance with their disease and their body," you will aid them. "If, however, you miss the right measure (*hamartanêis tou kairou*) in either direction," harm occurs (*Affections* 47).[50] Experts alone can reliably ascertain what befits each context (*Physician* 13). In fact, the centrality of context dependency is the reason that medical knowledge cannot be rapidly acquired (*Places in Man* 41).

Affections is unusual among Hippocratic writings for its emphasis on patients' capacity for discernment:

> Anyone who is intelligent must . . . have the personal understanding necessary to help himself when he suffers from diseases, and be able to understand and to judge what physicians say and what they administer to his body. . . . The layman must understand as much about [diseases and their causes] as befits a layman; and what it is fitting for the expert to understand, administer, and manage, about these matters, both what is said and what is done, let the layman be able to contribute his view with a certain amount of judgment. (1)

That *Affections* encompasses the notion of due measure and shows marked appreciation of patients' discernment—and this in a work likely aimed at physicians, not a popular audience[51]—makes it particularly important among Hippocratic writings as a backdrop for the *Statesman*'s handling of medicine.[52]

Having set forth the relevant features of the *Statesman*, we now embark on the first phase of our investigation of the *Laws*, its explorations of human nature, particularly the level that the best among us may attain. I argue that the *Laws* contains no infallible philosopher-rulers, as Plato has given up the *Republic*'s view that a human

---

[49] See also chaps. 5–7, along with further remarks on contextually right handling of fractures in chaps. 19, 30. On dislocations and reductions, see *On Joints* 8, 11; *Instruments of Reduction* 40.

[50] Even healing may be "untimely" (*akairôs*, *Epidemics* VI 3.23), presumably because the "recovery" is merely apparent.

[51] Controversy obtains on this point. On doctors as the audience, see Potter (1988a, 4); for the treatise's direction at laypeople, see Edelstein (1987b, 100n20).

[52] On Jouanna's (1999, 374) placement of *Affections* in the 380s, the dating is perfect for an impact on the *Statesman*.

being can be unerring in understanding or character, let alone both. If Magnesia contained philosophers à la Kallipolis or near counterparts thereto, they would be on or comprise Magnesia's nocturnal council. Therefore, in arguing that the *Laws*' optimal city does not include such figures, I devote special attention to it.

5. *PHUSIS* AND (IN)FALLIBILITY: THE *LAWS* AND *REPUBLIC* CONTRASTED

Recently the view that Plato became more pessimistic about the best sociopolitical condition has been vigorously challenged. As Schofield (1997, 216–17) describes the view he targets,

> in the *Rep*[*ublic*] Plato's hopes are high, and they are invested in the prospect of rule by philosopher kings. . . . By the time of the *Laws* Plato's disillusionment is complete. He has concluded that it is not humanly possible for any absolute ruler to combine political knowledge or expertise with a virtuous commitment to the common good. . . . Instead he works out a plan for what is acknowledged to be a second-best alternative to the ideal advocated in the *Rep*[*ublic*]. Its governing principle is the rule of law.

According to Schofield (219–20), this stance is rightly contested: "The *Rep*[*ublic*] already makes it clear that we should *not* be hoping for the ideal; and it already indicates the need for an approximation such as the *Laws* actually provides" (italics in original).[53] Schofield concedes (240–41) that in the *Laws*, Plato gives up the idea that a fusion of philosophy and political authority is needed for the genesis of the just city but insists that "the role of wise persons (represented in the *Laws* by the Nocturnal Council) . . . in *maintaining* the institutions of the good city once established" is not substantially different from that in the *Republic* (italics in original).

Schofield is right that an optimism-pessimism disjunction is too simplistic.[54] In addition, Schofield (1997) and Laks (1990) usefully emphasize the regulative status of the *Republic*'s ideal of unity. I diverge from them, however, on how to interpret the *Republic*'s ideal thus construed and the implications of its status as regulative for that dialogue's tie to the *Laws* regarding human governance. On my reading, the *Republic*'s ideal does not in fact make evident "the need for an approximation such

---

[53] Cf. Laks (1990).

[54] Cf. Laks (1990, 212).

as the *Laws* actually provides" (Schofield 1997, 219–20). With the state's functioning not genesis in view, I argue that the *Laws* makes an independent approach to unity qua regulative ideal. As to the fostering of this unity, the nocturnal council diverges substantially by key measures from philosopher-rulers in Kallipolis; hence it is highly problematic to view it as comprising philosophers or true approximations thereof.

As we saw in Chapter 4, Plato seeks for Kallipolis a civic unity that far surpasses the mere aggregation of its components (462c9–d7, cf. 464b). The first two innovations of *Republic* V—women as belonging by nature to any group in Kallipolis, and the disallowing of private property and families for the two higher groups—are interwoven so as to stress their purpose of fostering unity (466c–d). This unity, where nothing is strictly speaking mine as opposed to shared (462b–c), will be sought "so far as practicable" (464d3–4).

Though these two factors, or "waves" (457b–c, 473c), make great contributions to *eudaimonia*, the most fundamental shift that would best enable the outcome that Plato has in view is select individuals' combining philosophical insight and ultimate political authority (473b–d). Once reacclimated to the "Cave" (i.e., the less rarified, spatiotemporal plane) following advanced education covering mathematics, astronomy, musical harmony, and dialectic (philosophical method à la the *Republic*), each of these rare persons "will know what each of the 'idols' is and whereof it is a semblance because [he has] seen the Beautiful, the Just, and the Good" (520c4–5). Rational control of feelings and desires by those who possess this insight is such that they have been "struck free of the leaden weights" represented by desires stemming from the appetitive element (519a–b) and, by ready extension, the soul's spirited aspect as well. Once the requisite *paideia* is complete, "Would you not entrust the state exclusively to them?" (487a8). Plato's answer is a resounding yes.

Seamless unity in the *Republic* is presented as a regulative ideal (464d3–4, "so far as practicable"). To the question posed at 466d (cf. 471c)—can a community operating thus "be brought about . . . and in what way is it possible?"—Plato's answer at the close of Book VII is "in no other way than that described—when genuine philosophers . . . becom[e] masters of the state" (540d3–5). I therefore diverge from Kamtekar (1997, 250), for whom the *Republic*'s claim that philosopher-rulers can exist not merely as approximations "is not the linchpin of [Socrates'] presentation—and indeed, it seems to be of relatively minor political significance." In the *Republic*, governance by philosophers is indeed the crux of the sociopolitical grid most closely approximating full-scale *harmonia*.

I argued earlier that philosophy is the authoritative praxis in Kallipolis, indeed by implication the sole *technê*, because it alone truly meets the *Gorgias*' subject-matter, understanding, and goodness conditions. The *Laws* might seem powerfully continuous with the *Republic* based on its early comment that "insight into the nature and disposition of a man's soul will rank as one of the most useful aids available to the art (*têi technêi ekeinêi*) that is concerned to foster a good character—the art of statesmanship (*politikês*), I take it?" (650b6–9). As we will see, however, the grasp of character at issue here is not sufficient to ensure moral steadfastness in Magnesia's officials as was philosophers' apprehension in Kallipolis. That Magnesian high officials' apprehension does not guarantee their moral reliability shows that their praxis cannot be a *technê* as the *Gorgias*' model is deployed in the *Republic*.[55]

The topic of human motivation greatly occupies Plato in the *Laws*. In Book IV he maintains that "human nature . . . is never able to take full control of all human affairs (*anthrôpeia phusis oudemia hikanê ta anthrôpina dioikousa autokratôr panta*) without being filled with arrogance and injustice" (713c6–7).[56] In Book IX (875a–b), Plato elaborates the ground of this contention, noting that the possibility of a genuine political *technê* hinges on the guiding presence of one who could always be relied upon to subordinate his own interests to the welfare of Magnesia, the polity in his care. Having stipulated that "the proper object of true political skill is not the interest of private individuals but the common good" (a5–6), he indicates that "even if a man did get an adequate theoretical grasp of the truth (*deuteron de, ean ara kai to gnônai tis hoti tauta houtô pephuken labêi hikanôs*) . . . he might then attain a position of absolute control over a state. . . . In these circumstances . . . he would never devote his life to promoting the welfare of the community as his first concern. . . . His human nature will always drive him to look to his own advantage and the lining of his own pocket" (b1–7).

Since moral frailty did not block philosopher-rulers' quest in the *Republic* to maximize unity through *aretê*, "adequate" understanding at *Laws* 875b2 must mean something different from its sense when applied to those figures. Quite significantly, 875b–d distinguishes between adequacy (*hikanôs*, b2) and genuineness (*alêthinos eleutheros te ontôs êi kata phusin*, d1–2) in apprehension, where only the latter—not

---

[55] From this perspective, the contrast between *technê* and *nomos* in the *Statesman*'s handling of best practice is noteworthy. As we saw, its construction of political expertise and authority is intermediate between the *Republic* and *Laws*, if anything tilting toward the latter. The *Statesman* contrasts governance by *technê* with that grounded in law (297a4–5; cf. 295c–296c, 296e–297b, 299b–e, 300c–d). On this topic see Nightingale (1993, 285n27; cf. 1999, 113n51). The *Statesman*'s recognition that governance by law may be choiceworthy ties it generally to the *Laws*. The specific rationales, however, differ; notably, the latter alone independently takes unity as a regulative ideal whose attainment is best promoted through the provisions contained therein.

[56] The way was paved for the discussion in 710d–714b by Plato's explanation of how Sparta thrived, while the autocratic governing structure of Argos and Messene caused their downfall (690d–693c); cf. Vlastos (1957, 237n28). Unless otherwise noted, translations of the *Laws* are from Saunders (2004), with alterations.

possible for human beings—guarantees incorruptibility. The authentic understanding (*epistêmê*, c6) that *Laws* 875d pointedly makes inaccessible to human beings is precisely what the *Republic* had put under the head of adequacy for philosopher-rulers (see further Section 7.5 below). What follows offers abundant testament to Plato's conviction of the human fallibility even of the best among us, who occupy Magnesia's highest offices, including the nocturnal council.

6. THE TOUCHSTONE OF MAGNESIA'S QUEST FOR UNITY

The *Laws*' model is described as "second best" (739b3). The optimal setting by comparison with which Magnesia falls short is regularly taken to be that of Kallipolis. For Kamtekar (1997, 251), Magnesia aims to approximate as fully as possible the *Republic*'s approximation of ideal unity: "After summarizing the ideal city, which, as in *Rep*[*ublic*] 462a–e, holds all things—possessions, feelings, talents—in common for the greatest possible unity, the Athenian Stranger says that people should keep this state in view and try to find the one that most nearly resembles it (*Laws* V, 739a–e)."[57] "This state" and "it" in Kamtekar's formulation reflect an assumption that the *Republic*'s route is itself the *Laws*' regulative ideal. One must distinguish, however, between the ideal of unity tout court and the *Republic*'s attempt to approach it as fully as possible for a human community. Both dialogues stress that a virtuous existence maximizes unity. Appearances to the contrary notwithstanding, rather than the *Laws*' seeking to approximate the *Republic*'s own approximation, they seek the same regulative ideal—possession across the community of "an absolute and unremitting unity" (*Laws* 664a5–6)—through distinct sociopolitical routes.[58]

In a key passage from *Laws* V, we are told that if all things were to be truly held in common, "what is called 'private' will have been eliminated without residuum from human existence" (739c5–6).[59] This remark directly follows a backward glance toward the *Republic*'s fostering of unity by precluding private property and nuclear families (739c4–5). Now, at the time of the *Republic*, Plato may have thought that

[57] See also Schofield (2010, 15–16); Kraut (2010, 61–62); Barker (1960, 340–41n2—by comparison, the *Laws*' approach is "only a *pis aller*"); Pangle (1980, 459–60); Mayhew (1997, 136n2; 2007, 110). The contention of Guthrie (1978, 349) that the *Laws*' second-best state is one "lacking the perfect communism of the *Republic*" requires qualification in light of producers' crucial omission therefrom. The *Laws*, like the *Statesman*, is one of those unusual cases in Plato, all post-*Republic*, where Socrates is not the central character; here, that function is given to the Athenian Stranger.

[58] Laks (2000; 2001) too challenges what may initially appear to be an incontrovertible reliance on the *Republic*; cf. Bobonich (2002, 10–12).

[59] My translation.

Kallipolis achieved unity "so far as practicable" (464d3–4) despite the fact that it sought *harmonia* through the dissolution of the nuclear family and private property for rulers and auxiliaries alone. That this cordoning off of rulers and auxiliaries from producers, far and away Kallipolis' largest group, is not viewed as significant there is evinced by its lack of mention (416c–417b, 464a). Plato of the *Laws*, however, is clearly aware that while eliminating private possessions and similar measures taken with just a portion of the citizenry in view is one route toward the unity he still envisions, it is not the only one worth venturing.

Contra the *Republic*, many important measures in the *Laws* are attempts, revolving around pedagogy aimed at virtue, to integrate all citizens equally into Magnesia;[60] that is to say, they are taken with a view toward maximal unity across the entire citizen population. In the *Laws*, Plato is pointedly unwilling to tolerate the community's cleaving in two. Hence, all citizens learn to hold the same views through a single route, which is to say that they are rationally persuaded to accept the same arguments.[61] While the interpersonal ties of Kallipolis' guardians were vigorously regulated (see especially *Republic* V and VII), this was ostensibly far less so for producers.[62] In contrast, the *Laws* makes clear that little is private for Magnesia's citizens. Neither allotments of land nor one's person is to be viewed as one's own possession (877c–e, 923a–b); further, Magnesia's children "belong to the community rather than to their parents" (804d).[63] Though there are small pockets of individual discretion, the scope of what is tightly controlled leaves no doubt about the rigor that Plato continues to bring to the monitoring of individuals' existence (e.g., 780a, 788a–b, 790b, 793c–d). On Laks' (2000, 287) elegant formulation, "what we call 'private' is actually the scaffold of the entire legislative edifice."

On the widespread view reflected in Kamtekar (1997), *Laws* 739 is to be read wholly as a comparison with the *Republic*, one in which the *Laws* plays second fiddle. Although the passage's beginning calls this interpretation to mind, its continuation,

---

[60] Plato's high estimation of citizens in aggregate is reflected by numerous measures, central among them their role in the selection of officials—including *nomophulakes* (cf. Bobonich 2002, 379)—and eligibility to function as such. They must also approve any proposed legislative alterations (772a–d). Further, citizens' extensive *paideia* equips them, when serving as jurors, to assess the psychic condition of perpetrators as relevant to the selection of proper penalties (876c–d, cf. 957e–958a); on this topic see Saunders (1991, 184). In fact, the text of the *Laws* itself will be an educational tool (811c–e). For discussion see Bobonich (1996, 251, 253; 2002, 106–7).

[61] On this function of legislative preludes, see Bobonich (1991; 1996; 2002, 110–17). Cf. Woozley (2010, 391).

[62] On the tight regulation of producers' existence regarding property and economic standing, see Barker (1960, 245); Mayhew (1997, 134).

[63] This translation is from Guthrie (1978, 346), who aptly notes Plato's stress on "public weal" (342).

placed in the broader setting of the *Laws*, supports an alternative reading on which the idea in both dialogues is to approach the unity represented by the *Republic*'s finger analogy (462c–d) as closely as possible. This continuation notes precisely the unanimity of experience and affect that the *Laws* too seeks—but here through all citizens' rigorous education and extensive stipulations that are the basis of communal stability.

Since the *ergon* (function) of Magnesia's citizens is to operate well in that capacity (846d),[64] it is built into the fabric of daily existence that they know one another well (e.g., 738e, 751c–d, 771d–e). Further, they participate incessantly in the fostering of harmony through such activities as helping to bring disrupters of unity to justice.[65] In a manner not inferior to the *Republic* from the *Laws*' own vantage point (contrast *Republic* 417a–b), its measures taken together strive concertedly "to throw into a sort of common pool even what is by nature 'my own,' like eyes and ears and hands, in the sense that to judge by appearances they all see and hear and act in concert. Everybody feels pleasure and pain at the same things, so that they all praise and blame with complete unanimity. To sum up, the laws in force impose the greatest possible unity on the state (*kai kata dunamin hoitines nomoi mian hoti malista polin apergazontai*)" (739c7–d4).[66] Significantly, this summation reflects most directly the *Laws*' construction of how to foster the regulative ideal that the two dialogues share. That Plato's ideal continues to be regulative is signaled by his insistence that a wholly unified state would be one fit for gods or their progeny (739d) and by his designation of it as a *paradeigma* (e1). It is in the *Laws*, not the *Republic*, that *nomoi* (laws) themselves are the paramount agent through which unity is produced. *Laws* 739 is indeed quite important, but not for the reason many have thought. On my interpretation, the passage's unfolding signals Plato's shift—passes the baton as it were—from the *Republic*'s account of how unity qua regulative ideal is achieved to that reflected by the *Laws*' own distinct provisions.[67]

---

64 See also 807a, c–d, 847a. Though citizens have some responsibility for their allotments (808a–c), slaves work the land and "provide them with sufficient produce . . . to keep them in modest comfort" (806e1–2).

65 On the salience of citizens' mutual familiarity, cf. Morrow (1993, 129). One who does not permit "the wicked to do wrong" is more than twice as highly regarded as one who merely refrains from wrongdoing himself (730d). Crime is an assault on civic unity (cf. Pangle 1980, 470), and the *Laws* is replete with testimony of Plato's commitment to citizens' central role in bringing wrongdoers to justice: 742b–c, 745a, 754e, 774c, 799b, 824a, 844c, 845d, 846a, 856c, 866b, 868a–b, d–e, 871b, d–e, 878d, 879a–b, d–e, 880b, d, 881b–d, 882a, 907e, 909c, 910c, 913e–914e, 917d, 919e, 920d, 932b, d, 935c, 938a–b, 941e–942a, 947e, 954e–955a. Moreover, citizen jurors have a salient function as the venue of first resort in private offenses (766e–767b, cf. 956b–c) and in the beginning and final stages of crimes against the public (767e–768a).

66 For emphasis on unanimity in the *Laws*, see, e.g., 654c–d, 656b, 659c, 663a–c, 664b, 689a.

67 Cf. Laks (2001, 109).

7. MAINTAINING MAGNESIA: THE NOCTURNAL COUNCIL AS PHILOSOPHER-RULERS OR CLOSELY AKIN THERETO?

According to Kamtekar (1997, 251),

> it is true that no-one in the city of the *Laws* is given the kind of absolute power philosopher-rulers have in the *Rep*[*ublic*]. . . . On the other hand, the law in the *Laws* is interpreted and improved upon by the Nocturnal Council, a philosophically-trained body. . . . Further, the sovereignty of law is a form of rational rule which approximates the wise rule of philosophers. . . . This is true in more than one way: the laws are framed by a rational process and have the rational end of maximizing happiness, and their preambles rationally persuade citizens to abide by them.

Though she offers no examples, Kamtekar also asserts that "institutions in the city of the *Laws* approximate institutions in the *Rep*[*ublic*]'s city" (ibid.).

On my account, the same worry about corruptibility adduced by Schofield (1997, 240–41) in discussing Magnesia's genesis deeply impacts Plato's treatment of its operations. I argue below that the *Laws*' picture of how unity is best promoted so diverges from the *Republic*'s that it calls into question any idea that Magnesia represents the closest possible approximation of the *Republic*'s approach. As a result, one must either give up the idea that the philosopher-ruler specifically is what the *Laws*' model approximates or conclude that the "approximation" is so attenuated that the caliber of authority described in the *Republic* is not substantially recognizable in the *Laws*' provisions. Since the nocturnal council of Book XII is the feature of Magnesia on which claims about the approximation of philosopher-rulers rest,[68] my treatment of departures from the *Republic*'s scheme concentrates on it.

Laws XII contains two brief accounts of the council's composition. On the first (951d–e), it is to comprise "priests who have won high distinction," including all *euthunoi* (examiners, 946b–c);[69] the ten most senior *nomophulakes* (guardians of the laws); and the supervisor of education, himself picked from the *nomophulakes* (766b), plus his predecessors. In addition, each senior member brings along a younger man between the ages of thirty and forty whom he deems most suitable for membership (951e, cf. 952a–b). At 961a–b, though Plato claims to be repeating what he previously said, the council's composition differs from the earlier list: the ten eldest guardians of the laws are mentioned first, followed by "all who ha[ve] won awards of

---

[68] Prior to Book XII, the council receives brief mention at 10.908a, 909a.

[69] See Morrow (1993, 503); Barker (1960, 403); Pangle (1980, 506).

distinction" (a3–4). Instead of the director of education, we find mention of observers who have journeyed abroad to discern whether other cities' operations are superior to Magnesia's (961a). Each senior member is, moreover, to attend with a younger man of at least thirty years of age "but only after selecting him as particularly well qualified by natural abilities and education" (961a–b). The senior membership must then ratify the younger man's acceptance (961b). Plato's earlier description of the council is more revealing about what praise and censure attend choices, stressing that "if one of the protégés invited to attend is judged to be inadequate, the whole council is to censure the man who invited him" (952a7–b1). Further, if those granted admission "turn out worse than most other young men, they should suffer correspondingly greater disgrace" (952b). Among full, or senior, members of the council, only guardians of the laws appear on both lists.

7.1 Revising the Law

As Kallipolis' thriving rests on philosopher-rulers' insight and character, laws do not figure significantly in the *Republic*. Plato even disparages those who rely on laws in their quest for optimal sociopolitical results (425e). In contrast, Magnesia's thriving is guided by the vast provisions of its legal code. One claim for the nocturnal council's similarity to Kallipolis' philosophers rests on its allegedly major role in revising Magnesia's laws. That a major task of the council is to revise the laws requires, of course, that the *Laws*' framework permit substantial shifts therein. While it is hard to detect a wholly consistent position, on balance the evidence points to a highly restrictive view of legislative change.

Consider the following scenario. At 797a–799b, which indicates his general vantage point,[70] Plato stresses that keeping children's play utterly uniform conduces to "the conventions (*nomima* [cf. *nomôn*, 797a8]) of adult life [being] left in peace without alteration" (797b3–4). He continues: "When the laws under which people are brought up have by some heaven-sent good fortune remained unchanged over a very long period . . . the soul is filled with such respect for tradition that it shrinks from meddling with it in any way. Somehow or other the legislator must find a method of bringing about this situation in the state" (798a8–b6). This passage provides the rationale for those pedagogical strictures, including praise of Egyptian practice, set out at 656c–657a. In fact, 798d refers back to the line taken there with approval. Bobonich (2002, 402) claims that one cannot generalize from here to other cases because Plato is particularly conservative where *mousikê* is concerned. But this is called into question by the reasoning behind Plato's insistence on rigidity: One should be

---

[70] Cf. Klosko (2006, 250).

wholly invested in legal constancy. Because early upbringing is crucial to the kind of person one becomes, children's *paideia* must be scrupulously monitored so that the proper values are instilled.

It is against this backdrop that 772a–d, on sacrifice and dance, should be read. As Klosko (2006, 251) points out,[71] the passage's broader context (769d–772d) suggests a wider scope of application. Even on the narrow interpretation, however, the rationale provided for the fixity of children's education (797a–799b) implies a similar attitude toward the legal code in general. Elsewhere, in fact, the Stranger either stresses that the period prior to finalization will be limited (846b–c, 957b) or prescribes the provision of detail whose subject matter is evidently circumscribed (828b, 835a, 855c–d). As to approval procedures for laws' emendation, Klosko (1988, 82–83) argues persuasively that Plato undoubtedly envisions the process stipulated for sacrifice and dance—unanimous approval from "all the officials, the entire citizen body, and all the oracles of the gods" (772c7–d2)—or else one of similar rigor. Plato's remarks in the *Laws* as a whole thus support the view that he intends legal changes subsequent to the initial adjustment period to be rare and governed by a rigorous procedure.[72] I therefore cannot agree with Morrow (1993, 501–2, 510–11) and Bobonich (2002, 399–400)[73] that Plato intends the council to make regular, substantial legislative adjustments. In addition to the council's lack of authority to ratify straightaway legal alterations it might envision, there is, as Morrow (512–13) concedes, no "evidence that Plato intends to give it power to override [existing] law. Its members, most of them officeholders, are always subject to the numerous checks that Plato's law provides."

Schofield has recently claimed (2006b, 320) that if Barker and Klosko erred regarding the strength of philosophers-rulers' aversion to law in the *Republic*,[74] this gravely damages their portrayal of its political philosophy as "absolutist." Philosophers' authority is "absolute" in the sense of "final," however, even on a slightly weakened version of Barker and Klosko's thesis. Even if *nomoi* (laws)—including procedures not codified in writing—exist, shifts under philosophers' aegis in the *Republic* will be unilateral and may be substantial. This is not to say that anything goes; for instance, philosophers would never allow unredacted existing poetry (e.g., Homer's *Iliad*, Pindar's epinician odes) in Kallipolis either for children or for occasions intended to reinforce communal unity. Platonic metaphysics with the Good,

---

[71] See also Klosko (1988, 82).

[72] Cf. Klosko (1988, 82–83; 2006, 250–51; 2008); Barker (1960, 352–53); Stalley (1983, 81–82); Nightingale (1993, 290, 300; 1999, 118).

[73] Cf. Guthrie (1978, 368–69).

[74] On this view, law is irrelevant: Barker (1960, 237, 322); Klosko (1981, 379; 1984b, 174, 184).

grasped by philosophers, at its pinnacle would preclude any such operational shift. Moreover, Plato's presumption of their incorruptibility makes it impossible for him to conceive of philosophers' acting thus from a craving that stems from their souls' subrational elements.[75] But nothing prevents them from, say, coming to realize that greater flexibility in applying the Principle of Specialization within the producer group may be beneficial, or, for that matter—assuming that this is absent from Plato's original vision—from deciding to make the early curriculum available at least in part to producers. Hence, while I do not maintain that *nomoi* are wholly irrelevant in the *Republic*, philosopher-rulers' insight, powered by the Good, qualifies them to adjust "even key features of the state" (Klosko 2008, 473n30; see *Republic* 497c–d).

The statement that philosophers' authority is unrestricted by law is ambiguous. What Plato opposes is subordinating the agency of those with knowledge of the Good—which is needed for realizing any particular good (*Republic* 534b8–c5)—to anything else, *nomoi* (laws) included. The key issue is not whether Plato hates all *nomoi* on principle or whether he thinks there will be none in Kallipolis but rather what the ultimate touchstone is for determining what is best and so must be done. In the *Republic*, that touchstone is philosophers' insight and character, not *nomoi*. From that standpoint, Schofield's (2006b, 324n24) concession that "the *Republic* puts its trust in wisdom and sound character" is huge. Schofield does not address the significance for his argument of the *Laws*' elaborate checks and balances—including a role for ordinary citizens in bringing high officials to justice—and of Plato's motivation for them.

7.2 Magistrates' Corruptibility

Passages in the *Laws* that comment directly on human nature amply document Plato's concern with corruptibility. One need not rely exclusively on these, however, since his worry about the moral failings of even the best figures prominently in the *Laws*' constitutional framework and legal provisions. The council's constituent magistrates may display such shortcomings in the very official roles (e.g., guardian of the law) that qualify them for inclusion in that body.[76]

Not surprisingly, supervisory relationships in Magnesia operate hierarchically, with higher officials supervising lower ones.[77] However, they also operate laterally, with high officials overseeing one another. This element will be our focus here, since

---

[75] For *akrasia* as responsible for moral failings even of Magnesia's best—which shortcomings were not envisioned for Kallipolis' philosopher-rulers—see Bobonich (2002, 271–73; cf. 369–70, 441).

[76] Cf. Klosko (2006, 254).

[77] There is abundant evidence of this (e.g., 762c–d, 784a–c, 945a, 946c–e).

it bears directly on the standing of the nocturnal council—and hence on whether Magnesia includes a philosophical presence à la Kallipolis. As for oversight in the *Laws*, Plato insists that "apart from the officials whose decisions (like those of kings) are final, no judge shall hold court, and no official shall fill his position, without being liable to be called to account for his actions" (761e5–6). Noting contrasts with the Spartan system, which offers the closest contemporary parallel for high officials' intertwining, Morrow (1993, 550) maintains that "the ingenious system [Plato] proposes—without parallel . . . in any constitution of his time—is clearly an expression of his determination that every official shall be subject to accounting before a body that is legally competent to judge him."

As Plato recognizes, it lies in the nature of things that some venue's decision must be final in each case. This is precisely the import of his proviso, "apart from the officials whose decisions . . . are final," at 761e. Although the decision making "buck" must always stop somewhere, no one official or group in Magnesia is the invariable arbiter.[78] Such a strategy makes sense only if Plato now believes that anyone, including those in the highest positions, may go astray.[79] The state's mission is overarchingly moral in the sense that it aims at unity through virtue alone.[80] Shortcomings—including negligence, itself morally culpable, and vice—in higher Magnesian officials' execution of their duties gravely jeopardize that mission. The *Laws* therefore makes provision for their detection and addressing.

The dialogue's handling of guardians of the laws and orphans is just one manifestation of Plato's concern that "adequate" theoretical grasp joined to ultimate authority inevitably leads to the subordination of shared concerns to self-interest, including "the lining of [one's] own pocket" (875b)—and the power in these officials' hands is by Platonic design not even absolute.[81] "Everything to do with the protection of orphans should be the concern of the fifteen eldest guardians of the laws" (924b8–c1, cf. 926c), who must look after these charges "as though they were their own children" (926e7). Initially we are told that while disputants who claim that guardians of the laws are not up to the task may bring them before the select judges, the penalty for losing these suits is "censure and disgrace" (926d6)—no provision for winning is mentioned. This is perhaps what one would expect given the heft attached in Magnesia to the role of guardian of the law.

---

[78] Cf. Morrow (1993, 250–51), whose subsequent discussion (549–51) brings out well the mutual checks and balances operating on the guardians of the laws, examiners, and select judges.

[79] As Laks (2000, 284) observes, limited periods of service and a prohibition against second terms are also intended to prevent corruption.

[80] Cf. Guthrie (1978, 335, 368).

[81] See Stalley (1983, 8).

Plato, however, continues (928a–d): Guardians of the laws who actually do fail to properly care for these children may be brought before the select judges—the highest court of appeal—who will try them and assess the appropriate financial penalty (928b–c). Moreover, orphans themselves, having reached adulthood, can bring officials before these judges, who may convict them of culpable neglect (c7) or purposive injustice (*adikia*, d1). Punishment for injustice includes removal from the post of guardian of the law altogether (d2–4).

If the kind of malpractice *nomophulakes* (guardians of the laws) perform is like that of others involved in orphans' care, namely theft of assets from their charges (928b8–c2), then this crime is quite significant for what it reveals about the character of those who belong to this elite body. In the *Republic*, Plato locates the desire for financial gain under appetite (581a6–7), and in the *Laws* he stresses that possessions, including money, constitute the lowest class of good (697b, 743e–744a, 870b). Yet it is precisely guardians of the laws who anchor the nocturnal council. Book XII recurs to these senior officials' "overriding duty . . . to devote their lives to the care of children" (959d8–e1)—the very duty in whose execution they may falter in a legally and morally culpable way. Though Plato's focus here is on orphans, as Morrow (1993, 549) observes, "we may safely infer that the action would lie for malfeasance in other spheres of their duty."

Why on the deepest level is such conduct a moral failing? As Plato's great stress on *paideia* throughout the *Laws* makes clear, how Magnesia treats its children is pivotal to the entire communal endeavor. It is precisely for this reason that the care of orphans is entrusted to the guardians of the laws—and the most senior of these to boot. Misconduct regarding children shows agents' failure to fully appreciate the moral mission of the state and the proper route to its fulfillment. It can occur only if officials, guided for instance by greed or envy, believe something else to be more important than this duty even though there is nothing to which it is justifiably subordinated. In contrast, although philosophers in the *Republic* are inferior to the Forms (e.g., they are not eternal), this is not a character flaw that would impede their ability to rightly govern Kallipolis. Therefore, no provision was made for illuminating, measuring, and penalizing their misconduct.

Additionally, the *Laws*' selection procedures for office take into account potential misconduct stemming from bias. Since the start of life is the crucial determinant of adult citizens' character,[82] Plato dubs the director of education the most important

[82] On Plato's formulation, *paideia* is "the initial acquisition of virtue by the child, when the feelings of pleasure and affection, pain and hatred . . . are channeled in the right courses before he can understand the reason why" (653b1–4; cf. 672c, *Republic* 402a). On children's impressionability, see 659d, 696a, 729a–c, 765e–766a, 782d–e, 788a–b, 792d–e; cf. *Republic* 377a–b, 378d–e, 395c–d. The *Laws* takes further the *Republic*'s insistence that human beings are particularly impressionable early on by launching their upbringing prenatally (789a–e, cf. 792e).

position in the state (765e, cf. 813d). The one occupying this role must therefore be the "finest all-around citizen" (766a7–8). Particularly intriguing is an element of the selection process (766b). Rather than voting openly, as is the norm for Magnesia's elections, participants cast their ballots secretly for the guardian of the laws they deem finest. Electors then subject the top vote-getter to *dokimasia* (scrutiny) before he takes office. While guardians of the laws voted at the earlier stage, they are expressly excluded from participation in the *dokimasia* (b7). On the one hand, this may reflect Plato's confidence that *nomophulakes*' involvement in the nomination and voting processes will help the state choose the right person. On the other, that the remaining guardians of the laws—who arguably know that individual best due to their shared magistracy—are excluded from the *dokimasia* could suggest Plato's worry that something untoward might otherwise occur. It is certainly a departure from his procedure involving corrupt *euthunoi* (i.e., magistrates' assessors upon completion of their terms of office), where those who preside include all other such officials past and present (947e–948a). Given the tremendous prestige tied to the post of educational director, one wonders if Plato was worried that envy—whose presence in the soul constitutes *adikia* (injustice) whether it "lead[s] to any actual damage or not" (863e–864a, cf. 869e)—might corrupt guardians' judgment of what is best for the state as a whole.[83]

Plato stresses examiners' high moral standing (945c–e). Still, like other high officials, they fail to be arbiters across the board. While their designated function is to assess magistrates' conduct once their terms of office are closed (946c), officials who believe they have been handled unjustly by examiners may bring them before the court of select judges (946d). Plato thus provides for the possibility that examiners will be biased in their assessments. If bias is found, the wronged officials may bring suit against them (946d–e).[84] Examiners' character must be exemplary as befits the key nature of their position. Even if it passes muster initially, selection for the role of examiner does not inoculate that character against deterioration: "If an examiner relies on his election to protect him and goes to the bad (*kakos genomenos*), thus showing he's only too human after all, the law will order a charge to be brought against him by anyone who feels inclined to prosecute" (947e6–9). Those standing

---

[83] Moreover, though *nomophulakes* forge a preliminary slate of candidates for generalships (755c), which are the voting province of those with current or prior military service, Plato incorporates a mechanism through which others may propose alternative names (755c–d). The same procedure pertains to the selection of company and cavalry commanders (755e1–4, 756a6–7). While a proposed replacement may not be superior, the procedure allocates that decision to electors (755d).

[84] As Morrow (1993, 549) stresses, the penalty for losing one's suit is stiff. What is key for present purposes is the code's express provision for the fact that the plaintiff may win.

in judgment here are the guardians of the laws, all other living examiners past and present, and the court of select judges (948a1–3). As with senior guardians of the laws and misconduct involving orphans, the penalty for examiners' conviction of a moral failing is removal from office, along with the loss of honors already received and those to accrue at death (a6–8).

Despite the air of finality that may appear to surround them,[85] select judges are themselves subject to others' assessment. As Morrow (1993, 549) observes, since they constitute an official body, select judges, like other officials, undergo *euthuna* (examination). And like guardians of the laws and examiners, they may exhibit injustice in the conduct of their official duties: "If anyone accuses a judge of having knowingly returned a false verdict," he must bring the accusation to the guardians of the laws (767e). Plato allows for two grades of penalty between which guardians decide based on the gravity of the offense. Showcasing this innovation, Morrow (548n10) remarks that "there is . . . no historical counterpart in the procedure of any Greek state, certainly not at Athens, where the judicial power was exercised anonymously by the dicasts in the popular courts." The foregoing discussion illustrates the *Laws*' great concern to interweave mutual sitting in judgment of and by even the highest officials—including *nomophulakes* (guardians of the laws) and *euthunoi* (examiners), who figure prominently on the nocturnal council.

7.3 The Nocturnal Council's Fallibility as a Judge of Character

As its membership is drawn from several distinct (though somewhat overlapping) venues, the council's very composition reflects the model of checks and balances deployed so liberally up to Book XII. Plato stresses, moreover, that members of this body may err in their selection of junior members, who are to be singled out by their backers as suitable based on natural aptitude and strong character shaped by education. As a check on faulty judgments concerning virtue made by single members, every nominee must be approved by the entire membership. On one prominent estimate,[86] the council will be comprised of approximately one hundred individuals—a large body indeed compared with philosopher-rulers in Kallipolis, of whom just one would suffice (*Republic* 502b3, 540d4).

Even with this safeguard, some may get through who, despite having pursued the studies set for them by the older members (952a6–7), fall short—and not by a hair's breadth, as they may turn out to be inferior to most others of their generation (b4–5). While these men are young compared with full-fledged members of

[85] See Laks (2000, 282).

[86] See Barker (1960, 403n1); Klosko (1988, 76).

the council, who must be at least fifty, they will be at least thirty years of age and hence possess characters well established through the meticulous education that they, with other citizens, receive. It seems especially problematic, therefore, that members of this elevated group may err individually and even en masse—gravely at times—in assessments of their caliber. Moreover, since older members count on the "joint efforts" (965a3) of themselves and their protégés, including the latter's views of what is significant in communal happenings and their input in discussions (964e–965a), senior councilors could well rely on interpretive and theoretical contributions from junior members who turn out to be deficient. This uncertain ability to judge correctly how elements of the spatiotemporal realm are faring with respect to virtue and goodness more generally is antithetical to the *Republic*'s account of philosopher-rulers.

The failing most prominent in the earlier dialogue, in contrast, was producers' status as irrational stumbling block to Kallipolis' thriving. *Republic* IV's account of self-control (*sôphrosunê*) presents the appetitive element as able to recognize a modicum of rationality (431c9–d2). Elsewhere stressing their lack of discipline, Plato envisions producers as operating just shy of pandemonium (425c–d, 589d–590d). His paramount worry in the *Republic* is this lowest group's corruption (489d–e, 490d–e), which stems from members' susceptibility to entanglement in, hence dominance by, the highly disruptive desires that comprise the soul's lowest element (442a–b).[87]

On Schofield's (2003, 10) account, the *Statesman* features "a community where there is no intrinsic difference in nature any more between ruler and ruled—all of us are human." While the *Statesman* is well launched toward this result, Schofield's comment fits better as a description of the *Laws*.[88] Diverging from Kamtekar (1997, 251), who ties rational governance inextricably to philosophy, I submit that rationality and philosophical authority are far more detached here than in the *Republic*,[89] where they beautifully align. Thus, the *Laws*' emphasis on rational persuasion—concerning which scholars have singled out legislative preludes—is not a comment on the necessity or reality of philosopher-rulers' approximation. Instead, it reflects Plato's clear recognition that ordinary citizens have a substantive capacity to appreciate rational appeals, and hence that positive sociopolitical outcomes need not hinge on deception and flat-out commands in the fashion of Kallipolis.

---

[87] Cf. 485d12, 584c3–4.

[88] Cf. his contention (13) that the *Laws* lessens the distinction between high officials and other citizens. Schofield (2006a, 97n92) notes that the *Republic*'s producers are no longer citizens in the *Laws*, since craftwork will be practiced by metics. Notwithstanding this altered sociopolitical label, which looks prima facie like a demotion, we will see in Chapter 6 that by key measures, metics' position in Magnesia is superior to producers' in Kallipolis.

[89] Cf. Pangle (1980, 433); Bobonich (2002, 217).

7.4 Magnesia's Own Cognitive Resources Are Insufficient

As if the marked limits on authority and concern about shortcomings in human *phusis* were not enough—and consistent with these—the council's power as a theorizing body is not absolute and self-contained: outside feedback is recognized as a salient avenue through which illumination may occur. That internal deficiencies will not necessarily be recognized from within Magnesia is indicated by Plato's provision for observers (951a–d) to visit other cities with Magnesia's enhanced functioning, not genesis, in view. The hope is that they will stumble across rare individuals of the highest caliber—natural marvels in any type of state, good or bad (951b4–7). Because it is essential to communal stability that one grasp the purpose behind the city's laws versus having a familiarity with them due purely to habituation (b3–4; cf. 960d, 962a–b), citizens deemed incorruptible by the guardians of the laws must travel far and wide in search of these individuals (951b7–c1). When choosing citizens for this role, *nomophulakes* make judgment calls and mainly rely on prospective observers' reputations (951c8). Not surprisingly, given the account of fallibility in Section 7.2, we learn that those singled out as incorruptible by guardians of the laws may not really be so (952c5). If baseness is displayed, the relevant observers are precluded from assuming further public duties, with death as the penalty for disobeying that prohibition (c7–d2).

These observers report back to the nocturnal council (951d, 952b), and the city should be prepared and eager to incorporate from elsewhere what is deemed superior to its own provisions (951b–c, 952b).[90] Strikingly, what inaugurates a discussion ostensibly meant to valorize the council's standing is its role of listening to what returning travelers—the execution of whose charge is needed to maintain communal thriving (951c3–4)—have learned from *other* locales. There is, moreover, provision for a class of visitors who may have something notable to offer concerning what is admirable (*kalon*) and will be admitted to Magnesia without prior invitation (953c–d). Compared with the *Republic*, where philosophers' self-sufficiency as knowers of the Good was axiomatic, Plato's not assuming that those best equipped to grasp the telos of what has been forged will be found within the city's borders is remarkable and goes against Schofield's claim that the provisions for Magnesia's maintenance are essentially the same as those for Kallipolis.[91]

---

[90] Cf. Pangle (1980, 505).

[91] On conduct involving other venues in the *Republic*, see 469b–471b. Granting that behavior toward other Greeks will evince "a restraint which they need not show to the outer world" (Barker 1960, 307) is a far cry from contending that Kallipolis could learn something about how best to run itself from other locales. Though Barker notes the *Laws*' inclusion of foreign contact (402, 404), he fails to see that it casts doubt on his contention that the nocturnal council is in essence the *Republic*'s philosopher-rulers (406, cf. 402). Morrow (1953, 249) downplays implausibly the role envisioned for observers, stating that the council's concern upon their return is to ascertain whether any has been corrupted, not to consider the possible merit "of [their] new ideas."

7.5 *Cognitive Adequacy and the Council*

Overall, Plato's discussion of the council seems to set the bar for cognitive adequacy fairly low. We are told that its plane of awareness must surpass that of ordinary folk (964d3–5).[92] While a broad comparison involving adequacy also occurs in the *Republic* (472c1–2), its mention there precedes Plato's unambiguous, sustained effort to show the categorical uniqueness of philosophers' superlative cognitive state. As previously observed, *Laws* 875b–d distinguishes between mere adequacy (*hikanôs*, b2) and genuineness (*alêthinos eleutheros te ontôs êi kata phusin*, d1–2) in apprehension, which alone ensures incorruptibility: "If ever by divine grace someone adequate by nature were born (*tis anthrôpôn phusei hikanos theiai moirai gennêtheis*), and had the chance to assume absolute power, he would have no need of laws to control him. Knowledge (*epistêmê*) is unsurpassed by any law or regulation; reason, if it is genuine and really enjoys its natural freedom, should have universal power.... But as it is, such a character is nowhere to be found, except a hint of it here and there" (875c4–d3). The adjective *hikanos* (adequate) in c4, which occurs in a different context from the adverb *hikanôs* (adequately) in b2, signals the higher caliber of *phusis* required for untrammeled apprehension. The *epistêmê* (c6) that 875b–d expressly locates beyond human capacity is what *Republic* VI–VII (506a with 534b–c) had placed under the heading of adequacy in discussing philosophers' grasp of the Good and its translation into practice.[93] Thus, for the *Republic*'s philosopher-rulers, adequacy and authenticity coincide. But the *Laws* denies precisely this equation where human nature is concerned. The superlative condition that Book IX dubs adequate for what transcends the human it puts out of reach for us, and nothing else in the text suggests that this barrier may be surpassed.

In Book XII's discussion of the council, Plato states that "if our guardians are going to be genuine guardians of the laws they must [1] have genuine knowledge of their real nature (*dei tous ontôs phulakas esomenous tôn nomôn ontôs eidenai ta peri tên alêtheian autôn*); they must be articulate enough to explain the real difference between good actions and bad and [2] be capable of sticking to the distinction in practice" (966b5–8). This passage reprises the two factors stressed at 875a–b: intellectual

---

[92] Since the *Epinomis* is inauthentic, it is not legitimately used as independent support for an account of *Laws* XII that privileges what is alleged to be an elevated cognitive state of the nocturnal council, one serving to tie it closely to philosopher-rulers' in the *Republic*. See, e.g., Saunders (1962, 45–46). Barker (1960, 407–8), having noted that the *Laws* "comes to an end, halting ... on the threshold of the last room which remains to be explored," assumes that the *Epinomis* is at least Platonic "in spirit." In my view, it is hermeneutically questionable to assume direct continuity between the two works and use details from the latter to support a favored interpretation of the former that one cannot directly substantiate by reference to it.

[93] Relevant phrases in the *Republic* include *kata doxan* (according to opinion) versus *kat' ousian* (according to being, or reality; 534c2); and *ouk epistêmêi* (not by knowledge, c6).

attainment and reliability in its implementation. Observing that this is what genuine praxis requires is quite different from saying that the conditions can be met. Though the *epistêmê* referred to at 875c6 would protect against corruptibility, the adequacy possible for human beings fails to offer this assurance. While this is not stated expressly, it would seem that the cognitive state of the *Laws*' best falls somewhere between the attainment of its own ordinary citizens and that of Kallipolis' philosopher-rulers.

Such a placement is suggested too by Plato's treatment of the advanced curriculum that is offered to members of the council only after they have joined—in contrast to Kallipolis, where candidates' response to the rigors of advanced education determines whether they are suited to enter the city's highest echelon. Those on the council must "master" theological proofs (966c–d), in particular those involving the soul's priority over matter and the rational direction of cosmic motion (966d–e, cf. 967d–e).[94] These folks will endorse the proofs' conclusions and trace the steps through which they are reached (966e). Thus formulated, their undertaking sounds broadly like that of mathematicians on level three of the *Republic*'s Divided Line, who operate with *dianoia* (reasoning) rather than *noêsis/epistêmê* (understanding) since they move from assumptions to conclusions, not from them to first principles (510b–511d). Rather than saying, with some,[95] that dialectic à la the *Republic* does not appear in *Laws* XII because its centrality to the advanced curriculum can be assumed, I submit that its absence makes sense given the level of cognitive activity that Plato describes.[96] If the nocturnal council can be spoken of as "philosophical" at all—which is highly doubtful—it is not so in a sense reasonably approximating that of philosopher-rulers in the *Republic*.

[94] Saunders' rendering *kata tên mousan* (967e2) as "with the eye of a philosopher" is not obviously supported by the passage and Plato's discussion of the council more generally. Notably, even after completing these studies, those admitted as junior members—whose original selection was ratified by senior members in aggregate—may reveal themselves to be morally inadequate (952b).

[95] See, e.g., Morrow (1993, 505–6, 573–74, 575n4).

[96] Cf. Versényi (1961, 75). Barker's (1960, 233) stress on the marked difference in level between the *Republic*'s preparatory studies and dialectic is apropos, since it foregrounds the salience of dialectic's omission from the *Laws*: if *auto to agathon* remains the telos of the advanced curriculum, and mathematics paves the way on a lower tier for the dialectical inquiry that sets one up most directly for that glimpse, an omission of its mention is unlikely. According to Saunders (1962), who views the council's studies as "coincid[ing] to a large extent" with those of philosopher-rulers (45, cf. 43), scholars are wrong to worry whether they are identical: "If Magnesia is a 'second-best' state it is natural that the education there prescribed will also be 'second-best'" (45n3). Saunders assumes, however, that the *Laws*' scheme is an approximation having the *Republic*'s own as its reference point. If one views Magnesia's framework as aiming separately at unity taken as a regulative ideal, then the divergence of the sets of studies bears significantly on one's quest to pinpoint differences between the two approaches based on their respective constructions of human nature.

8. CONCLUSION

Klosko (1988, 84–85) and Guthrie (1978, 369n3; cf. 370–71) conclude that philosophers are present in *Laws* XII: Klosko stresses discontinuity with the earlier books, while Guthrie, following Morrow, takes the discussion to constitute "for P[lato] the crown and climax of the whole work." My argument supports instead the claim of Versényi (1961, 78) that philosophy in the *Republic*'s sense is not found in the *Laws*.[97] Unity attained through virtue remains the guiding telos of the *Laws*' community. The route to it, however, differs substantially from that envisioned in the *Republic*. It stretches the notion beyond all reasonable limits to call the *Laws*' unity an approximation of the *Republic*'s and its infrastructure vis-à-vis maintenance, above all the nocturnal council, the approximation of philosopher-rulers for which the earlier dialogue calls. Kallipolis' philosophers rule sequentially insofar as they alternate active governance with periods of abstract reflection (*Republic* 520c1–2). This, combined with Plato's stating that even one philosopher-ruler would suffice for Kallipolis to exist (502b3, 540d4), reflects his robust confidence in philosophers' insight and incorruptibility. In the *Laws*, Plato's lack of such trust in anyone leads him to favor collectivity, including rigorous checks and balances, as the modality of high officials' and the council's functioning.[98] Even operating together, Magnesia's best may err.

Plato's reduced expectations concerning human nature at its best have far-reaching implications for the structure of society at every level. The shift in his view of human nature's upper limit opens Plato's eyes to the substantial rational capacities of ordinary citizens[99] and fosters greater appreciation of what nonphilosophical professionals, among them good physicians, actually do. This point bears on the final disposition of Plato's earlier rivalry with medicine for paramount authority on human nature and thriving. Let us turn now to the *Laws*' handling of medicine and its sociopolitical milieu.

---

[97] Cf. Bobonich (2002, 393).

[98] On this contrast between the *Republic* and *Laws*, cf. Laks (2000, 272–73); on the *Laws* specifically, cf. Bobonich (2002, 381).

[99] Cf. Klosko (2006, 218).

6

Medicine in the *Laws*: A Rivalry Dissolved

I. INTRODUCTION

Up through the *Republic*, Plato conducts substantive rivalries with rhetoricians/sophists, poets, and physicians. These disputes are carried out in light of the *Gorgias*' *technê* framework, under whose highly normative guidelines the former two endeavors never make the grade.[1] In contrast, having overtly valorized medicine, contra knacks like cookery, as a *technê* in the *Gorgias*, Plato targets medicine's preeminence in the *Symposium* and is committed by implication in the *Republic* to retract its very status as a *technê*.

The *Republic* defends philosophy's position as the *technê* par excellence, claiming that its practitioners' grasping the Good equips them to oversee all other activities. Plato's critical and laudatory accounts are flip sides of his project to secure philosophy's role as the arbiter of *phusis* and *eudaimonia*. Medicine cannot be a self-standing *technê* in Kallipolis, since (1) judgments of the whole person are made at moments of decision bearing on health; (2) reaching pertinent assessments necessitates insight into the Good, which only philosophers possess; and (3) their decisions about what is best will sometimes interfere with doctors' implementation of what is practicable, medically speaking.

Though Plato's rivalries with rhetoricians/sophists and poets continue in the *Laws*, his final work, the doctor does not compete with any official emblematic of Platonic

[1] For a defense of this claim about poetry, see Levin (2001).

constructions of *phusis* and *eudaimonia*. Why is this dispute over governing authority laid to rest even as others continue? First, Plato's appreciation of good medical practice is substantially enhanced by comparison with the *Republic*. By key measures, centrally including the domain of virtue, Magnesia's metics (i.e., resident aliens) surpass producers in Kallipolis, which improvements necessarily apply to good physicians as members of this class. Plato lauds sound medical practice specifically through quite positive accounts of the doctor-patient tie in the *Gorgias*' rigorous terms. His esteem for medicine is also reflected in a legal provision for doctors to constitute a jury and in doctors' limited involvement with phenomena bearing on the soul (*psuchê*).

Second, constitutional and legislative measures for Magnesia establish many checks and balances to promote justice, with no one person or official body always the arbiter. The *Republic*'s oversight framework was strictly top-down, with philosophers ultimately prescribing what happens in all arenas, including medicine. But in Magnesia the philosopher-ruler is often replaced by citizen jurors who assess the state of perpetrators' souls (876c–d, cf. 957e–958a). Magnesia's extensive web of oversight roles makes it quite likely that conduct evincing psychic incurability will be brought to light outside the medical arena. This takes the weight off the healthcare setting as the crossroads where decisions about the whole person must be made. Contra the *Republic*, no one disrupts doctors' implementation of the medically feasible on grounds of justice. These two major shifts with a bearing on medicine stem ultimately from the *Laws*' position that since no one's incorruptibility is assured, no activity can function any longer as a *technê* à la *philosophia* in Kallipolis.

The *Gorgias* makes clear that the first of these two factors steering the enhancement of medicine's standing is insufficient on its own, for that dialogue at once praises medicine and underscores its inevitable subordination to what justice requires, determinations of which exceed its purview. Though it is evident that medicine cannot be preeminent among human endeavors, the *Gorgias* leaves open whether and how considerations of justice will impinge on medical practice itself. The *Republic* addresses the issue such that medicine loses the rank of self-standing *technê*. In contrast, fusing high esteem to checks and balances, the *Laws* enables its restoration. As we saw in the previous chapter, the *Republic*'s transition to the *Laws* is mediated by the *Statesman*, which points ahead to the latter in key respects. Only in the *Laws*, however, does Plato's lauding of medicine clearly comport with his own guiding notions of *phusis* and *eudaimonia*.

2. THE *LAWS*' OPPOSITION TO RHETORICIANS/SOPHISTS AND POETS

To help accentuate the difference between what happens with poets and rhetoricians/sophists on the one side and doctors on the other, let us briefly consider the

Laws' handling of the first two rivals. As we will see, not only do Plato's clashes with these pursuits continue in the *Laws* in light of the *Gorgias*' *technê* conditions, but this final dialogue adds new dimensions to his critiques.

In a set of scathing remarks (937e–938c), Plato castigates those steeped in rhetoric for purporting to practice a *technê* when in fact they do no such thing. The "immoral practice" targeted here "masquerad[es]" as a *technê* when it is merely an *empeiria* whose telos is practical success and whose devices for its promotion "are available . . . to anyone offering a consideration [i.e., adequate remuneration] in return" (937e3–938a2). This passage—particularly the *technê-empeiria* dichotomy and the notion of masquerade—hearkens back vividly to the *Gorgias* (464b–465e).[2]

New in the *Laws* is Plato's expression of disdain through a legal code fixing strict penalties for rhetoric's pursuit (938a–c). Applying his penology, where states of mind are key, to rhetoricians, Plato's stipulations here distinguish punishments based on motive (938b–c).[3] In fact, Plato's own judicial framework, which stresses the pedagogical background and rational conduct of juries, arguably has as a key impetus his staunch opposition to rhetoric's place in Athenian court procedure.[4]

While his opposition to rhetoric is prominent in his account of judicial procedure, Plato's *agôn* with poets strongly impacts his handling of education.[5] The state he envisions, rooted in law, is the only genuine *mimêsis* (representation) of "the finest and noblest life" (817b4)—the very thing that poets claim to provide. As in the *Republic* and *Gorgias*, poets are chastised for extolling pleasure (*Laws* 802d), which makes their creations pernicious to all, but particularly to the young (810b, 811a). The Athenian Stranger enrolls the *logos* unfolding under his aegis (i.e., the *Laws* itself) as a competitor for highest authority regarding *eudaimonia*—a role traditionally granted poets. On Plato's formulation, this *logos* has itself come to appear "just like a literary composition" (811c9–10) that accomplishes what poets promise but cannot deliver: ever keeping *aretê*, rightly construed, firmly in view.

---

[2] On the dangers of prose compositions, see also 810b–c, 858c–e, 885d, 890a, 957c–d.

[3] For wide-ranging stress on Plato's calibration of punishments on this basis, see Saunders (1991, 249–51, 298, 317, 353), according to whom Plato "enlarges the passing references to states of mind in the orators into a potentially comprehensive psychic map" (352).

[4] See also Saunders (1991, 180).

[5] For emphasis on the *Laws*' tie to the *Republic*'s critique of poetry's corruptive impact, see also Stalley (1983, 127–30).

Poets are also criticized in Plato's repudiation of atheism (885d–886c, 890a, 899d–e, 941b–c). Given the *Laws*' attention to theology, rationally construed,[6] apropos of education, his challenge to poets in this setting reinforces Plato's earlier insistence that the dialogue itself be viewed in a competitive light. In the *Laws*, as in the *Republic*, poets' failure to satisfy the goodness criterion on *technai* stems from their inability to meet the other core *technê* requirements: they lack insight regarding *aretê* (virtue) and a properly ordered subject matter on topics ranging from the existence and nature of the divine to fitting conduct in martial affairs.[7] Poetry's failure to promote thriving, premised on these flaws, excludes it as before from the ranks of *technai*.

At the dialogue's close, Plato brings the two targeted groups together in a powerful recurrence to their deficiencies where flourishing is concerned (964c4–6). To the end of his life, Plato was convinced that, their own pretentions notwithstanding, both groups fall profoundly short in the promotion of human welfare.

That Plato's opposition to sophistry/rhetoric and poetry would continue unabated makes very good sense. Not only do both involve values fundamentally opposed to his own, but those values correlate with sociopolitical priorities and institutional structures highly divergent from those he favors. The *Gorgias* attests to this scenario concerning the former by embedding a harsh critique of rhetoric in an equally strong castigation of Athenian democracy, in which rhetoric had a prominent role. While the latter's sociopolitical tie is less direct, martial bravery à la Homer, for instance, meshes best with an aristocratic-style system, that is, with institutions favoring an elite nobility. This puts Homeric-style perspectives at odds not only with democratic milieux but also with settings, not strictly democratic, in which is embedded a single notion of *aretê* broadly applied, as is the case with Magnesia. In contrast, while medicine has distinctive guiding notions, as befits its occupation with health, apart from doctors' professional need to work toward that goal without real interference from without, medicine does not directly correlate with or imply particular sociopolitical values or institutions.

---

[6] Mayhew (2010) rightly stresses the rational nature of the *Laws*' "divine": "*Nous* is what makes the gods gods. . . . A human soul with reason is not a god, though at its best it may be called godlike or said to become like god" (206). While the *Laws*' account of the divine *phusis* is not wholly clear, "any hypothesis that dismisses Reason as a candidate for Plato's chief god or demotes the place of Reason in his theology is likely to be mistaken" (216).

[7] See 719c–d regarding the former condition; concerning the latter, see 817a–d, 829c–e, 858c–e, 885d, 886c, 890a, 899d–e, 941b–c.

Though the *Laws* retains the *Gorgias' technê* framework as the lens through which sophistry/rhetoric and poetry are viewed, Plato's plan for how the text itself is to function in Magnesia constitutes an innovation: "Are we to read the poets and others who have recorded in prose or verse compositions their advice about how one should live, to the neglect of the compositions of the legislators? Or isn't it precisely the latter that deserve our closest attention?" (858d1–4). The *Laws* itself is Magnesia's core pedagogical text from childhood to the end of life and the touchstone (*paradeigma*, 811b8, c6, d6) against which the suitability of all other linguistic constructs will be judged (811b–812a, 817a–d, 858c–859a, 957c–d).[8] Thus, far from softening his opposition to sophistry/rhetoric and poetry at the close of his career, Plato's *agôn* (rivalry) with them is vigorously renewed.[9] Strikingly, in contrast, Plato's earlier *agôn* with medicine disappears.[10]

3. MEDICINE IN THE *LAWS*

In Kallipolis, if a person's capacity to execute his naturally appropriate function is seriously jeopardized, this is straightaway sufficient to render his existence objectively lacking in merit. Therefore, in some scenarios involving health, doctors must not offer treatment even if it would be medically reasonable to do so, as when people require care in order for a conclusion to be reached about whether their illnesses are chronic, terminal, or neither. Further, if someone's soul is irreparably corrupt, doctors may not undertake medical treatment, however practicable, to promote the good of health. In assessments bearing on health, ultimate pronouncements are philosophers' as sole experts on the Good. Intervention by these infallible few effectively remove doctors, as medical decision makers, from the equation. This impingement results in medicine's loss of the rank of freestanding *technê*.

---

[8] On the *Laws*' function as educational text, see Bobonich (1991, 377–78; 1996, 251, 253; 2002, 106–7); Adomėnas (2001); Görgemanns (1960, 12–17, 104). On legislative preludes as rationally persuading citizens to accept the same conception of thriving, see Bobonich (1991; 1996, 251, 279–80; 2002, 97–119). Cf. Pangle (1980, 447); Adomėnas (2001, 38, 47); Schofield (2006a, 319–20). On *paideia* as a lifelong endeavor, whose continuation past youth includes choruses and civic festivals, see Brisson and Pradeau (2007, 113–14, 116).

[9] According to Naddaf (2000), Plato "intends the laws themselves to be put into verse and performed as songs and dances" (346), through which performances Magnesia becomes the true representation of "the finest and noblest life" (349; 817b4). On this account, the code's triumph through poetry's supplanting is more pointed still.

[10] Book X (888d–889e) mentions the placement of medicine among the highest *technai*, since its activity cooperates with *phusis*; viewed thus, medicine takes precedence over legislation, which is merely a human construct. This positioning stems not from doctors themselves, however, but from atheists, identified here as natural philosophers and sophists. On Plato's opposition to these "modern pundits" (886d2–3), see Mayhew (2008, 76–94); Guthrie (1978, 361–62).

The *Laws*' distinction between "free" and "slave" physicians—generally treating free people and slaves, respectively[11]—at 4.719e–720e evinces a greater appreciation than the *Republic* of what good doctors actually do. The kind Plato disdains, who "pick up the skill empirically," lack the genuine insight (*theôria*) that sound physicians have both acquired themselves and teach to others (720b). This specious doctor cares naught for patients' input via *logoi* (rational accounts) and, lacking understanding, is unable to contribute *logoi* of his own. On Plato's formulation, such a one "never gives any account of the particular illness of the individual slave, nor is he prepared to listen to one. He simply prescribes what he thinks best in the light of experience, as if he had precise knowledge, and with the self-confidence of a dictator" (*oute tina logon hekastou peri nosêmatos hekastou tôn oiketôn oudeis tôn toioutôn iatrôn didôsin oud' apodechetai, prostaxas d' autôi ta doxanta ex empeirias, hôs akribôs eidôs, kathaper turannos authadôs*, 720c3–7). In contrast, a real practitioner of medicine deems it crucial both to solicit and to offer *logoi*, providing such instruction during treatment (e.g., about his procedures and their bearing on the telos of health) as is accessible to nonprofessionals. Broadly put,

> his approach is to construct a thorough case-history by consulting the ailing one and his friends. In this way he himself learns something from the sick and at the same time gives the individual patient all the instruction he can. He gives no prescription until he has gained the ailing one's consent. Then, using persuasion to foster his ongoing cooperation, he tries to complete his restoration to health (*tauta exetazôn ap' archês kai kata phusin, tôi kamnonti koinoumenos autôi te kai tois philois, hama men autos manthanei ti para tôn nosountôn, hama de kai kath' hoson hoios te estin, didaskei ton asthenounta auton, kai ou proteron epetaxen prin an têi sumpeisêi, tote de meta peithous hêmeroumenon aei paraskeuazôn ton kamnonta, eis tên hugieian agôn, apotelein peiratai*). (720d2–e2)

Though other indications reveal pretenders to expertise, their lack of motivation and ability to offer (or solicit) *logoi* is thus an unmistakable sign of ignorance on their part. The doctor with rational mastery of his field knows intimately its telos of health (961e–963b).[12] In *Laws* IV (720c–e), as in the *Gorgias* (465a, 501a), the

---

[11] In Hippocratic accounts, the same practitioners handle cases irrespective of patients' age, sex, and sociopolitical standing (i.e., citizens of their own and other cities, foreigners, and those working in service to others). In contrast, in Magnesia inferior practitioners usually treat slaves (720c1–2), while true doctors for the most part (*hôs epi to pleiston*) handle free folk (d1–2), namely, citizens and foreigners, who would ordinarily be residents (i.e., metics). Plato's comments bearing on slaves elsewhere in the *Laws*, anticipated by the *Statesman* (311c), evince a higher view of slaves than the *Republic* and the Athens of his own day.

[12] Cf. 902d, 903c–d, 965b.

capacity to give an account (*logon didonai*) of one's procedures and their relevance to the end in question is the most salient indication that one has the pertinent insight.

In *Laws* IX, Plato considers further the methodology of the superior (i.e., genuine) kind (857c–e).[13] Again he sharply juxtaposes "one of those doctors who lack a theoretical framework and practice medicine by rule of thumb" (*tis iatros tôn tais empeiriais aneu logou tên iatrikên metacheirizomenôn*, c7–8) against the knowledgeable physician whose insight allows him to offer the requisite *logos* of what is transpiring and of the context in which it unfolds. Such a physician, Plato adds here in Book IX, "would be using *logoi* almost like a philosopher by engaging in a discussion that ranged over the source of the disease and pushed the inquiry back into the whole nature of the body" (*tou philosophein engus chrômenon men tois logois, ex archês te haptomenon tou nosêmatos, peri phuseôs pasês epanionta tês tôn sômatôn*, 857d2–4).[14] Plato's approach to what the doctor knows here harks back to *Gorgias* 501a, where, deriding cookery, he stresses that medicine "investigates the nature of what it treats and the cause of what it does, and can offer a *logos* of each of these things" (*toutou hou therapeuei kai tên phusin eskeptai kai tên aitian hôn prattei, kai logon echei toutôn hekastou dounai*).[15]

Scholarly discussions of *Laws* 857c–e often draw attention to Plato's turn of phrase *tou philosophein engus* (almost like a philosopher, 857d2) in lauding favorable medical practice. Plato's language here is indeed positive. Far from using the occasion to invoke a continuing struggle for preeminence between philosophy and medicine, Plato stresses a limited parallel, or analogy, in method. This is not tantamount to saying that the comparison point is philosophy in the *Republic*'s technical sense. As others have observed,[16] the verb *philosophein* is quite rare in the *Laws*. The other, participial, occurrence involves materialist constructions of divinity (12.967c8), and the noun *philosophia* does not appear at all. This passage in Book IX, with its notion of pressing "the inquiry back into the whole nature of the body" (857d2–4), ties *tou philosophein engus* not to Platonic philosophy or any other specific philosophical approach but more generally to reflective efforts to discover what is truly natural, hence foundational. *Tou philosophein engus* is complimentary to doctors, since it links good physicians' methodology, particularly their self-conscious quest to grasp the natural and primary, to the broad intellectual orientation of philosophers. That

---

[13] As in Hippocratic writings, it is sometimes ambiguous whether inferior practitioners are bad doctors or not physicians at all. In the *Laws*, one failing to meet the requisite conditions is ultimately a nondoctor simpliciter.

[14] Cf. *tauta exetazôn ap' archês kai kata phusin* (720d2–3).

[15] My translation.

[16] See Morrow (1993, 573). Cf. Pangle (1980, 497); Nails and Thesleff (2003, 20n38).

philosophers themselves differ on what specifically fits the bill in this regard is beside Plato's point here in *Laws* IX.

Poor practitioners, in contrast, are wholly oblivious to their own limits and envious of good ones who have consistently better results. This is the likely source of the former's deprecation of the latter at *Laws* 857d1–e1. In the *Laws*, practitioners who lack understanding are not truly doctors at all, even if people, speaking loosely, call them such (720a6–8). As noted in Chapter 2, Hippocratic authors find reliable assistants effective in manual aspects of treatment without suggesting that they grasp the nature of health or anything past anatomical basics that sophisticated laypeople might be expected to know. On these accounts, good assistants of true experts are superior to bad "doctors," since at least the former operate under the guidance of knowledgeable physicians. Plato's formulation at 720a6–8—which demarcates real doctors from "their assistants" (*tines hupêretai tôn iatrôn*)[17]—suggests that Magnesia's so-called slave doctors are, like Hippocratic assistants, subordinate to doctors. The *Laws*' defective operators are actually inferior to Hippocratic assistants insofar as failing to recognize their limits leads those who would by rights work under experts' eyes to eschew those reins, embarking instead on independent praxis. In fact, the hubris of defective operators is front and center in their deriding of real doctors' painstaking efforts at 857d1–e1. On the *Laws*' account, then, inferior practitioners lack knowledge of health and its causes, and evince the failure to appreciate their own limits for which realization the *Gorgias* lauded helmsmen (511d–512d).

Insofar as Plato derides anyone in *Laws* 857c–e, it is ignorant medical poseurs who imprecisely assimilate anything smacking of abstract inquiry into essences, and conveyance of these, to what are stereotypically viewed as other abstruse, hence useless, activities. Charlatans' negative estimate of good practitioners in no way invalidates Plato's laudatory description of the latter's apprehension of health and capacity *logon didonai*. On the contrary, his discussion of medicine in Books IV and IX, combined with positive remarks elsewhere in the *Laws*, makes clear that Plato's characterization of exemplary physicians stands. Far from reflecting poorly on medicine tout court, 857c–e casts poor operators alone in unflattering terms. The dialogue's sole passage addressing medicine and "philosophizing" thus contains no trace of Plato's earlier construction of the practice per se as rival, with justice requiring doctors' subordination, qua medical decision makers, to philosophers.

Further evidence of the *Laws*' positive regard for medicine is Plato's return to valorizing it as a *technê* along the lines of the *Gorgias*' construction. While the *Laws*' handling of medicine when showing the role of legislative preludes foregrounds the

---

[17] See also *rhastônên houtô tôi despotêi paraskeuazei tôn kamnontôn tês epimeleias* (c8–d1).

understanding criterion, that involving subject matter is pertinent too, since what ignorant poseurs fail to comprehend is the *phusis* of health (720b).[18] Plato's later reference to the physician's grasp of "the whole nature of the body" (857d3–4) reaffirms the salience of this requirement. As for the goodness condition, early in the *Laws* he had stressed that pleasure was not the telos of medicine (684c). Since, as this chapter argues, doctors may implement the medically feasible straightaway, their agency qua physicians to promote the good—as defined by the subject matter of their field—has no political impediment. Thus the *Laws*, like the *Republic*, uses the *technê* framework both to contest and to valorize activities. The *Republic* denies the rank of *technê* to all three of philosophy's rivals—rhetoric/sophistry, poetry, and medicine—pointedly lauding it, in sharp contrast, as the *technê* par excellence.[19] In the *Laws*, Plato remains staunchly opposed to rhetoric/sophistry and poetry, and philosophy à la Kallipolis disappears. What is praised through the *technê* framework here is medicine, the remaining member of Plato's earlier trio of competitors.

It is not just doctors whom the *Laws* views more positively than did the *Republic*. Also striking about the *Laws*' handling of medicine is what it shows about patients' capacities. Though the *Republic*'s carpenter sees on his own that treatment should not proceed, a mark in his favor there, what he acknowledges does not involve health and medicine per se but stems instead from his noting an impairment of his ability to practice his craft. Not only does this recognition fall short of the more than rough grasp of medical remediation that the *Statesman*'s patient needs to adjust the prescriptions of his absent doctor, it is nowhere near the strongly collaborative tie that will obtain between good doctors and their patients in Magnesia.

On the *Laws*' model of the clinical tie, the doctor's account is comprehensible to the patient. Moreover, the fact that Magnesia's patient and doctor exchange *logoi* (i.e., rational accounts; 720c–d, 857d) assumes a high level of reciprocity, which bidirectionality is based on shared human aptitudes. Plato does not conclude from the fact that the patient will likely not come in understanding everything needed for

[18] The issue of what the *Laws*' medical analogy reveals about shifts in Plato's view of medicine is distinct from the question of how the analogy illuminates the role of legislative preludes. Since analogies always operate against a backdrop of difference, it is not surprising that points of divergence, even significant ones, have been claimed to exist; for foundational work on this aspect of metaphor, see Richards (1936, 87–138). Engaging the controversy about the value and limits of the *Laws*' medical analogy from a political standpoint falls outside my purview here. For discussion see Görgemanns (1960, 37–38, 44–46, 53–54, 82–83); Pangle (1980, 447); Laks (1990, 223–24; 1991, 422–27; 2001, 111–13); Bobonich (1991, 367–71, 379, 386n83; 1996, 250–51; 2002, 8–9, 97–100, 105, 447–48); Nightingale (1993, 286–88, 293–94; 1999, 117–19); Stalley (1994, 169–70, 176); Thanassas (2005, 49–51); Klosko (2006, 243–44); Schofield (2006a, 84–85).

[19] That the *Republic*'s account commits Plato to the view that philosophy alone meets the *Gorgias*' conditions is not directly relevant for present purposes, since, as argued in Chapter 4, this is not a stance that he opts to adopt but rather one whose needful embrace by him is implied.

the encounter that he is incapable of it. This confidence is warranted, as the patient's education from childhood on, while not specifically transmitting this, has prepared him both intellectually and ethically to receive the apprehension bearing on health that the doctor conveys. Applying his epistemology and allied *technê* theory here in a new way, Plato presents as strong the patient's capacity not merely to absorb information but for insight. This ability suffices to enable his grasp of the doctor's diagnosis and account (*logos*) of how possible treatments foster health.

In the *Laws*, which lacks philosopher-rulers, a citizen-patient not only may but typically would have a deeper and more comprehensive grasp of human values than his doctor, a metic. This makes him better equipped than the doctor to place the latter's medical assessments and recommendations in the context of thriving. Plato's idea that patients may assume this superior role is not a bland abstraction, as there are at least two ways in which a free doctor's patient in the *Laws* may instruct him concerning values. First, the dialogue's revamped Principle of Specialization no longer identifies one's naturally appropriate function, hence communal and human merit, strictly through an occupational function narrowly construed (846d, 850b, 881b, 913d–914a, 917d, 932d). While free physicians contribute more to communal thriving than merely occupational performance, they are more likely to see people's value through the lens of specific functions they perform. A doctor may view the fact that a citizen has a chronic ailment preventing him from sustaining the rigors of generalship, for instance, as tantamount to the loss of his human value. The patient would then have to remind his physician that people's merit is not reducible—as Plato had thought in the *Republic*—to their capacity to perform highly circumscribed roles.

In addition to educating his doctor on the finer points of the Principle of Specialization as operative in Magnesia, the patient may instruct his physician on goods' hierarchical typology, including relations within each class. The *Laws* operates with a threefold ranking of goods: (1) psychic, (2) bodily, and (3) material—strictly in that order.[20] Free doctors will have sufficient awareness of justice and virtue generally to help maintain communal unity. Since, however, their purview is a bodily good not that native to the soul, one would expect them to incline at times toward fostering the pursuit of health where that would be unsalutary from a higher and more comprehensive vantage point. Thus, the doctor's medical knowledge, itself adequately expressible to the patient through their mutual exchanges (*logoi*), is complemented

[20] Plato notes health's place atop the second class (631c) and its significance with virtue in view (775d–e, cf. 732e–734e). Although health is first among external goods (i.e., bodily and material *agatha* taken together), to the unjust even *hugieia* is "a curse" (661b).

by the latter's typical superiority in the wider sphere of values relevant to *eudaimonia*. The resulting orientation is a modality that I call "a functionally complementary and ultimately balanced asymmetry."

The *Laws*' stress on the patient's capacity to give and apprehend *logoi* takes for granted his ability to attain the highest plane of collaboration accessible to expert and layman. The free doctor—unlike the philosopher in Kallipolis vis-à-vis all nonphilosophers—assumes that, through a series (720d6–e2) of reciprocal exchanges, the patient can be brought up to speed in the pertinent time frame on factors relating to diagnosis, treatment options, and the latter's rationale with a view toward the telos of health. The physician represents the parent in Plato's parent-child analogy at 720a due strictly to his medical expertise—which is, after all, the impetus for the patient's consultation of him in the first place—not because patients are categorically inferior where epistemic gifts and values apprehension are concerned. On the contrary, Magnesia's citizens, having received more extensive *paideia*, will typically surpass their metic doctors in broad cognitive attainment and in their capacity to locate health-related exchanges in the wider setting of *eudaimonia*.

In presenting a stance of this kind, Plato of the *Laws* takes a position on a prominent debate in medical writings about how far laypeople's abilities extend.[21] *Hippias Minor* (365d) notes a propensity on the part of patients to deceive their doctors. To Socrates' query, "Do you say that liars, like sick people, don't have the capacity to do anything, or that they are able to do something?" Hippias replies, "They most assuredly are able to do many things, and especially to deceive people." While Hippocratic treatises consistently laud medicine when undertaken by true experts, they diverge markedly on the capacities of patients (i.e., medical laypeople). Some express confidence in patients' ability to follow instructions reliably and even, within limits, to apprehend medical accounts and assess doctors' performance. Others, however, suggest that patients can be relied on neither to heed instructions nor to fess up to their deviations from what doctors prescribe. Authors' differing expectations of patients' abilities reflect different notions of the doctor-patient tie, particularly whether it can and ought to be collaborative. Showing what Hippocratic authors find patients able to offer by way of aid in the clinical setting helps to illustrate their range of views.[22]

---

21 While Wehrli (1951) notes rightly that the *Laws* "takes up an issue that was the subject of lively debate in medical writings" (179), he overstates the extent of common ground (179–80).

22 Although a clean distinction between physical and mental contributions is impossible in practice, for analytical purposes I typically present the classes as separate. Since my purpose here is conceptual, I also do not emphasize multiple categories' pertinence at a single juncture.

Many of patients' contributions rest on *aisthêsis* (sense-perception). Thus, doctors rely on patients' input regarding water's temperature (*Use of Liquids* 1) and inquire whether their sputum tastes "sweetish" (*Diseases* II 47) or "foul" (III 15). Physicians also ask about pain (*Prorrhetic* II 42; *Regimen in Acute Diseases*, Appendix 22). Further, patients' sensations of tightness or looseness are welcomed when bandages are first applied (*In the Surgery* 18).[23]

Another type of patient input involves *kinêsis* (motion). Some motion occupies patients alone, as when *On Joints* (37) deems them likely to succeed best in the manual manipulation required for dealing with a fractured nose. Patients may also aid their doctors in the preparation of cooling agents (*Diseases* III 17L), the induction of vomiting (*Internal Affections* 44), and the removal and replacement of suppositories (*Fistulas* 3). Further, a patient can facilitate the doctor's procedure by "standing, sitting, or lying so as to maintain most easily the proper posture" (*In the Surgery* 3).[24] Often patients' motion essentially comprises their nonresistance to others' manual manipulations. While doctors may perform manual work (*Internal Affections* 23; *Regimen in Acute Diseases*, Appendix 57; *On Fractures* 13), most often it is done by assistants (*On Fractures* 8, 15, 19; *On Joints* 2–3, 5, 76; *Instruments of Reduction* 38; *Hemorrhoids* 2).

Closer to the *Laws* is patients' aid in the form of verbal input, as when their medical histories are sought (*Prorrhetic* II 42; cf. *Prognostic* 3) and perhaps in addition those of families (*Prorrhetic* II 2).[25] According to *On Wounds in the Head*, though reliance on patients' reports should not be doctors' first choice (14), physicians may request chronologies of symptoms and other pertinent happenings, as when patients are asked how their injuries occurred and what transpired directly subsequent thereto (10–11). Doctors may also seek information about the patient's regimen when well (*Regimen in Acute Diseases* 28). *Affections* (37) instructs doctors to cast a wide net regarding patients' verbal contributions: "When you come to a patient, you must question him thoroughly about what he is suffering, in consequence of what, for how many days, whether his cavity has passed anything, and what regimen he is following." The author's instructions to doctors assume that the patient is truthful, has a sound memory, and is consistently attentive to all aspects of his condition.[26]

---

[23] For patients' input involving *aisthêsis*, see further *On Fractures* 5–6, 8–9, 16, 26, 48; *On Joints* 50; *Prognostic* 16; *Critical Days* 3. On the patient as data collector through all five senses, see *Epidemics* IV (43), which describes a kind of complementarity: the patient's observations are based on sensation, i.e., involve the readily apparent, while the doctor's stem from an awareness penetrating beyond surface phenomena.

[24] On hollow splints and patients' movement, see *On Fractures* 16.

[25] In what follows (4–5), *Prognostic* notes patients' carelessness and errors in following medical recommendations. The author leaves open the possibility that individual patients could provide good medical histories but fall short in their obedience to doctors' instructions.

[26] Authors do not, however, take the existence, let alone co-presence, of positive qualities for granted; for instance, *The Art* (11) notes patients' "careless neglect," while *On Joints* (37) chastises them for impatience.

Affections is arguably the Hippocratic treatise that is most confident about medical laypeople's capacity to grasp doctors' accounts, assess what doctors say and do, and properly regulate their own behavior for healing's sake. According to *Affections*' opening chapter,

> any intelligent man must, on considering that health is of the utmost value to human beings, have the personal understanding necessary to help himself in diseases, and be able to understand and to assess what physicians say and what they administer to his body, knowing these matters to a degree reasonable for a layperson (*andra chrê, hostis esti sunetos, logisamenon hoti toisin anthrôpoisi pleistou axion estin hê hugieiê, epistasthai apo tês heôutou gnômês en têisi nousoisin ôpheleesthai; epistasthai de ta hupo tôn iêtrôn kai legomena kai prospheromena pros to sôma heautou kai diaginôskein; epistasthai de toutôn hekasta es hoson eikos idiôtên*). . . . The layman must understand as much about [the causes of illness] as befits a layman. And what it is fitting for the expert to understand, administer, and manage about these matters—both what is said and what is done—let the layman be able to contribute an opinion with a certain amount of judgment (*peri de toutôn kai tôn legomenôn kai tôn poioumenôn hoion t' einai ton idiôtên gnômêi tini sumballesthai*).[27]

The potential rewards for the ailing are great indeed, as "by understanding these things, the layman will be less likely to fall into . . . diseases that tend, from minor provocations, to become serious and chronic" (33).[28]

By Hippocratic standards, *Affections* displays a positive view of ordinary people's intellectual capabilities. Not only is there less of an expert-lay gap than medical authors often find to obtain, but laypeople acting as *Affections* prescribes are deemed superior to many practicing as physicians. This is true also in the *Laws*, since free patients surpass "slave" physicians not only ethically but in their intellectual sophistication. *Affections* stresses repeatedly that patients must carefully monitor both

[27] Cf. the chapter's close: *Êdê oun hopothen toutôn hekasta dei ton idiôtên epistasthai egô phrasô*; *Regimen in Health* 1 (*Tous idiôtas hôde chrê diaitasthai*).

[28] *Affections*' confidence in laypeople's capacity for understanding and evaluation contrasts with other medical writings' critique. From that standpoint, it is far more likely that patients disobey doctors' commands than that those prescriptions err (*The Art* 7). Patients' reports will be flawed, since they operate via *aisthêsis* and *doxa* (cf. *Laws* 720c6 on inferior practitioners) rather than knowledge (11). Patients also exercise "careless neglect" such that "it is only when ailments have established themselves . . . that patients are ready to submit to treatment" (ibid.). What is more, they are wont to shift doctors willy-nilly (*Precepts* 7; with Jones 1923a, 323n2). The comment in *Regimen in Acute Diseases* (6) that laypeople cannot adequately distinguish excellent from inferior medical practitioners puts it directly at odds with *Affections*.

doctors' speech and their deeds, which may be taken to imply that a gap between the two is not uncommon.[29]

Though broadly speaking the *Laws* aligns itself with *Affections*' positive attitude toward patients, Plato goes further still by making doctors and patients collaborators, not adversaries as *Affections* implies with its cautionary words. In addition, the *Laws*' account shows parity, albeit asymmetrical, with the doctor's expertise grounding medical decisions and the patient generally superior in his grasp of values and *eudaimonia*. All the while, however, the Magnesian parties are united by appreciable intellectual abilities enabling fluid exchanges of *logoi*. The *Laws* embeds the doctor-patient tie in a unified sociopolitical milieu where citizens and metics receive genuine *paideia* (i.e., pedagogy directed at the instilling of key human values). Further, it insists that metic doctors, like their citizen patients, possess the salient virtue of *sôphrosunê*—and that in a nonperfunctory way (see Section 5 below).

Stress on these features of the *Laws*' account shows also that despite what scholars regularly assume, its construction of the link between doctor and patient diverges markedly from the *Republic*'s. Not even hinting that good practitioners' cognitive resources may be inadequate to deal with all the situations they confront, the *Laws* demarcates cases in which both parties are ignorant of the nature of health (the so-called slave doctor-patient relation) from those in which the doctor, possessed of understanding, seeks to persuade and educate the patient as to what treatment is fitting and why. Praise alone does not eliminate tension between medicine and some other, overarching authority. However, the *Laws*' lacking an *agôn* with medicine is not fortuitous. Elaborate checks and balances in Magnesia's framework tout court obviate the need for moments of decision bearing on health to carry the weight of justice. Crucially, the notion that what is medically feasible (*dunaton*) may not be best with justice in view—and hence must not be done by doctors—leaves the picture due to shifts in sociopolitical, legislative, and judicial structures. Let us turn now to those changes.

4. MAGNESIA'S ORDINARY CITIZENS FRONT AND CENTER

As we saw in Chapter 5, in the *Laws* no one, even the best, is incorruptible; hence, Magnesia contains neither philosopher-rulers nor close approximations thereto. People of the highest caliber, who constitute the nocturnal council, do not possess clear, direct insight into ultimate reality as did the finest in Kallipolis. Instead, their cognitive state best corresponds to that of mathematicians (i.e., *dianoia*) in *Republic*

---

[29] For other reservations about doctors, see chaps. 3, 13, 33.

VI's Divided Line (510b–511d). Human beings are at last on a single continuum where cognitive ability and character are concerned.[30]

Plato's diminished confidence in the best people's capabilities leads him to implement elaborate checks and balances across the spectrum of official and nonofficial duties. In marked contrast to the universal oversight role given to philosopher-rulers in Kallipolis, Plato quite deliberately declines to make a single venue the arbiter for Magnesia. Duties' wide dispersion features (1) high magistrates overseeing both lower authorities and one another; (2) officials monitoring citizens and other members of the community; (3) citizens keeping tabs on (a) officials and (b) nonofficials, centrally including other citizens; and (4) in some instances, noncitizens being authorized, indeed obliged, to react to the conduct of others, including citizens, their sociopolitical superiors. I address (3b) in what follows and (4) in Section 5.[31]

Ordinary citizens' direct, salient contributions to communal thriving span a range of responsibilities, among them bringing wrongdoers to justice and serving on juries, both of which fall under (3b). While I comment selectively on this issue, my concern here and in Section 5 is not to compare the *Laws*' provisions with those of Athens but rather to put the *Republic* and *Laws* head-to-head on issues bearing on medicine.[32]

Though each of Magnesia's 5,040 allotments is assigned to one citizen family, citizens' own energies will not be devoted to farming (739e–740a).[33] Their *ergon* (function) is being citizens, which is a full-time job (846d, 807c–d). A central way in which citizens promote communal welfare is by bringing wrongdoing to light.[34] One who refrains from wrongdoing himself will be highly regarded. More highly esteemed for his virtue (*aretê*), however, is one who also refuses to let others' misdeeds go unpunished (730d). Citizens' lack of mutual familiarity, which allows right ascertainment of others' character, would jeopardize such a project. To enable the effective detection and assessment of wrongdoing, Plato therefore places a premium

[30] For extensive defense of the claim that Plato's view of ordinary citizens is dramatically enhanced in the *Laws*, see Bobonich (2002), who attributes the shift to "a more complex account of how our psychic capacities interact and of how non-sensible items are accessible to thought" (12).

[31] Concerning (3a) see, e.g., 846b, 907e. That Plato's provisions for citizens' recourse include the highest officials is evident from his treatment of guardians of the laws and orphans (928a–d); in addition, if scrutineers deteriorate, anyone may bring charges against them (947e–948a). According to Morrow (1993, 251), in making officials accountable to the public, Plato "goes even further than his native city had gone, further perhaps than any other system of law, ancient or modern, has ever attempted to go." Regarding high-low supervision under (1), see, e.g., 762c–d, 784a–c, 945a, 946c–e. On high officials' mutual oversight and for further discussion of citizens' recourse against them, see Chapter 5.

[32] For extensive discussion of the *Laws*' relationship to Athenian praxis, see Morrow (1993).

[33] These allotments belong to the state, not to individual family lines (740a, 877d–e, 923a–b).

[34] For stress on citizens' role in law enforcement, see also England (1921, 494).

on citizens' knowing each other well (738e). Religious festivals (771d–e), common meals (806e–807a), and the existence of tribes (including their function as courts, 768b–c) are among the means through which he promotes this outcome.

Settings in which citizens in the *Laws* monitor one another for the sake of justice through law enforcement span minor to quite major, and cover both relatively localized crimes (e.g., assault) and offenses against the state (e.g., subversion). The *Gorgias* insisted, though without elaboration, that the obligation to remediate injustice covers not simply the duty to confess one's own injustice but also each one's preparedness to report that of others, including family members (480c–d). This is a small but salient harbinger of the *Laws*' full-blown emphasis, marked in elaborate legislative provisions, on Magnesian citizens' duties to report injustice. Metics and even slaves have important responsibilities in this regard. My aim in what follows is not to give an exhaustive catalogue of the *Laws*' contents but rather to illustrate the range of contexts that it addresses.

Plato's discussions of reporting often feature language of obligation (e.g., 742b–c, 846a, 873e–874a, 910c). Where his language is not expressly such, as in statements of the form "anyone who wishes may . . . ," the strong presumption is that one who learns of a transgression must report it to authorities. Given the pivotal role of education across the life span in fostering respect for established law, which is pivotal to thriving, it is implausible to read as anything other than strictly obligatory Plato's contention, for instance, that if anyone disobeys existing regulations concerning music and dance, and resists expulsion, he is subject to an impiety charge "at the hands of anyone who wishes to bring it" (*tôi ethelêsanti parechein*, 799b8). Elsewhere Plato observes that if anyone, having killed in anger and as yet unpurified, enters locales public and sanctified, "anyone who wishes (*ho boulomenos*) should prosecute both the killer and the relative . . . who allows the killer to do this" (868b1–3). While couched in the language of permission (*ho boulomenos*), the harm to communal welfare of such failures to act makes clear that latitude exists concerning who may report but not about whether someone who witnesses the conduct brings it to magistrates' attention.[35] Given flourishing's crux of virtue and unanimity, Saunders' (1991) rubric of "back-up provisions" (350)—which include "penalties for those who fail to prosecute when they should"—is misleading. By downplaying unjustifiably the import of these measures, Saunders suggests a firmer distinction between central and subsidiary contributors than exists in Plato's scheme.

Because grave harm stems from extremes of wealth and poverty (728e–729a), citizens must report anyone who violates Magnesia's strict requirements involving the

---

[35] For other illustrations, see 745a, 754e, 844c, 866b, 868d, 869a, 871b, 878d.

declaration of assets and limits on their possession (745a, 754e).[36] As for harm to persons, the regulations are extensive and include numerous references to citizens' duty of notification. Involuntary killings (866b), killing in anger (868a–b, d–e), and premeditated homicide (871b, d–e) generate this obligation, as do wounding in anger (878d, 879a–b) and assault (879d).

Legislative requirements also bear on judicial matters distinct from jury service. Contract violations, for example, must be reported to the tribal courts (920d). In addition, misuse of the courts to foster injustice generates an obligation to report (938a–b) such that "anyone who wishes should indict [the perpetrator] on a charge of perverse pleading or criminal advocacy." Given the pivotal tie between avarice and wholesale disarray, both within and without, once again what is literally optional must be in reality no such thing. Moreover, it is requisite that magistrates be notified when parties' or witnesses' court appearances are blocked (954e–955a).

There exists not only an obligation to report wrongdoing but also a positive duty to aid, as when bystanders' failure to assist those chastised by willful bachelors results in their acquiring "the reputation of being . . . rotten" (774c2). Elsewhere Plato describes age-indexed obligations to aid other Magnesians in cases of assault (880b, d). Moreover, when a sane person assaults another family member, "the passerby must render assistance" (881b4–5). The same applies if a slave assaults a free person, whether citizen or foreigner (882a).

In the *Gorgias* and *Republic*, psychic incurability, discerned by an expert in justice, renders a person's existence unworthy of continuation. Though the *Laws* is far more invested than the *Republic* in the remediation of offenders wherever possible, Plato's certainty that it is unjust for the psychically irreparable to go on living receives special emphasis there. Conviction of crimes featuring psychic irreparability warrants a sentence of death (862e–863a), and citizens play a central role in bringing such offenses to magistrates' attention.[37] Anyone "who is any good at all" must, for instance, "denounce the plotter [of subversion] to the authorities and take him to court . . . a majority vote being sufficient for the death penalty" (856c2–5). Temple robbery (854e) and stealing public property (942a) are crimes against the state falling in the same class of offense.

---

[36] Other pertinent examples involve buried treasure and others' property tout court (913d–914e). Plato also requires that misconduct involving allotments or the city's territory more generally be reported (843b, 844c, 845e, 846a–b).

[37] Unless mitigating conditions exist, a citizen's commission of grave crimes shows incurability, as despite his extensive *paideia*, he pursued a life of vice (854e). Short of this, punishment with improvement in view is called for (854d–e, 957d–e; cf. 731b–d). For discussion see Saunders (1991).

Murder of parents (869c) and intentional killing of fellow citizens (871b, d–e) also merit a sentence of death. The court handling intentional homicide of fellow citizens is the same as that presiding over temple robbery, and once again death is the sentence for conviction (871d). If the perpetrator slips away from Magnesia and later returns, "the first relative of the deceased who comes across him—or, indeed, any citizen—should either kill him with impunity or tie him up and hand him over to the judges who tried the case so that they may carry out the execution" (871d8–e2).

Relevant settings include, in addition, daring to serve as a witness following a third perjury conviction (937c); a first or second conviction for unjust courtroom behavior due to greed and contentiousness, respectively (938c); corrupt observers' disregard of the prohibition against their again assuming public duties (952d); and bribe-taking by officials (955d).[38] The case of observers shows that those invested with high positions may display behavior evincing irreparability. In addition, Plato's account of officials' challenging unsuccessfully the results of their scrutiny (946d–e) makes clear that death is one penalty that *euthunoi* had open to them at the original point of sentencing (e1–3).

Citizens play an important role as jurors in connection both with private offenses (766e–767b, cf. 956b–c) and with crimes against the state (767e–768a).[39] Having received the *paideia* that the *Laws* voluminously describes, citizens will be equipped to make the requisite psychic determinations:

> In a country where . . . jurymen-to-be have received a good education and been examined by all kinds of tests, it is right and proper to grant them discretion on most points to do with the punishments or fines that convicted criminals should suffer. . . . [They are to] give each individual crime a penalty appropriate both to the damage done and to the wickedness that is at the root of the actual deed. We believe, in fact, that the people for whom we are legislating may well turn out quite conspicuously able judges of these matters. (876c3–d6)

Such comments clearly illustrate Plato's high level of confidence in ordinary citizens. He recurs to this judicial role near the dialogue's close, singling out here findings of incurability warranting death (957e–958a).

---

[38] Incurable offenders figure, moreover, in Book X's handling of atheism (909a).

[39] Given Plato's attempt to minimize the public-private divide (780a, 788a–b, 790b, 793c–d, 804d, 942a–d; cf. Laks 2000, 286–87), and his conviction that all wrongdoing stems from a condition deleterious both to oneself and to the community, all crimes are in some way offenses against the state. On this point see Shuchman (1963, 29). Morrow (1993) maintains too strong a public-private distinction for Magnesia, as when he asserts the guarding of orphans and vulnerable parents to concern "clearly private interests" (278). See also Schaps (2001, 147), according to whom Plato's expectation for Magnesia is that "each citizen, in pursuing his own private good, not encroach upon others."

Though Plato cites a range of crimes whose commission evinces incurability at least in part to guide jurors in these and any other situations they confront, his provisions are not a recipe. Since many times the deed itself is insufficient to determine the proper judicial response, Plato's expectation is that jurors will have ample occasion to look beneath the surface of the act to discern pertinent contextual factors, crucially including the perpetrator's psychic condition.[40] For instance, was a progenitor's attacker mad or sane (881b)? Did a particular homicide stem from anger (867c–869e) or forethought (871a–872c, 873a–c)?[41]

Given the dialogue's overall stress on checks and balances, and Plato's confidence in ordinary citizens, it is reasonable to conclude that their intended responsibilities surpass what is noted expressly.[42] Citizens' contributions beyond the *Laws*' voiced provisions would of course include their juridical role in addressing crimes whose commission under pertinent conditions shows psychic irreparability. Citizens' role vis-à-vis justice, along with officials' contributions, ensures, or nearly so, that those in this psychic state are discovered and handled through proper channels—ones that do not include the health-care setting.

5. NONCITIZENS' ENHANCED POSITION IN MAGNESIA

The *Laws* never identifies good doctors' sociopolitical position apart from their being *eleutheroi* (free; 720b4, d1, 857d1), which Greek term covers both citizens and aliens. Citizens' *ergon* of being such precludes their serving as physicians, since this would involve the impermissible pursuit of a twofold role. The caliber of respect accorded by Plato, along with the fact that forging needed ties with the patient and his intimates requires a sustained communal presence, indicates that doctors must be metics (i.e., resident aliens), not foreigners who are merely passing through. Is my claim that the *Laws* lauds medicine once again as a *technê* in the *Gorgias*' normative terms not however rendered implausible by the fact that at the very juncture in question, the sociopolitical standing of doctors suffers what appears to be a demotion from citizen-producer to metic?

Commentators often assume that producers' reclassification as metics reflects a lowering simpliciter of their standing.[43] This shift, however, is not a demotion in real terms. The *Laws*' heightened confidence in ordinary citizens extends to noncitizens

[40] For valuable discussion of Plato's great expectations of citizen jurors here, see Saunders (1991, 184–85, 187–90, 354).

[41] On the category of killing in anger as "a Platonic innovation," see Saunders (1991, 156; cf. 225, 250).

[42] Cf. Saunders (1991, 298, 335).

[43] See Sabine (1973, 88); Stalley (1983, 111); Laks (1990, 225).

too, including those classed as producers in Kallipolis. Though it does not totally overhaul Plato's orientation toward those who functioned as producers, the *Laws* testifies both to an improvement in metics' status compared with citizen-producers', which elevates doctors as members of this group, and to a marked enhancement involving medicine in particular. Regarding the latter, having concentrated in Section 3 on the *Laws*' valorization of exemplary praxis, at the close of the present section I consider Plato's provision for doctors' own jury service. Although this innovation is small in scope, it is important when one compares the *Laws* with the *Gorgias*, where medicine and judging are wholly separate endeavors, and with the *Republic*, where doctors like other producers foster justice strictly through performing well their occupational roles.

Due to their insight into the Good, anything Kallipolis' philosophers impose to maintain order is justified simply by virtue of their having decided it. When Plato's expectations of human nature at its best are lowered, the automatic rationale for this modus operandi falls by the wayside. Strict limits are placed even on high officials' actions in Magnesia. What is more, noncitizens enjoy key, express protections. The fact that Kallipolis' producers occupy the far end of a spectrum that is actually a chasm separating them by nature, as it were, from philosophers grounds Plato's unwillingness to grant them "[any] capacity for public service except their trades" (Sabine 1973, 64). Even the process of craftwork will be closely monitored (*Republic* 401a–d). In Magnesia, not only are noncitizens assigned such duties, but metics themselves are involved in the formulating of provisions bearing directly on their occupational praxis, including pecuniary matters. Let me now expand what was said about producers in Chapter 4 as a foundation for my defense of doctors' elevated standing qua metics in the *Laws*.

In Kallipolis, "the desires of the inferior multitude [will be dominated by rulers'] desires and wisdom" (*Republic* 431c10–d2). The question is, how will this primacy be secured? Plato's presentation of *sôphrosunê* as it involves producers (389d–e) clashes with his descriptions of the appetitive element's force and how that element is prone to operate, leaving one inclined to the view that reason will in their case often have to be imposed by philosopher-rulers, that is to say, from without.[44]

Turning adversarial, Plato stipulates at 415d–e that rulers choose as auxiliaries' base of operations the spot that best enables their putting down of threats to the

[44] As Plato's express comments on the topic are scanty, commentators often base positive inferences about producers' capacity for *aretê* at least in part on justified claims concerning auxiliaries, their sociopolitical superiors. See, e.g., Kahn (2004, 350–52); Stalley (1994, 161, 167); Vlastos (1978, 93–94). On Vlastos' line of reasoning, if producers' standing is not the fruit of *paideia*, 430b on untutored belief does indeed apply to them.

city, both internal rebellions and external attacks. He thus provides for the possibility that producers en masse or in substantial numbers may revolt against the polity of which, at least technically, they are citizens.[45] Following on the heels of 586d–587a, which stresses the divide between philosophical and other *psuchai* (cf. 527d–e),[46] 590c–d is quite negative regarding producers' souls, contending that "it is better for everyone to be governed by the divine and intelligent, preferably indwelling and his own, but if not, imposed from without, so that we all so far as possible may be akin and friendly because our governance and guidance are the same" (d3–6). As at 415d–e, no limits are placed upon allowable forms of external imposition for the sake of communal harmony.[47]

Given the appetitive element's mass and power (431b–c, 439b–d, 589d, 590a), reason and *thumoeides* (spirit) together are needed to prevent its inundating the soul (441e–442b).[48] These two aspects of *psuchê* should "preside over the appetitive part that is the mass of the soul in each of us and by nature most insatiate when it comes to wealth. They will keep watch upon it, lest by being filled and infected with the so-called pleasures associated with the body and so waxing big and strong, it may not keep to its own work but may undertake to enslave and rule over the classes that it is not fitting it should, and so overturn the entire life of all" (442a5–b3).

This alliance of reason and spirit is made possible by their own natures and the *paideia* (education) comprising *mousikê* (poetry and music) and *gumnastikê* (physical training) that cultivates this association in the souls of budding philosophers and auxiliaries. It is all but certain that producers do not also receive this *paideia*.[49] While auxiliaries' cognitive state and character fall well short of philosophers', Plato depicts their *orthê doxa* (true belief) regarding *andreia* (courage), instilled through this early *paideia*, as reliable and sufficient to enable their collaboration

---

[45] On this possibility, cf. Laks (1990, 220).

[46] On the magnitude of the gap, cf. Bobonich (2002, 7), though I contend that the distinction between auxiliaries and producers qua "non-philosophers" in their capacities for *aretê* is greater than he suggests. For stress on the distinction between types of nonrulers, see also Annas (1981, 117).

[47] Schofield's (2006a, 273–74) view that 590c–d does not apply to Kallipolis is called into question by 590d5–6, where the telos of rulers' imposition of reason from without is that "we all so far as possible may be akin and friendly because our governance and guidance are the same," which is precisely Plato's aspiration for Kallipolis, and by comments elsewhere in the dialogue that mesh with the notion of producers' *psuchai* in 590c–d.

[48] Cf. 439e–440b, 589a–b.

[49] Though Plato does not assert that producers do not also receive this *paideia*, his pointed disjunction between "the guardians having the education we've described" and "the cobblers educated by the art of cobbling" (456d9–10) is tantamount to such a claim (cf. 466e–467a). On this topic see also Hourani (1949). In addition, as Reeve (1988, 186) observes, Plato specifies repeatedly that guardians are its target (386b–c, 387c, 394e–396b, 398e, 401b–d, 402b–c, 404a–b). Moreover (188), Plato's definition of "true musicians" as "able to recognize . . . self-control, courage, liberality, and high-mindedness . . . and their opposites, in all the combinations that contain them" (402b9–c5), simply does not apply to the lowest class in Kallipolis.

with philosophers in keeping the city safe (429e–430b).[50] While auxiliaries' possession of this trait is justifiably though qualifiedly dubbed *andreia*, "for mere right opinion about the same matters not produced by education, which may manifest itself in a beast or a slave . . . you would use a term other than 'courage'" (430b6–9). This remark about the status and efficacy of true belief thus construed applies by extension to the insubstantial possession of any other *aretê*, including *sôphrosunê*.[51]

As I argued in Chapter 5, a striking development in the *Laws* is that foreigners as a class are not intrinsically inferior to Magnesians in their capacity for insight. Unlike the *Republic*, where consultation of those outside Kallipolis on matters of great import would have been unthinkable, Magnesia provides two routes, observers (*Laws* 951a–d, 952b, 961a) and visitors (953c–d), through which the nocturnal council may receive salient input from abroad. These visitors will be nonresident aliens, whom Athens and the *Laws* regard less highly than metics. The claim that foreigners may know better than Magnesians what is best in human institutions and practices reflects a dramatic elevation in Plato's view of the cognitive aptitude and character of people not native to the community whose elucidation and lauding are his prime concern.

Further evidence of Plato's confidence in foreigners' capacity for virtue, including an ability to withstand temptation, is evinced by his claim that children's teachers will be metics who provide "complete courses of instruction in military matters and *mousikê*" (804d1–3). Such education is mandatory without exception: "Children must not be left without teachers . . . any more than flocks and herds must be allowed to live without attendants" (808d2–4, cf. 804d). This formulation vividly captures Plato's view, often expressed, that human beings are most impressionable at this stage of character formation.[52]

Since Magnesia's prospects for thriving crucially depend on children's *paideia*, Plato's selection of metics as their teachers is significant. That his expectations of their ability to affirm what is best are not low is shown by their role in deploying the *Laws* as children's core educational text (811c–812a). Plato requires that metic teachers "learn this material and . . . endorse [the educational minister's] own high opinion" of it, thereby warranting the city's pedagogical trust in them (811e–812a). Not only do Kallipolis' producers lack this role, but given their fundamental untrustworthiness, it is unimaginable that Plato would assign it to them. Whitehead

---

50 Cf. 440d, 458b–c.

51 Cf. Saunders (1962, 47–48). Taylor (1997, 48n17), who attributes to the *Republic* a "pessimistic moral psychology" (43), effectively opposes Vlastos' contention (1978, 84–85, 93–94), based on what clearly obtains for auxiliaries, that 430b6–9 applies to neither group of nonrulers.

52 See 765e–766a, 782d–e, 792d–e; cf. 659d–e, 696a, 729a–c, 788a–b.

(1977, 132) claims that Plato deprecates the job of teaching. This, however, would be glaringly at odds with his insistence that "children's games affect legislation so crucially as to determine whether the laws . . . survive" (797a7–9) and emphasis on the pivotal import of early *paideia* to communal thriving. As I have argued, Plato's provision for metic teachers reflects his significant confidence in members of that group. The *Laws*' handling of teachers, unlike the *Republic*'s treatment of producers, shows him committed to a middle ground between the poles of inner governance and order imposed from without.

Notably, unlike what occurred with producers in the *Republic*, the *Laws* indicates that noncitizens receive *paideia*, not merely training directly required for the performance of their crafts. Book I speaks of play, including that of noncitizens who will pursue crafts in adulthood, as aiming to "channel children's pleasures and desires toward the activities in which they . . . will have to be absolutely perfect when [they grow] up" (643c7–d3); for instance, "the carpenter must learn in his play how to handle a rule and plumb-line, and the soldier must learn to ride a horse" (643c4–5). All children—those of citizens, metics, and slaves—are brought to play at the same venues (794a–b). Plato's discussion here of children's punishment (794b–c) is motivated by play's telos of character formation (793e, cf. 792d–e). Given the foregoing, it is clear that the play of noncitizen children does not aim merely to facilitate circumscribed occupational training.[53] Moreover, all members of the community are to participate in choruses from childhood on.[54] Plato's stress here on participants' "find[ing] perpetual pleasure" (665c6–7) in their performances relates to his earlier insistence that "there is one element you could isolate in any account you give [of children's *paideia*], and this is the correct formation of our feelings of pleasure and pain. . . . Call this 'education,' and I . . . think you would be giving it its proper name" (653b6–c4). Saunders (1991) contends that metics receive occupational training alone (215), hence no genuine *paideia*, yet stresses that "licensed" teachers "approach quite closely to citizens" (214). As Plato stands firmly behind building good character through early *paideia*, it is to be expected that metics, having some capacity for *aretê*, will receive guidance in this direction when they like other human beings are most impressionable. Plato's esteem for metic teachers and this manifestation of a broader concern for metics' upbringing are thus mutually consistent.

More generally, the *Laws* stresses that virtue is not the exclusive province of citizens, including even slaves in this expansion (e.g., 936b, 777e, 919c–d). In a

---

[53] For 794a–b as encompassing noncitizens, see also Morrow (1939, 44; 1993, 328); Guthrie (1978, 349).

[54] See 665c; Morrow (1939, 44).

notable passage, Plato observes that when the legislator wants to dampen an appetite (*tina epithumian*, 838d4) such as that for sexual indulgence, "he must try to make everyone—slave and free, women and children, and the entire state without any exception—believe that [the circumscription of sexual activity] has sacred backing" (838d6–8). This law, introduced for sexuality (d8–e1), is then extended to related desires. In particular, it is commended because it also "discourages excesses in food and drink" (839a8–b1). The Big Three *epithumiai*—a key soul-based trio from the *Gorgias* on—are thus expressly encompassed. Noteworthy is Plato's emphatic mention of those able to appreciate the law as spanning "slave and free [the latter term covering citizens and metics], women and children, and the entire state without any exception" (*doulois te kai eleutherois kai paisi kai gunaixi kai holêi têi polei kata ta auta*, 838d7–8). Moreover, his reference to the "spontaneous unanimity" (*to toiouton ethelontas legein pantas*, e2–3) resulting from a shared conviction about these *epithumiai* suggests a real contribution by noncitizens to Magnesia's unity here that is not, as may occur in Kallipolis, imposed through force from without (*Republic* 589d–590d).[55] In keeping with his belief in noncitizens' capacities of a kind where virtue is concerned, Plato stresses that the telos of punishment for all deemed curable—both citizen and noncitizen—is their moral improvement (854d–e).

Regarding self-control and metics specifically, while Athens' resident aliens paid an annual tax of twelve drachmas[56]—with exemptions a rarity[57]—Magnesia's metics are asked solely to evince *sôphrosunê* (self-control, 850b). Whitehead (1977, 68n122) posits as the backdrop here for the *Laws* that "*kosmiotes* and *sophrosune* is evidently a *cliché* coupling." This is far from "a *cliché* coupling" for Plato, however, whose account of *aretê* and *eudaimonia* in the *Gorgias* equated *sôphrones* (self-controlled people) with *kosmioi* (orderly ones; 493d2 with d7). Regarding the *Laws*, Whitehead (131, 137n25) wrongly depreciates Plato's inclusion of *sôphrosunê* as, apart from professional expertise, the sine qua non of one's admission to Magnesia

[55] Cf. *Statesman* 311c. The *Laws* does not relax Plato's view of the Big Three as essentially deleterious beyond the circumscribed, strictly monitored exploitation of negative affects through drinking games that serve moral education, viewed by Plato as a lifelong affair. On drinking games, see 639d–653a, 673e–674c. Though the measure itself is new, Plato's goal, as always, is to maximize self-control (673e) and communal unity (640b–d). Having emphasized drinking games' poor management to date (639d–e), the Athenian straightaway (640a) begins his corrective account, central to which is that their director must not imbibe (640d) in order that suitable order and discipline be maintained. On the *Laws*' pedagogical use of affects like shame, see Frede (2010).

[56] See Morrow (1993, 148).

[57] See Whitehead (1977, 12–14).

as a metic.[58] Given Plato's focus on *aretê* (virtue) and specific legal provisions—including metics' consultation in setting profit margins—his stress on *sôphrosunê* here is surely not pro forma. Thus construed, the *Laws*' positive stance toward noncitizens' capacity for *aretê*, especially that of metics, diverges markedly from his palpable worry about producers' ability to attain any meaningful semblance of *sôphrosunê*.

Moreover, the *Laws*, building on the *Statesman*, displays an appreciative attitude toward craftwork itself:[59] "The class of craftsmen who have enriched our lives by their arts and skills will have Athena and Hephaestus as its patrons while Ares and Athena will be patrons of those who protect the products of these craftsmen (*dêmiourgoi*) by . . . the techniques of defense. . . . Both classes are in the continuous service of land and people" (920d7–e5). At 921d, Plato links generals, along with "other experts in military techniques," to craftsmen in the familiar sense: "These persons are just as much craftsmen (*dêmiourgois*) as ordinary workmen, though of a different kind."[60] His folding of such folk into the broad genus of "craftsmen" (*dêmiourgoi*) is noteworthy and goes some way toward combating the negative weight that Whitehead (1977, 131) gives to Magnesian metics, unlike those in Athens, not performing martially. While the Principle of Specialization applied to citizens includes military service, the role of craftsman precludes it. Rather than tying traditional craftsmen to martial activity via performance, the two specialties' association here lauds craftsmen's own.

Moreover, numerous provisions of Magnesia's legal code itself show greater confidence in and respect for noncitizens, particularly metics, than Plato had displayed regarding Kallipolis' producers. The dialogues differ in that the *Republic* does not contain formal legal provisions. This difference is, however, insignificant here since the issue is what the *Laws*' supplying of them regarding noncitizens—especially metics, including doctors—reflects about shifts in Plato's view of what those dubbed producers in Kallipolis are capable of, entitled to, and so on.

Metics are to aid other Magnesians based on their professional expertise, as when Plato stipulates that "a passerby with the knowledge and ability to expose [one who

---

[58] Based on the argument of this chapter, I diverge from the claim of Bobonich (2002, 69) that in the *Laws* Plato "explicitly expresses a very bleak view of the ethical capacities" of those who functioned as producers, including metics, whose value in Magnesia lies merely in their labor (cf. 378) and who are otherwise "excluded from the city." Saunders (1962) rightly contends that Plato's estimate of producers' psychic abilities is low (47). However, his deprecatory estimate of Magnesia's noncitizens (43, 55), central to which is his close assimilation of metics and slaves (43n1), is called into question by the evidence involving virtue that I present.

[59] Regarding the *Laws* on this point, cf. Schofield (2006a, 97n92); Morrow (1993, 145).

[60] Cf. 643c–d, where Plato links children's play at once with craftwork and military skill.

sells a defective item] should prove his case before the authorities and . . . may then take the faulty article for himself (*pheresthô to kibdêleuthen*)" (917d1–3). Those in this position include metics who, due to their grasp of crafts or retail practices, share a responsibility regarding justice that transcends their direct involvement in them. Whitehead (1977, 139n53) dismisses this duty to expose as supporting metics' occupation with gain alone. Whitehead's account, however, fails to do justice to the defectiveness of items coming into metics' possession—which would seem to exclude prospective ownership as sufficient motivation—and to the fact that they cannot be blindly gripped by wealth if Plato treats testimony from them as central when setting profit margins.

As we saw above concerning the Big Three *epithumiai* (838d–839b), noncitizens have responsibilities involving communal unity apart from their professional engagement. Other such duties are lodged with them, as when it is stipulated by law that a metic who assists a parent or grandparent assaulted by a child who is not insane will sit up front at the games (881b)—this being decidedly nonpecuniary recognition. In addition, anyone, free (i.e., citizen or foreigner) or slave, who observes it must report mistreatment of parents if the victim himself is unable to do so (932d). Moreover, both free persons and slaves are obliged to report the theft of buried treasure. Free persons thereby gain a reputation for *aretê*, with the opposite reputation produced by failures to act (913d–914a). While Plato does not specify what would constitute "some notable service to the state" (850b6–7) allowing extensions of metics' twenty-year sojourns in Magnesia, the grounds will certainly include the sorts of things detailed above.[61] The aforementioned scenarios have noncitizens' acting, sometimes physically, against their sociopolitical superiors and involve others' greed. Mutatis mutandis given guardians' (i.e., philosophers' and auxiliaries') lack of families in Kallipolis, such a scenario involving producers and their superiors was not envisioned, and a fortiori not provided for, in the *Republic*.

Further, Plato's stipulations regarding homicide of foreigners show a measure of respect for the value of those existences. As Morrow (1941, 40) observes, "Platonic law gives the life of the foreigner the same protection as that afforded the citizen." Measures concerning voluntary homicide, including the right to bring suit, apply

[61] Those permitted to remain, perhaps for life, "must be allowed to enjoy to the full whatever concessions the state bestows" (850c2–3). On the intriguing suggestion of Morrow (1939, 102), the twenty-year sojourn "was intended by Plato to be a period of probation, permitting the state to select intelligently its permanent *metic* population." On the rare occasions that Athenian metics became citizens, the shift served mainly as "a tool of international diplomacy" (Whitehead 1977, 159). As the Principle of Specialization precludes the assumption of a second *ergon*, extensions of residency are the *Laws*' functional equivalent—and here the motive is not expediency but true recognitions of merit.

whether the killing happened or was merely planned (871e–872b). The same respect is shown by Plato's provision for self-defense, including situations where foreigners protect themselves from citizens (869c–d, cf. 879d–e). As at 932d, the paramount distinction is between slave and free, with citizens and foreigners, in particular metics, comprising the latter class.[62] The *Republic*'s counterpart, which is unthinkable, would involve Plato's moving toward parity by recognizing the import of existences across what is there a vigorous guardian-producer divide.

The *Laws* deviates from Athenian practice here in a way favorable to metics, our own focus of attention, since it handled intentional killings of foreigners and citizens in separate courts and did not differentiate penalties for involuntary versus deliberate acts against the former.[63] Saunders (1991, 250–51) aptly stresses the salience of the *Laws*' innovation: "According the foreigner the same protection from homicide as a citizen, by punishing a person who kills a foreigner on the same basis as one who kills a citizen, strengthens the distinction between slave and free man that is fundamental to the code."[64] As he (236, 238) observes, moreover, Magnesia's provisions concerning sureties (871e–872b) represent a move toward equality in the legal treatment of foreigner and citizen. In yet another such move, there is no trace of the citizen *prostatês* (sponsor), who was crucial to metics' ability to negotiate life in Athens, including its judicial system. Plato's conscious elimination of this figure "considerably enlarged the extent of the metic's legal capacity" (Morrow 1941, 42).[65]

Importantly, metics themselves are consulted on certain legislative and judicial matters. The *Republic* will not legislate about business affairs (425c–d). Insofar as Kallipolis has regulations, philosophers are their exclusive source (425d–e). The *Laws* not only legislates about such things, but practitioners are consulted in the formulation of provisions bearing directly on their work. Plato notes, for example, that "market wardens and guardians of the laws, having ascertained from experts the details of the adulterations and malpractices of sellers, should record in writing rules that specify what vendors must and must not do," which regulations will be on display outside the office of the market wardens (917e–918a). In addition, those excelling in sanctioned pursuits are to meet with the guardians of the laws

---

[62] On this topic, cf. 729e–730a, 865a–866d. Slaves too are offered express legal protections (872c, 932d).

[63] See Morrow (1941, 40); Whitehead (1977, 93–94); Saunders (1991, 107, 238).

[64] On Magnesia's legal provisions more generally as "accentuat[ing] the distinction between slave and freeman"—and this despite their also giving slaves a broader role in law enforcement than accrued to them in Athens—see Morrow (1939, 127–28).

[65] On the Athenian *prostatês*, see also Whitehead (1977, 90–91); Hunter (2000, 16–17). As Hunter observes, the Athenian requirement, including enslavement for lacking this figure (19), reinforced what was a marked citizen-metic distinction (17).

to determine "what ratio of expenditure to receipts will give the retailer a decent profit," which provisions are then displayed publicly and implemented (920b–c).[66]

Plato's reliance on practitioners' input here is striking indeed, given the importance he places on Magnesia's precluding wealth and the lust for same.[67] Those applying for admission to the city as metics will doubtless be a self-selecting group, since Plato's provisions "effectively purge [the pertinent] occupations of the potential for 'exorbitant gain' . . . that is the reason for supposing commerce to be morally dangerous in the first place" (Meyer 2003, 211). Indeed, "in the controlled economy of Magnesia, the livelihood of the craftsmen places them at no greater risk of [becoming obsessed with wealth] than the citizen farmers" (ibid.). Plato's insistence on metics' *sôphrosunê* is not only not pro forma but illustrates the superiority of their self-control to what Kallipolis' producers may reliably attain. In the *Republic*'s terms, Plato would be giving a say to producers, deeply prone to governance by appetite, including a desire for wealth, when the ground rules of their work were forged. Given Plato's mistrust of their psychic orientation, his allocating this responsibility to them is inconceivable.

Plato makes multifaceted provision for noncitizens' role in court (e.g., 932d, 937a–b, 938b–c, 954e–955a). Stressing equity among *eleutheroi*, Plato stipulates that "whenever an alien prosecutes an alien, the trial should be held under the same rules [as those for citizens]" (949c4–5).[68] This parity between foreigner and citizen in the conduct of suits would correspond to equality between producers and guardians in the outlets they had for claims of improper treatment. Once again, a measure incorporated in Magnesia would be unthinkable in Kallipolis.

Finally, within the metic class there is evidence that exemplary doctors stand above others, including craftspeople who generate material goods and traders who purvey them.[69] First, one may recur to Plato's description of medicine's distinguished practice, discussed in Section 3, which foregrounds its satisfaction of the *Gorgias*' *technê* criteria. In addition, while the foregoing provisions regarding metics cover physicians as members of that larger group, a striking measure involves doctors specifically. They will constitute a jury (916a–b) when controversies arise

[66] Cf. Morrow (1993, 144).

[67] Cf. 918a–e, where Plato observes that the practice of "retailing [and] trade" (d6–7) is not inherently corrupting and automatic evidence of vice in its practitioners.

[68] See Saunders (2004, 526, sec. 25, n15).

[69] Edelstein (1987b, 87) observes that the typical Hippocratic doctor, qua "businessman," was viewed as "the equal of the other craftsmen and thereby occupies a low position in society." The *Laws*, in contrast, marks doctors off from craftspeople qua artifact producers, etc. (see, e.g., 903c5–6). By so doing, Plato arguably attempts from a different vantage point what Hippocratic authors themselves at times assayed, as evidenced, e.g., by *Regimen* I's marked privileging of medicine over *technai* such as cobblery (15) and basket-making (19).

concerning the sale to nonspecialists of slaves with "consumption, stone, strangury or the so-called sacred disease [i.e., epilepsy] or some other mental or physical complaint that is chronic and difficult to cure and that the ordinary man could not diagnose" (*ean tis andrapodon apodôtai kamnon phthoêi ê lithôn ê strangouriôn ê têi kaloumenêi hierâi nosôi ê kai heterôi tini adêlôi tois pollois nosêmati makrôi kai dusiatôi kata to sôma ê kata tên dianoian*, a4–7). Both cases where experts sell to laypeople and those where both parties fall under the latter head "should be heard before a bench of three doctors appointed by joint nomination of the parties," with recompense in guilty verdicts tied to whether the vendor was an expert or a layman (b5–c3).

Since metics consulted about financial strictures (917e–918a, 920b–c) are not also appointed as enforcers of justice, Plato's assigning this role to doctors renders them unique among noncitizens. Where slaves' vendors are medical laypeople, doctors will sit in judgment of citizens, their sociopolitical superiors. Physicians' jury service constitutes an advance by comparison with Athenian praxis, for, as Aristotle observes (*Politics* 1278a37–38), metics possessed no *timai* (offices), including "*to dikazein*, the right to sit on a jury. . . . No amount of lesser concessions compensate for [such] basic exclusions" (Whitehead 1977, 70). As doctors are among producers in Kallipolis, in the *Republic*'s terms, the *Laws*' provision would have doctors exercising power over guardians, whose authority over producers is depicted there as absolute. Thus, doctors' comprising a jury, like the aforementioned stipulations involving metics generally, would be unheard of in the *Republic*. Finally, as noted above, this instance of physicians' involvement in determinations of justice represents a clear expansion of their duties from the *Republic*'s staunch refusal to have doctors promote this value beyond performing their naturally fitting occupational role. More generally, at *Laws* 916a–b, for the first and only time in Plato, doctors participate in the task of judging.

Furthermore, since disturbances of *dianoia* (here, "mental functioning") are a mitigating circumstance in criminal proceedings[70]—as at 881b, where it matters vis-à-vis justice whether a progenitor's attacker is mad or sane—given Plato's confidence in good physicians, their role as jury in 916a–b, and the great salience of motive to his penology, they will likely be called upon in especially difficult cases to aid juries in discerning offenders' states of mind.[71] In such cases, possible defendants once again include citizens.

---

[70] *Dianoia* here has a broader meaning than when the term is used of mathematicians' cognition as treated in the *Republic*'s Divided Line (510b–511d), where it involves stepwise reasoning from ultimate principles to particular conclusions.

[71] On the extension, see also Amundsen and Ferngren (1977, 212).

Taken in sum, the foregoing developments in Magnesia result either in doctors' sole placement at the top of the metic class or in their sharing of this honor with the teachers who preside over children's *paideia*. Either way, physicians' standing is notable and far surpasses the regard shown them in Kallipolis.

6. THE *GORGIAS*' UNCERTAINTY RESOLVED

In the *Republic*, philosophers' oversight is required in cases of serious illness, including those where time and effort are needed to discern how far, if at all, a condition is remediable. Since during this period the individual could not perform his naturally fitting occupational role, as with conditions known to be terminal or chronic, treatment should not be provided. The second type of case where philosophers supervise involves psychic irreparability. While individuals in the former class will not be treated, those in the latter are to be killed (409e–410a). In both cases, philosophers' assessments of patients' standing ground conclusions about whether technically feasible measures comport with what is best for both the individual and the community (*to . . . ariston . . . autois te tois paschousin kai têi polei*, a5–6). The result is that doctors are sometimes precluded from deploying their expertise to foster health, as when diagnostic periods yield curable conditions or psychically defective persons have treatable medical conditions.

While putting individuals to death is discussed in the *Laws*, letting die is not considered. The one conceivably relevant passage is 761c–d, where Plato states that young men are to establish "in every quarter gymnasia for themselves and senior citizens, including warm baths for the old folk,[72] and lay up a large stock of thoroughly dry wood. All this will help to relieve those who are ill, and farmers wearied by the labor of the fields—and it will be a much kinder treatment than the tender mercies of an ignorant physician (*iatrou dexin mê panu sophou beltiona suchnôi*)." For those who are ailing, warm baths' soothing properties will likely be of greater aid than the measures of inferior practitioners.[73] Plato's formulation, "a much kinder treatment than the tender mercies of an ignorant physician" (d3), makes clear that 761c–d does not encompass the sound doctors of 719e–720e and 857c–e, whose apprehension of health is lauded and who would surely know what was feasible in the relevant types of cases. The thought here appears to be that since poor practitioners lack the knowledge of health that grounds reliable provisions of benefit, it is safer for patients if measures taken aim to soothe (i.e., comprise palliative care) irrespective of whether this was all that could be done to improve the condition of elderly folk

[72] In modifying Saunders' rendering I follow England (1921, 573).

[73] For this line of interpretation, see England (ibid.).

and those tired and sore from working the land.[74] Since Plato's comment at 761c–d is restricted to poor operators, he is not led to make the medical practitioner as such dependent on someone else. Whatever limits on treatment may be implied here, Plato indicates no lack of confidence in physicians' ability to reach fitting diagnoses, prognoses, and treatment regimens.

Further, there is reason to think that the *Laws* is more generous than the *Republic* regarding what would count as impairments meriting treatment. According to Burkholder (1978, 34), Plato must revise the Principle of Specialization since it "radically underestimates the extent to which re-education can develop latent talents." While Burkholder's comment, made of the *Republic*, also applies to the *Laws*, it ignores the fact that the latter's version of the principle is more generous. Nowhere in the *Laws* are we told, as with the carpenter in *Republic* III, that what is feasible with healing in view should not be done. Though an argument from silence is not decisive, this particular silence fits with the *Laws*' revised Principle of Specialization, which does not identify one's naturally appropriate function, and hence one's communal and human merit, with an occupational role narrowly construed. Even when an elderly person can no longer foster communal welfare directly, there is no suggestion that his life lacks value altogether, as would be the case in Kallipolis. In fact, an indirect way in which such lives continue to possess value is through the opportunity they provide for the young to cultivate filial respect (930e–932a) as part of character formation. The penalties for neglect of parents—those "treasures old and frail" (931a5)—are serious indeed (932a–d). Unstinting regard for one's progenitors also fosters the reverence for elders generally that Plato stresses (690a, 714e). As for direct contributions, being a citizen of Magnesia encompasses a wide range of activities. An incapacitation (temporary or permanent) for some contributions (e.g., the rigors of certain official positions) need not mean a lack of fitness for all (e.g., bringing wrongdoers to authorities' attention). Insofar as factors beyond the strictly medical figure in such treatment decisions, the *Laws* gives one no reason to think that they cannot be addressed by good doctors from within the clinical tie on my account of it in this chapter.

The *Republic*'s rigid notion of how a person fosters Kallipolis' welfare is at odds with Hippocratic writings. The *Laws*' more generous notion is appreciably closer to what one finds in medical authors, who regularly take for granted that individuals'

---

[74] The Hippocratic Corpus notes palliative care in extremity (*Diseases* III 1). For baths of water or vapor as a treatment in medical writings, see *Diseases* II 12–14, 47, 67, 73; III 2–3, 12, 16; *Regimen* II 57; III 72; IV 89; *Regimen in Acute Diseases* 68; *On Joints* 47; *Internal Affections* 1, 10. Some doctors would diverge from Plato's suggestion that baths can do no harm. On context dependency in their provision, see *Regimen in Acute Diseases* 65–67; *Internal Affections* 39–40.

physical impediments associated, for example, with amputations and clubfoot do not deprive those so afflicted of their human worth. Moreover, such impairments need not do away with people's ability to undertake useful work. Some may, with adjustments, be able to perform the same tasks as before: "Manual exercise contributes greatly to good flesh-development in hand and arm. In fact, taking all sorts of handiwork, the weasel-armed are ready to do with this one most of what they can do with the other arm, and do the work no less efficiently than with the sound limb" (*On Joints* 53). If the impairment renders pursuit of the same work infeasible, other jobs may be found. For instance,

> in adults, when the shoulder is dislocated and not reduced, its point is less fleshy than usual and this part assumes a lean habit. Still, when they cease to suffer pain, though as regards all such work as requires raising the elbow outwards from the side they are unable to do it as before, any work such as involves moving the arm either backwards or forwards along the side they can execute. For they might work a bow-drill or saw, and might use a pick or spade without much raising of the elbow, and so with all other tasks that are done in such attitudes. (12)[75]

Concerning *psuchê*, although the *Laws* is more nuanced than the *Republic* and *Gorgias* in its handling of impairments, it is equally stern on the irreparably corrupt. It would be best if there were no occasion for putting vicious, recalcitrant individuals to death (627d–e), and Magnesia's institutions, resting on an edifice of law, aim to keep those cases to a minimum. By comparison with the *Gorgias* and *Republic*, the *Laws* adds both to the scenarios that properly elicit remedial efforts and to those warranting death. The *Laws*' foregrounding of attempted salutary work pre-condemnation puts it at odds with the *Republic*, which gave the impression that philosophers, with unlimited room to judge people psychically incurable, would often if not always reach those decisions quickly. The *Laws*' account is closer in spirit to the *Gorgias* (see especially 480a–c), which stressed remedial efforts, without, however, showing what these would comprise. Although the *Gorgias*' psychic *technai* included preventive and restorative endeavors, legislation and judging respectively, that dialogue did not address the role of legislation. The *Laws* fleshes out the *Gorgias*'

[75] Jouanna (1999, 112–17), who lauds Hippocratic doctors' "humanism" (116), discusses both doctors' treating slave and free and their work with ordinary craftspeople. On doctors' care for those who serve others, see *Epidemics* I 15, 21; II 4.5; IV 9, 13, 32–33, 38, 50–52; V 19, 25, 35, 41, 85, 87. A foreigner is attended to in *Epidemics* IV 17. For craftspeople or their family members as patients, see *Epidemics* IV 20e–f, 23, 29; V 1, 45, 59; VI 3.8; *Prorrhetic* I 123.

distinction via the twofold nature of Magnesian *nomoi* (laws). While the preludes to individual provisions and the code itself motivate people to self-willed obedience via rational persuasion, the text of the laws not only stipulates how violations will be handled but arguably attempts to stave off violations by detailing the penalties on tap for those who do not comply.

Even with Magnesia's vast framework in place, exigencies are bound to arise, and the city's legal code makes provision for them. The *Laws* retains Plato's earlier distinction between reparable and incurable psychic conditions. Further, as before, the lives of the incurable—harmful to themselves and the community—will be terminated on grounds of justice: "The cases that are reparable we must cure. . . . But suppose the lawgiver finds a man who's beyond cure—what legal penalty will he provide for this case? He will recognize that the best thing for all such people is to cease to live—best even for themselves" (862c–e).

In the *Laws*, Plato displays a more nuanced appreciation than before of what good medical practice involves and substantially deepens his recognition of ordinary people's cognitive gifts. Magnesia's quite different and elaborate setup for fostering justice takes the weight off moments of decision bearing on health as the venue where judgments about psychic injustice must be made. With the number of households relatively small, widely dispersed responsibilities in place for promoting justice, and conduct veiled from public view being minimized as far as possible, a doctor's healing one who turns out to be psychically incurable is no longer a grave threat to society, as the person's injustice is meant and bound to be noticed by officials or community members—including doctors themselves as metics. In the *Laws*, unlike the *Republic*, there is no occasion for interference in medical decision making from without. Hence, the doctor is freed up to decide and straightaway implement what he considers to be of potential aid.

As one would expect based on this altered framework for detecting injustice, on the *Laws*' account of medicine—contra the *Republic*'s, where judges (i.e., philosophers) were poised to intervene (409e–410a)—the psychic domain thus construed is not a focus of treatment decisions. Unlike the *Republic*, the *Laws* clearly demarcates psychic failings involving virtue, for which people remain accountable, from liabilities comprising disruptions of *dianoia* (mental functioning), among which are delirium, senility, and insanity (881b, 916a–b, 925e–926b, 928e–929e, 934c–d). As we saw in Chapter 2, the latter class of psychic conditions is often referenced in medical writings.[76] The *Laws* not only distinguishes disruptions of mental functioning

[76] In the earlier chapter, delirium and madness were addressed. While medical writers pursue "mental disorder" generally, which they explain physiologically (see Drabkin 1955, 226, 229), one finds virtually no reference to dementia in the aged (see Finley 1981, 170; cf. Karenberg and Förstl 2006, 6).

(*dianoia*) from *adikia* (injustice), but in keeping with the dialogue's concern to calibrate punishments to offenders' psychic standing, disturbances of *dianoia*, unlike vice, are a mitigating factor at sentencing (864d–e). As Saunders (1991, 159) observes, Plato is at pains to distinguish "recompense, which is non-penal," from the "penalty proper." Penalties are not imposed on those whose *dianoia* is disrupted, since they do not meet the criterion that "the state of mind identified caused the offender to offend while in full possession of his faculties, with full and deliberate intent, without over-persuasion, and 'in character'" (190).

As with Magnesian doctors and jury service, an ostensibly small innovation comprising medicine and disruptions of *dianoia* reflects a notable extension of doctors' competence compared with the *Gorgias* and *Republic*. While the *Gorgias* clearly separated *technai* addressing bodily conditions from those occupied with soul (464b–c), the *Republic*'s handling of judges' oversight of medicine and psychic conditions (409e–410a) did not distinguish causative scenarios past that binary. The *Laws*' extension of doctors' sphere to include a portion of what falls under *psuchê* is thus important intra-Platonically. What is more, doctors, as metics, may help uncover *adikia*.

Medicine in the *Laws* thus makes palpable inroads respecting justice and *psuchê*. As previously observed, the dialogue's innovations support either our location of medicine atop the metic group or our identification of it as sharing that rank with children's metic teachers, whose use of the *Laws* as their pedagogical text reflects Plato's high estimation of them.

In the *Gorgias*, "injustice, lack of discipline, and all other kinds of psychic corruption are the very worst thing of all" (477e4–6)—far outpacing misfortune and misery tied to disease (477e–480d). As medicine's purview does not include justice, whose realization is vital to thriving, it cannot reside at the pinnacle of *technai*. What the *Gorgias* leaves uncertain is whether this state of affairs will be addressed through a direct curtailing of medical enactments from without (*Republic*) or indirectly, via sociopolitical shifts that eliminate medicine as a place where injustice is singled out (*Laws*).

In the *Laws*, as in the *Gorgias* and *Republic*, a life is not worth preserving if that would undermine justice,[77] and in its legal provisions a distinction between curable and incurable criminals figures prominently. What has shifted in the *Laws*, compared with the *Republic*, are the sociopolitical mechanisms through which Plato expects psychic injustice to be illumined. In Magnesia, the unjust—including those incurably so, whom Kallipolis would execute when found in the health-care setting—are to be singled out through other, strongly complementary agencies.

[77] See 707d, 727c–d, 854c, 874d.

Only in the *Laws*, then, is medicine presented as operating in a sphere unto itself in the sense that what the good physician deems medically practicable he may implement straightaway. Burkholder's (1978, 32n12) contention that "the physician himself must decide whether a patient would benefit from treatment" thus applies not to the *Republic* and *Laws* but solely to the latter. Plato's final dialogue resolves the *Gorgias'* uncertainty in medicine's favor, allowing it truly to be a self-standing *technê*. Having shown the *Laws'* centrality to Plato's own handling of medicine, I shall now argue that it provides a collaborative model of the doctor-patient tie and its social embedment that warrants fuller inclusion in contemporary reflections.

7

Plato's Legacy to Contemporary Bioethics

1. INTRODUCTION

For the first time in the history of bioethics as a discipline, the possible contributions of ancient philosophy are receiving notable attention. While this turn began with bioethicists (Kuczewski and Polansky 2000, ix), specialists in ancient philosophy have now entered the discussion.

Thus far Aristotle, particularly his concept of *phronêsis* (practical wisdom), has been the primary focus of attention.[1] Aristotle is often misappropriated, however, as when *phronêsis* is celebrated for favoring elastic context dependency over objectivism and hence is lauded as an antidote to rigidity about governing principles and doctrinal asymmetry favoring medicine's practitioners. In contrast to Aristotle's frequent mention, not only does Plato's *agôn* with medicine remain underappreciated by scholars of ancient philosophy, but his promise is nearly untapped by those working to illuminate what ancient philosophy can offer bioethics regarding the clinical tie and its societal embedment.

A persistent difficulty confronting proposed alternatives to extremes of autonomy and paternalism has been surpassing the notion of pronounced intellectual and values asymmetry favoring doctors. In the next two sections of this

[1] Though recourse to Aristotle has centered on broad grounds involving *phronêsis* and communitarianism, he has also been tied to specific topics (e.g., abortion, regarding which see Megone 2000; Kuczewski 2000).

chapter, I discuss two prominent contemporary proposals, both of which evince marked paternalism, and show recourse to Aristotle as inapposite. Subsequently, I argue that reflection on Plato yields four criteria that a genuinely collaborative model must meet and suggest how the *Laws* addresses them. It is thus via Plato, not Aristotle, that ancient philosophy is helpful as a reference point once one rejects paternalism and recognizes that tying autonomy in our sense to antiquity is anachronistic. While Plato's discussions will not solve our own quandaries, they suggest how we might retain asymmetry of a kind without capitulating to familiar oppositional modalities. The result is that the *Laws* merits fuller inclusion in bioethical discussions than it has heretofore received. Though I will concentrate on that dialogue, I also address what we may learn from the trajectory of Plato's engagement with medicine across the *Gorgias*, *Symposium*, *Republic*, *Statesman*, and *Laws*.

2. ENTRENCHMENT IN BIOETHICS' QUEST FOR ALTERNATIVES: TWO PROMINENT ILLUSTRATIONS

In 1959, Karl Jaspers, a prominent philosopher and political thinker, wrote of a crisis in medicine. Many since then have echoed that sentiment, attending particularly to a setting in which the principle of patient autonomy has come to the fore in medical practice.[2] As Emanuel and Emanuel (1992) observe, one may frame the tension between paternalism and autonomy, historically the mainstays of bioethical attention to the doctor-patient tie, as a contest—in Greek terms, an *agôn*—over whose values should trump, the doctor's or those of the patient: "This struggle forces us to ask, What should be the ideal physician-patient relationship?" (2221).[3]

In addition to the overarching contest between autonomy and paternalism, oppositional constructions of the doctor-patient tie are integral to both models.[4] Decision making under the sway of autonomy is always potentially adversarial (Pellegrino and Thomasma 1993, 129–30), as when the disclosure of risks to patients

[2] As Walker (2009b) observes, what is meant by "autonomy" is not often expressly considered (340). She contrasts "the standard view" with what she dubs "rational autonomy." What typically passes for autonomous decision making, "simply informing patients about treatment options and probable outcomes" (359), will often not meet this higher standard; it need not follow, however, that decisions arrived at thereby will be barred from implementation (360; cf. Walker 2009a). Handling of this concept is limited to what is required for the present study.

[3] Brody (1992) stresses a traditional, endemic agonism governing medicine seen through the lens of power. I coin the term "agonism" (versus simply using "antagonism") to bring out the ongoing relevance of the notion of *agôn*.

[4] For valuable emphasis on the inherence of tension between and within the models, see Koppelman-White (2009, 448, 452, 455, 457, 466).

(e.g., from surgical procedures) is pro forma and aimed squarely at circumventing doctors' legal liability (Katz 1984, 81–82). In addition, physicians may defer to patients' autonomy "as a way of evading moral responsibility" (Callahan 2012, 83). Moreover, an extreme preoccupation with autonomy foregrounds conflict in ways that devastate the idea of communal thriving (Pellegrino and Thomasma 1993, 131). With autonomy, clashes in values seem preempted in patients' favor even as doctors' values actually continue to govern the content and manner of what is conveyed (Pellegrino and Thomasma 1993, 56–57; Stalley 1980, 21).[5]

With paternalism, there is an extra level. Caretaking "metaphors" (e.g., that of parent and child) suggest that substantive discord is illusory and harmony of purpose real because the doctor's knowledge and experience, channeled by her good will, warrant patients' trust in the merit of her contributions.[6] On this scenario, opposed values and priorities—which occupy a third tier beneath this "accord"—evade direct awareness and hence critical engagement (see Katz 1984, 98–100).

While collaborative proposals avoiding the extremes of autonomy and paternalism are badly needed,[7] efforts thus far have failed to stake out genuine alternatives. To illustrate this state of affairs, I focus on accounts offered by Emanuel and Emanuel (1992) and Pellegrino and Thomasma (1993). Each combines stress on our need to transcend existing oppositional models with an articulation of its own optimal successor. Far from coming off as genuinely collaborative, however, both treatments evince values paternalism. If tilting is to occur in attempts to forge alternatives, this direction is unsurprising, for it fits with a current predisposition to downplay autonomy, which has had several decades to occupy center stage. This trajectory is unsurprising, too, from medicine's standpoint as a profession, since a notion of doctors' superior insight and relevant values' apprehension has been central to the profession's self-understanding from antiquity to the present day.[8]

Though, as I will argue, values paternalism is demonstrably its bent, the Emanuels' account is unclear about both the scope of values claims and values' metaethical standing: are they objectively binding, relativistic, or something intermediate between the two? As to standing, their "deliberative" (i.e., allegedly collaborative) physician's use of the term "best" in offering treatment recommendations (1992,

[5] Cf. Brody's (2009, 111) claim that a reliance on autonomy does not in fact dissipate "*problems of power imbalance*" (italics in original).

[6] For use of the term "metaphor" with regard to existing models, see Childress and Siegler (1984); Siegler (1985, 713).

[7] See, e.g., Brody (1992, 44, 66, 95, 123).

[8] Concerning antiquity, see especially Chapters 2–3.

2222, 2223) is ambiguous between "best for this patient given that regarding which he consulted me" and "best in a context-independent way whose merit I must bring the patient to see." This is, I submit, precisely the sort of obscurity that a truly collaborative model would shun. As their argument unfolds, the Emanuels tilt pronouncedly toward the second construction of "best"; thus, they indicate that, far from accepting values pluralism as manifested in society generally and through his dealings with a given patient, the deliberative physician seeks to "persuade the patient to adopt other values" (2224) so as to foster his "moral development" (2226). Since perspicuity and transparency regarding values' status is required for genuine collaboration, their absence from the Emanuels' account here is key.

Regarding the scope of values claims, the Emanuels do not fully appreciate how deeply continuous the patient's clinical situation is with the person's existence outside the examining room.[9] Aiming to stress a distinction in breadth between what doctors handle and human values tout court, they present the deliberative doctor as indicating "why certain health-related values are more worthy and should be aspired to" (2222).[10] On a range of occasions, however, the Emanuels work with a most expansive notion of what "health-related" values encompass[11] or jettison that limitation unwittingly. Respecting the latter, they claim that the hoped-for outcome is "a recommendation designed for the patient's specific medical *and personal* condition" (2224) and assert that the deliberative physician aims to "persuade the patient to accept this recommendation as the intervention that best promotes his or her *overall well-being*" (2225).[12] While the Emanuels reject the "interpretive" model for its exclusion of doctors' role in fostering patients' "moral development" (2226), their stress in its presentation on the doctor's helping the patient grasp how treatment choices impact "his or her identity" (2222) already shows the physician's role far surpassing "health-related" values on any circumscribed construction of that term. This unclarity about the scope of pertinent values is a reflection of just how difficult—indeed, impossible—it is to sustain that separation between values' spheres of operation to which the Emanuels expressly commit themselves when introducing the deliberative approach. In line with Plato, I submit that this point is significant, since recognizing the impossibility of such a demarcation is key to doctor-patient collaboration.

[9] This continuity was noted long ago by Peabody (1927). As Katz (1984, 96) effectively points out, the same applies to doctors' values.

[10] The locution "health-related values" appears several more times on that page, where they also identify the deliberative model as fostering "moral self-development relevant to health care."

[11] The term "expansive" is borrowed from Annas (1981, 13), who uses it of the *Republic*'s broad-based account of justice.

[12] Emphasis added in the foregoing two quotations.

While the Emanuels' description of this model foregrounds doctor-patient collaboration (2222), values asymmetry favoring the doctor is pronounced in their illustration involving a forty-three-year-old premenopausal woman with a 3.5-cm ductal carcinoma but no lymph node involvement or metastasis. The example is meant to "crystallize essential differences among the models [i.e., paternalistic, informative, interpretive, deliberative]" (2222). As they write in 1992, the medical community is uncertain whether chemotherapy benefits those whose cancer is node-negative (2223). Given this, several months of chemotherapy are a significant burden (2223). Having acknowledged that "the issue of chemotherapy is . . . fraught with conflicting data," the deliberative physician asserts that "balancing all the options, I think the best one for you is to enter a trial that is investigating the potential benefit of chemotherapy for women with node-negative breast cancer" (2223).

Having mentioned the high quality of care that study participants receive as a rationale for involvement in the clinical trial—and not considering whether the researcher-participant tie even counts as that of doctor and patient—the Emanuels defend at length a second rationale, that "to participate in a trial is altruistic" (2223). The "deliberative" doctor concludes that he has articulated "our current knowledge and offer[ed] my recommendation so you can make the best possible decision" (2223). Here, "best possible" clearly means best not merely or even primarily for this patient within her own doctor-patient tie—which optimality has not been shown—but rather best from the standpoint of scientific progress, that is, in a sense that is not ultimately about the situation that the patient seeks to address with the doctor's aid. The deliberative doctor's locution "best one for *you*" (2223) is therefore disingenuous. In fact, the Emanuels' construction fits well Koppelman-White's (2009, 451) depiction of paternalism as representing "the idea that physicians are in a better position than patients to reflect and determine the best course of action. . . . That is, the question of whether anyone has reason to act depends on whether that act, in fact, leads to what *really* has value" (italics in original). The patient's embrace of this value commitment to altruism might revise, even substantially, her self-conception and priorities. It is thus notable that the Emanuels' illustration of the deliberative model does not include discussing with the patient the ground and merits of shouldering an obligation to centrally consider others' welfare—here, unknown future persons—let alone consideration of how this revision of the patient's values would impact her priorities overall.

The Emanuels underappreciate the fact that their concerns about the inconstancy and incoherence of patients' values apply at least as well to physicians. The parties are linked, after all, as human beings inhabiting a particular historical, cultural, and sociopolitical context. They provide no reason for us to think that doctors are intrinsically better poised as human beings—or better equipped due to medical school training (1992, 2226)—to untangle others' or their own limitations concerning values development and values understanding. The Emanuels' confident envisioning of doctors as spearheading an enhancement of societal values (2226) is therefore unfounded.

Pellegrino and Thomasma (1993), too, emphasize a distinction between values and traits "internal to medicine" and the human plane tout court, claiming that they will concentrate solely on the former (134; cf. 85, 146–47). Like the Emanuels, Pellegrino and Thomasma have trouble sticking to that distinction: they contend that medicine aims to do more than restore the patient's status quo ante, hoping instead to bring him "to a state of higher *satisfaction and* health than had been reached previously" (86).[13] In addition, they observe that doctors' "own moral values"—unrestricted to the medical realm—naturally come into play in clinical care, with difficulties stemming solely from a triggering of values divergence between the parties such that the tie dissolves (97). Pellegrino and Thomasma recognize, moreover, that "in subtle ways, the virtues of the good person and of the good physician overlap. Educating for virtue in one domain undoubtedly influences the other" (176). This—with their acknowledgment of the physician's having traits "*qua* person" that are inevitably intertwined with her character as a "professional," the locution "the moral life" comprising both at once (178)[14]—renders Pellegrino and Thomasma's dissociation of these planes in their analysis misleading.

A quest for demarcation combined with an inability to make it stick goes back to the American Medical Association's original Code of Medical Ethics (1847).[15] This code takes it as gospel that doctors are the source of all values rightly governing medical practice (86, 90, 94, 103), including their conduct in the public sphere (e.g., courts, 105), and demarcates these from broader human values: medicine does not "assum[e] the office of moral and religious teaching, to add to the civilization of an entire people" (86). Soon thereafter, however, the code assumes a doctor's ability to assess "both the physical and moral state of his patient" and strongly implies mutual assessments of physicians' human, not merely professional, moral worth (88; cf. 86 and the binary virtue-vice, 95). This assumption is evinced also by the document's claim that "hasty generalization, paradox and fanciful conjectures, repudiated at all times by sound logic, are open to the severest reprehension on the still higher grounds of humanity and morals" (88–89). While the inner tension in Pellegrino and Thomasma's account is subtler, by nature it is quite similar.

---

[13] Emphasis added.

[14] Cf. Loewy (1986, 67): "The same basic person persists whether one is acting professionally or personally."

[15] For the code's grounding in Percival, a British doctor occupied with medical ethics, see Veatch (1981, 90–91); *Journal of the American Medical Association* 1965. All page references are to the Appendix of this document, which contains the "Introduction to the Code of Medical Ethics" and that code itself.

"Prudence"—stemming from Aristotelian *phronêsis* (practical wisdom), the sole intellectual virtue needed for good character—is the overarching virtue on Pellegrino and Thomasma's account (1993, 85–86, 90; cf. Pellegrino 2001, 576). As we will see further in Section 3, Aristotle's *phronimos* (person of practical wisdom) has a fine-grained capacity to see and instantiate what pertinent situations require (*Nicomachean Ethics* II, VI.5). According to Pellegrino and Thomasma, the doctor's overarching vision enables her to discern whether a patient's response to his situation is worthy of her endorsement.[16] If the doctor deems that response inadequate, paternalistic involvement is allowed. How is one to know, however, whether the situation before one fits the bill? Doctors' disagreement with patients' goals may, for instance, make them too quick to declare patients incompetent (Koppelman-White 2009, 451).

Pellegrino and Thomasma's (1993, 88) answer is simply that "in the concrete case, moral insight, or prudence as we have been describing it, is necessary if we are to do the morally best thing." Their reliance on prudence is accompanied neither by an express recognition that the distinction they draw between medical and broader values does not exist nor by a defense of the claim that doctors are specially equipped to be prudent. Pellegrino and Thomasma's own failure to demarcate the value spheres clearly despite their express goal to operate thus (85–86, 134, 146–47) suggests that one is dealing here not with virtues specific to medicine but rather—as Plato saw, indeed never doubted—with virtues simpliciter that people apply to all the realms in which they function. In that case, however, doctors emerge with no clear advantage regarding them. This is precisely the claim of Veatch (2012), whose stance, differently grounded from my own, I address in Section 11. The dominance of Pellegrino and Thomasma's physician on the metalevel means that ultimately *her* judgment determines whether the patient is acting in a fashion worthy of respect or whether, instead, his preference should be overridden.[17]

Though Pellegrino and Thomasma voice a "wish to underline the roots of any virtue theory within the community that supports the individuals" (7)—which

[16] Groll (2011) seems initially to relax this notion, but his own approach suggests a notable edge for clinicians regarding values generally (34). In addition, he blurs his own distinction (29) between "means-ends disagreements" and divergence on ends themselves. Groll claims that a doctor, like anyone else, "can see that it is crazy not to get a toe amputated on the grounds that God will cure [his] gangrene" (33). He presents this case (ibid.) as involving a clash about ends, the type of dispute he had earlier claimed was "beyond the purview of medicine and science," hence must be adjudicated "nonmedically" (30). Originally, however, this particular scenario involving gangrene was introduced as showing divergence on means to the shared end of health's restoration (28–29), in which connection doctors normally possess marked authority (29). By widening the scope of "means-ends disagreements" beyond that originally proposed, Groll invests doctors with greater values authority than had appeared to be his aim.

[17] Cf. Pellegrino (2001, 571–73), where doctors' superiority in judgment and character is also clearly evident.

sounds more promising than the Emanuels' approach respecting doctor-patient parity and the tie's societal embedment—the "moral community" whose existence they hope for throughout the book is that of the medical profession (3, 31–50, 154–57, 190). In addition, Pellegrino and Thomasma's belief in values asymmetry favoring medicine beyond the clinical setting is evinced by their claim that "were physicians to take moral leadership, the medical profession could be a model and an inspiration for the others" (39). They note, further, that "professional ethics must at times be independent of conventional morality. . . . If they use their moral power well, the professions can become paradigms of disinterested service that can raise the level of conventional morality" (144). Putting the point figuratively, they assert that fostering moral communities within professions would be "the leaven for raising the standards of conventional morality as well" (159). These statements regarding the public, the professions' impact on which would stem ultimately from medicine (39), are an expression writ large of Pellegrino and Thomasma's commitment to values asymmetry in the clinical setting, with the patient represented here by medical laypeople in aggregate.

In sum, neither of the two salient accounts treated here grounds a genuinely collaborative model. Despite the wishes of the Emanuels and Pellegrino and Thomasma to differentiate their views from prevailing oppositional approaches, both tilt markedly toward paternalism. For the present inquiry, attempts by Pellegrino and Thomasma are of special note for their appeal to Aristotle as a central guide. As the following section will show, Pellegrino and Thomasma's veering into paternalism as they invoke this ancient backdrop is no accident, instead dovetailing tightly with the cast of Aristotle's account in the *Nicomachean Ethics*.

3. AVOIDING SCYLLA AND CHARYBDIS: ARISTOTLE TO THE RESCUE?

Aristotle's ethics, especially the notion of *phronêsis* (practical wisdom), is often said to inspire an approach to clinical medicine, not to mention health policy and public discussion of priorities, that emphasizes context-dependent decision making: "Everywhere one looks in current bioethics literature, references to Aristotle and remarks about the need for practical wisdom abound" (Kuczewski and Polansky 2000, ix).[18] Illustrating this occupation, Thomasma (2000, 82–84) takes Aristotle as inspiration and support for his own favoring of contextualism over absolutes—including greater appreciation of patients' abilities and contributions—as the lens through which medical decision making should occur. Similarly, Montgomery

[18] Specialists in ancient philosophy who have entered the mix have also focused on Aristotle and operated with assumptions about Plato broadly like those of bioethicists.

(2000) takes Aristotle to inspire a needed turn to "a narrative . . . rationality" (59) featuring particulars and situational differences versus one's operating from a plane of generality (60, 62).[19] The foregoing examples, which are just the tip of the iceberg that is Aristotle's invocation here, suffice to set the stage for my critique of his deployment and subsequent defense of Plato's import.

I will argue that far from being a tight bioethical fit, Aristotle's notion of *phronêsis* and its accomplished possessor, the *phronimos* (person of practical wisdom), most naturally reinforces the very asymmetry in medical paternalism that contemporary attempts to find middle ground aim to avoid. I focus here on Aristotle's notion of context dependency, which is doctrinal and objectivist, and his view of the relation between intellect and exemplary character in the *Nicomachean Ethics* (hereafter, *NE*), his core ethical treatise (where "ethics" derives from *êthos*, meaning "character").[20]

The Doctrine of the Mean, introduced in Book II, Chapter 6, is key to Aristotle's account of moral virtue. By that lens for character assessment, "we can experience fear, confidence, desire, anger, pity, and generally any kind of pleasure and pain either too much or too little, and in either case not properly. But to experience all this at the right time, toward the right objects, toward the right people, for the right reason, and in the right manner—that is the median and the best course, the course that is a mark of virtue (*hoper esti tês aretês*)" (1106b18–23).[21] Aristotle continues:

> There are many ways of going wrong, but only one way that is right (*to de katorthoun monachôs*). . . . We may thus conclude that virtue (*aretê*) is a characteristic involving choice and that it consists in observing the mean relative to us, a mean that is defined by a rational principle as a man of practical wisdom would use to determine it (*hôrismenêi logôi kai hôi an ho phronimos horiseien*). . . . In respect of its essence and the definition of its essential nature, virtue is a mean, but as regards what is best and what is right, it is an extreme (*kata men tên*

---

[19] See also Callahan (2012, 166). For Schultz and Carnevale (1996), "clinical *phronesis*" involves "responsibly narrating and interpreting the patient's story of illness" (189, cf. 195) and includes "incorporating knowledge of the patient as person into the best ethical and clinical decision to be made in continuing dialogue with the person as patient" (194). This endeavor necessitates "*the joint participation involving a dialogue or conversation between both parties*" (196; italics in original).

[20] On Aristotle's account, doctors themselves would not number among *phronimoi*, but this point is irrelevant here since the goal of contemporary bioethics is the application *to* medicine of Aristotelian *phronêsis*. Though I dispute her contention that Aristotle can play a grounding role, Tress (2000) rightly observes that bioethicists incorrectly invoke him in connection with their stress on narrative to ameliorate asymmetry.

[21] Cf. 1112a5–7: "A choice is praised for being directed to the proper object or for being correctly made. . . . Moreover, we make a choice of things that we definitely know to be good." Translations of the *Nicomachean Ethics* are from Ostwald (1962), with some adjustments.

> *ousian kai ton logon ton to ti ên einai legonta mesotês estin hê aretê, kata de to ariston kai to eu akrotês*). (1106b28–1107a8)

Urmson's account (1980, 161) rightly stresses the mean's lodging in character, not action, and hence the level of discernment needed in the morally accomplished (i.e., the *phronimos*):

> In his definition [Aristotle] says that excellence of character is a settled state in a mean; thus an emotion or action is in a mean if it exhibits a settled state that is in a mean. The man whose character is such that he feels only mild annoyance at a trivial slight and is enraged by torture has a character that is in a mean between one that exhibits rage on trivial as well as important occasions and one that can coolly contemplate the greatest outrages. On each occasion his reaction exhibits a mean state, and thus his actions are on each occasion in a mean.
>
> To have one's emotions and actions in a mean, says Aristotle, is to feel and manifest each emotion at such times, on such matters, toward such people, for such reasons, and in such ways as are proper. To diverge from the mean in the direction of deficiency is as much not to experience and exhibit emotions at all when one should, or not about matters about which one should, or not toward people toward whom one should as it is to exhibit the emotions to the wrong degree. The same holds of the defect of excess, *mutatis mutandis*.

It is true that practical human endeavors (the most central of which are ethics and politics) do not admit of a priori, or deductive, specification across the board in the way of abstract work in mathematics (*NE* II.2, VI.8). This, however, is wholly consistent with ethics' involving objectively correct responses, arrival at which necessitates that "the agent . . . consider on each occasion what the situation demands" (1104a8–9). Aristotle reinforces this objectivity in his discussion of moral responsibility, which foregrounds an appearance-reality match in the case of virtuous folk. While

> in an unqualified sense and from the standpoint of truth, the object of wish is the good (*haplôs men kai kat' alêtheian boulêton einai tagathon*), for each individual it is whatever seems good to him. Thus, what seems good to a man of high moral standards is truly the object of wish (*tôi men oun spoudaiôi to kat' alêtheian einai*). . . . A man whose standards are high judges correctly, and in each case what is truly good also appears to him to be so (*Ho spoudaios gar hekasta krinei orthôs, kai en hekastois talêthes autôi phainetai*). . . . Perhaps the chief distinction of a man of high moral standards is his ability to see the truth in each moral question since he is, as it were, the standard and measure for such

> questions (*Diapherei pleiston isôs ho spoudaios tôi talêthes en hekastois horan, hôsper kanôn kai metron autôn ôn*). (1113a23-33)[22]

In contrast, appearance and reality regularly clash for ordinary folk, who "are misled by pleasure. For though it is not the good, it seems to be (*ou gar ousa agathon phainetai*)" (1113a34–b1).

In keeping with this appearance-reality talk, Aristotle stresses the exemplary level of attainment that the *phronimos* embodies. "It is," he insists, "extremely difficult to hit the mean (*tou mesou tuchein akrôs chalepon*)" (1109a34, cf. 1109a24–25). For instance, "Anyone can get angry—that is easy—or can give away money or spend it. But to do all this to the right person, to the right extent, at the right time, for the right reason, and in the right way is no longer something easy that anyone can do. It is for this reason that good conduct is rare, praiseworthy, and noble (*spanion kai epaineton kai kalon*)" (1109a26–30, cf. 1109b12–16). The extraordinary accomplishment of the *phronimos* warrants his being all other moral agents' regulative ideal (1105b5–9): "Acts are called just and self-controlled when they are of the kind that a just or self-controlled man would perform. The just and self-controlled man, however, is not he who performs these acts, but he who, in addition, performs them in the way that just and self-controlled men do."

Absorbing from Plato, his teacher of two decades, a recognition that people's development hinges on early moral influences, Aristotle is strict with children as well as adults. Our acts have an unrelentingly cumulative impact, for good or ill: "We must see to it that our activities are of a certain kind, since any variations in them will be reflected in our characteristics" (1103b22–23, cf. b30–31). Indeed, as "a given kind of activity produces a corresponding character . . . while an unjust or a self-indulgent man initially had the possibility not to become unjust or self-indulgent . . . once he has acquired these traits it is no longer possible for him not to be what he is" (1114a8–21). Because human goodness is rooted in character, not actions, moral education pivots on people's being raised "from childhood to feel pleasure and pain at the proper things, for this is correct education" (1104b11–13, cf. 1105a10–13). Aristotle's emphasis here, following Plato, is in keeping with his foundational, normative concern not merely with people's doing the right thing but with why they do so.

Though particular action-settings of course continue to differ, once virtue has been attained, the *phronimos* weighs each context as a moral agent and finds the single right response thereto. This happens through his fitting application of general

22 On Aristotle's account, males alone can attain consummate virtue. Discussion of this view, including a comparison to Plato, would take us far afield.

truths (more on this below). Thus, "virtue, like nature, is more precise and better than any art" (1106b14–15). Moreover, virtuous people do the right thing precisely because it *is* what's correct in that situation: "An act is not performed justly or with self-control if the act itself is of a certain kind but only if, in addition, the agent has certain characteristics as he performs it. First of all, he must know what he is doing; secondly, he must choose to act the way he does and choose the act for its own sake (*kai proairoumenos di' auta*); thirdly, the act must spring from a firm and unchangeable character" (1105a28–33). For instance, rescuing a drowning child from a lake at a modest risk to oneself reflects an agent's courage only if his motivation stems directly from the act's fitness to the situation, as opposed to his performing the courageous act because he anticipates a reward in the form of a "good" that lies on an objectively lower plane of merit (e.g., a sumptuous meal or financial compensation).

I turn now to the relation of intellect to exemplary character. Consistently preserving the mean necessitates the *phronimos*' understanding universals (i.e., his knowing concepts like justice and courage) and grasping *eudaimonia* (flourishing). On Sorabji's (1980, 205–6) formulation, "the man of practical wisdom deliberates with a view not merely to particular goals but to the good life in general. . . . A picture of the good life will save him from giving away too much, or too little, or to the wrong causes, in particular instances." Acknowledging Aristotle's claim that "in actions the initiating cause is the end at which we aim, as the hypotheses are in mathematics" (1151a16–17), Sorabji observes that the *phronimos*' launching point for deliberation is "his conception of the best . . . at which he is said to aim . . . and from which his reasoning is said to start. . . . This helps to explain the statement that as soon as we have practical wisdom, we must have all the virtues together" (207). The *phronimos*' broader understanding motivates and contextualizes Aristotle's stress on the match between what appears good and really is such in the case of virtuous folk (1113a23–b1).

Again we see the sophistication and subtlety of the *phronimos*' expertise. Aristotelian *phronêsis*, understood through its possessors in *NE*, supports the *phronimos*' closer proximity to the *Republic* than to the *Laws* from the standpoint of human (in)fallibility. As I argued in Chapter 4, the *Republic* evinces no Platonic worry that irrational yearnings will exist to infect philosophers' praxis. In keeping with this, Kallipolis' shift to timocracy—metaphysically inevitable due to participants' intrinsic lack of eternality—stems from a calculative error involving the timing of procreative activity (546a–547a). Aristotle's allowance of errors by *phronimoi* is similar. That he is concerned to tightly circumscribe error in the virtuous is evident in the moral centrality of genuine post hoc "sorrow and regret" (1110b18–25, cf. 1111a19–20) if such error occurs. Aristotle demarcates involuntary action due to reasonable ignorance of, for instance, the means through which one acts (1111a4–5), where the goal is appropriate, from culpable ignorance of moral truths (1110b28–33) and non-voluntary action due, for example, to anger (1110b25–27). While involuntary action due to ignorance reflects a cognitive error, it is not errancy of intellect involving one's grasp of virtue itself, nor does the misstep evince a moral failing. As Section 6 will show, with regard particularly to character flaws, contemporary discussions of fallibility—a notable example being the Institute of Medicine's 1999 report, *To Err Is Human: Building a Safer Health System*—have thus far been more in keeping with the *Republic* and Aristotle than with the *Laws*.

Since only *phronimoi* are resolute in their rightly motivated, hence pleasurable, virtuous action, superiority in knowledge and character lies squarely with them. As bioethicists referencing Aristotle have seen (e.g., Thomasma 2000, 75, 78–79), role-modeling is key to his account of *phronêsis*. Role-modeling is not itself a bad thing; indeed, it can be a precious boon. However, the superiority of Aristotle's *phronimos* is categorical, including the precedence of the *sôphrôn* (self-controlled person, i.e., the *phronimos* directed toward the Big Three) over the *enkratês* (one who is morally strong, i.e., a doer of right only after a struggle within).[23] The upshot is that *phronêsis* applied to medicine leaves the doctor as such superior.[24] Others will try, but fail, to be *phronimoi*, since even if people's actions pass muster, this does not on its own testify to virtuous character. If one's goal is fruitful alternatives to existing models, there is danger in making pivotal Aristotle's *phronêsis*, with its intellectual and ethical centers, as do Pellegrino and Thomasma (1993).[25] Even attempts to forge middle ground between objectivism and relativism, with truths applying not invariably but "for the most part" (see Thomasma 2000, 87), fail to truly attenuate doctors' categorical supremacy. *Someone* has to decide on applications of truths to praxis and determine where valid exceptions lie. On a model inspired by Aristotle, this someone will always be the physician.

What has been said here bears also on the topic of medicine's "self-policing," that is, on the question of whether the medical profession can and should be monitored by itself alone. Legitimate, indeed requisite, concerns that would arise on the *Laws*' account of human fallibility are unlikely to surface on Aristotle's model, since the *phronimos* is the one whom others must emulate for *eudaimonia*'s sake, and his errors, like philosopher-rulers' in Kallipolis, are essentially calculative rather than involving failures of insight or character.

---

[23] As Gould (1994, 176) observes, both conditions, as well as their opposites, are *hexeis* (i.e., established dispositions) rather than the latter's being a way station on one's developmental route to the former. Further comparison of the *sôphrôn* and *enkratês* in *NE* VII falls outside this project.

[24] See also Erde's (1997, 36) critique of Pellegrino and Thomasma.

[25] See also Thomasma (2000, 84–85).

Unlike many bioethicists, Pellegrino and Thomasma rightly look to Aristotle as inspiration for their own approach to clinical medicine and the medical profession's guiding role. The problem is that Aristotle's notion of *phronêsis* buttresses paternalism. While recourse to ancient philosophy is helpful in bioethics' quest for fresh approaches to the doctor-patient tie and its social embedment, Plato is the better choice. I contend not that Aristotle is irrelevant but that Plato, in particular the *Laws*, offers a better foundation for what bioethics currently seeks.[26] As will become clear, the ultimate difficulty with Pellegrino and Thomasma's account is not that it foregrounds virtue, an approach that I too endorse, but rather how their focus on virtue is deployed.

4. BIOETHICS AND PLATO THUS FAR

In bioethical discussions of fresh approaches to the doctor-patient tie, Plato has been either ignored or misappropriated. While Veatch repudiates the Hippocratic Oath and Corpus many times for omitting patient involvement (2009, 12–14, 34–35, 93), he leaves Plato unmentioned, citing Aristotle but once. Veatch's account thus suggests that he associates antiquity as a whole uncontroversially with paternalism—an impression reinforced by his unfavorable contrasting of ancient with contemporary education where citizens' understanding is concerned (115). Though Pellegrino and Thomasma (1993) cite Plato, they ignore him as a backdrop for their handling of the virtuous physician, instead grounding their model in Aristotle.

As we saw in Section 2, the Emanuels' deliberative physician seeks to "persuade the patient to adopt other values" (1992, 2224). They claim *Laws* 720 as an ancient precedent for the content and telos of persuasion as they construe it (2225). However, their use of the passage reflects a deep misconstruction of its broader place in the dialogue. Most fundamentally, the *Laws*' exemplary physician does not seek to persuade the patient to adopt "*other* values." As we saw in Chapter 6, if anything this tutelage goes in the other direction.

The stress on continuity in other approving Platonic citations veers into anachronism. For Siegler (1981, 68; cf. 65), "the ingredients essential for a physician-patient accommodation—mutuality, voluntariness, respect for autonomy, and communication and negotiation between physician and patient—are surely preconditions for the practice of morally acceptable medicine." Plato's account of "the best clinical medicine" at *Laws* 720 shows that "recognition of this fact is not a recent development"

[26] Further, genuine boons in Aristotle (e.g., his stress on early education qua attitude formation, and virtue as the crux of thriving) are centrally grounded in Plato. Defending this view would of course be a topic for another occasion.

(ibid.).[27] Autonomy is not of "recent" advent insofar as, philosophically, it goes back to the eighteenth century and Kant. The notion is, however, wholly absent from Plato's work. As Jennings (2007) points out, autonomy "is individualistic. . . . It is the self's reason, not that of a community or higher authority. . . . It speaks in the first-person singular rather than the first-person plural. It is a vision of free *I*s, not free *We*s" (81). While apprehending and living by the *Laws*' strictures requires much *of* individuals, it, like antiquity generally, does not contain the notions of "individualism" and "self-expression" (78) that belong to the fabric of autonomy. Plato would instead deeply approve Jennings' reminder that autonomy on its own is insufficient: "Other principles that remind us of our social natures and our interdependence as human beings . . . are also ideas of potent resonance. They are the words of civilization and moral order; they are the elements of an essential vision of the human good" (88).[28]

Unwarranted conflation occurs, too, when Balint and Shelton (1996, 888) deem paternalistic the *Laws*' doctor-patient asymmetry rooted in the former's knowledge. Conscious or not, one finds here an assimilation of Plato's account with the Hippocratic Oath. Katz (1984, 4–6) conflates Plato's views in the *Republic* and *Laws*, treating his notion of the clinical tie as authoritarian throughout. As a result, Katz fails to recognize intriguing ties between his own discussion and the *Laws* via its emphasis on the mutual exchange of *logoi*, whose existence, situated in Plato's epistemology, assumes a high level of patients' attainment.[29] Mentioning just the *Republic*, Brody (1992, 121n3), like Katz, attributes to Plato an authoritarian take on doctors' praxis. The passage he relies on, however, involves not medicine but the metaphorical use of medical language in a discussion of truth and falsehood in children's *paideia* (389b). Moreover, this view of medical practice is at odds with Plato's own handling of medicine in *Republic* III, where the carpenter, a mere producer, may overrule his doctor's recommendation if he deems it at odds with what the Principle of Specialization requires of him.

---

[27] Cf. Jaspers (1989, 253–54). Siegler (2000, S22), too, wrongly associates autonomy with the *Laws*; because it omits this feature, Dugdale, Siegler, and Rubin (2008, 551–52) is more plausible.

[28] See Jennings (2007) also for discussion of autonomy as it bears on bioethics.

[29] Conversely, Heyd's (1995) assertion of Plato's doctor-patient relation as "*interactive*" (381; italics in original) and "dialogical" (382) applies to the *Laws* but not the *Republic*. For conflation of the two dialogues' accounts, see further Entralgo (1969, 37–41). Stalley (1980) mentions nonanachronistically Plato's handling of medicine, including the *Laws*, but merely cites the dialogue's "slave" physician to raise the specter of technocracy run amok (22). Assuming a uniform standpoint throughout the dialogues, Lidz (1995) concentrates on Greek medicine's impact on Platonic ethics rather than focusing on Plato's handling of medicine per se. Schaffner (1979, 46) and Guttentag (1979, 117) cite Plato in what they deem salutary models of the doctor-patient tie but for his views on nonmedical topics.

Given his perennial association with authoritarian sociopolitical frameworks, Plato might seem the last person to invoke to avoid paternalism. Deeper recourse is possible, however. Further exploration of Plato, above all the *Laws*, stands to enrich reflections on the clinical tie that seek to build collaborative models avoiding the pitfalls of paternalism and autonomy. In claiming that Plato's orientation, not Aristotle's, offers a fruitful ground for moving forward, my aim is not to commend wholesale his own virtue-based approach to the clinical tie and its social embedment or to make specific proposals (e.g., for accountability structures).[30] Rather, I advance Platonic considerations that we would do well to ponder moving forward, weighing in Platonically, as I do so, on contemporary points of contention.

5. PRECONDITIONS OF TRUE DOCTOR-PATIENT COLLABORATION: GROUNDING AN APPEAL TO PLATO

Perhaps surprisingly, bioethics' grounding of true doctor-patient collaboration remains an elusive goal. Reflection on Plato suggests that necessary conditions of its foundation include

1. clarity regarding the kind(s) of truth values claims represent, along with the level(s) and directionality of those values claims;
2. the doctor-patient tie's firm embedment in society at large, which carries with it marked continuity between medicine and human existence generally on values' application;
3. the notion that both parties to the relation are equally equipped to participate, though not necessarily for the same reasons in equal proportions; and
4. widespread transparency regarding (1)–(3).

Irrespective of whether Plato ends up fully meeting all four criteria, which is not my contention here, disclosing steps taken by him can motivate further reflection. I discuss ways in which the *Laws* addresses these conditions, comparing Plato's approach with current views. As we will see, the dialogue's handling of conditions (2)–(4) stems from key Platonic insights regarding human fallibility, accountability, *paideia*, and certain goods' incommensurability.

Regarding (1), unlike the Emanuels' approach (Emanuel and Emanuel 1992) to the status of values claims, which is ambiguous, Plato's conviction that values are

[30] The modest exception comprises suggestions involving awards in Section 9.

objective is unequivocal.[31] While paternalism and objectivism are regularly correlated (Koppelman-White 2009, 450), Plato's account suggests that objectivism does not necessitate paternalism. This is a highly important point, since bioethical attempts to guarantee autonomy amid values pluralism regularly assume that necessity. Plato's defense of values' standing includes clarity about their trajectory, namely that there exists an overarching set of human values, which are applied not only by individuals to their own actions but also to all human pursuits, including medicine. The *Laws*' enhanced respect for endeavors other than philosophy, presaged by the *Statesman*, means greater acknowledgment by Plato of a range of technical specialties and their attendant skills. His approach, however, squarely opposes the notion, which remains prominent in medicine, that professions, including medicine, set their own values from within. Instead, overarching human values apply, as relevant, to all specific planes of expertise. We will return to the subject of (1) in Sections 11–12 when addressing, through the lens of Plato, how best to move forward from here.

6. BIOETHICS COMPARED WITH THE *LAWS* ON HUMAN FALLIBILITY

Plato's meeting of conditions (2) and (3) above stems most of all from his realization that a deep potential for fallibility is present in all, even the best, combined with his greater recognition of ordinary citizens' capacities for apprehension and *aretê*. As we have seen, Plato's relinquishing the view that a select few are truly infallible, intellectually and in character, leads him to institute an elaborate web of checks and balances across all dimensions of society: sociopolitical, official, and nonofficial. To set the stage for seeing Plato's merit respecting fallibility, let us consider how bioethics has addressed this crucial matter.

Fallibility has not yet been fully appreciated here. This is not to say that substantive acknowledgment of human limitations is absent. Gorovitz and MacIntyre (1975) stress epistemological constraints, closely tying inevitable fallibility to the modus operandi of any science centrally handling particulars.[32] Fallible character

[31] In the *Phaedo*, *Symposium*, and *Republic*, Plato argues extensively that Forms are the ground of human nature and thriving. As Cherniss (1965a) notes, his argumentation involving Forms' existence revolves largely around their explanatory force respecting core philosophical problems. While scholars do not concur on whether Forms remain operative in the *Laws* precisely as they did before, Plato clearly remains convinced that the views he holds on *phusis* and *eudaimonia* are correct in an absolute, context-independent way. The present inquiry does not require that I address Forms' standing in the *Laws*, since even if they remain, Magnesia's best cannot apprehend them; a fortiori, insight into Forms cannot steer their work.

[32] In a piece also focused on science, McIntyre and Popper (1983) argue for a more accurate view of knowledge as growing not by "accumulation" but rather through "the recognition of error," i.e., "correction" (1920).

may be all but reduced to intellectual constraints, as when Veatch (2012)[33] and Daniels (2008, 122) emphasize intellectual limits such that even moral fallibility is treated as largely if not wholly cognitive: "Humans are fallible animals. They perceive the moral reality from a finite perspective. Their reasoning is inevitably flawed" (Veatch 2012, 182).[34] Noting doctors' fallible understanding and psychic limitations, Katz (1984) hopes that their self-awareness will minimize associated damage (xxi, 89–90, 102–3).[35] More generally, he speaks of constraints, including "vulnerabilities," in doctors and patients that both must apprehend (102, 151)—a feat that he concedes may be especially hard for physicians (163–64). Though Katz's account references character (xxi), it gives precedence to limited knowledge and doctors' resisting its acknowledgment as the foundational stumbling block (163–64).

Accounts that more directly address character also fall short. Considering the psychology of error concealment, Banja (2005, 7) illustrates the persistence and dangers of medicine's self-exemption. He strives to keep "medical narcissism" distinct from "pathological" kinds (48, 57, 112–13). However, Banja demarcates healthy from unhealthy types of the former (79–80) and acknowledges that narcissism, as a trait, is lodged on a continuum between two virtually nonmanifesting extremes (222). His attempt to separate medical narcissism from pathological types is ultimately unconvincing. In many of the situations he describes, practitioners' "rationalizations," whose crux is "*reinterpret[ing]* the moral situation" (33; italics in original),[36] involve deceit of others to preserve self-deception about their own infallibility. Banja's discussion illustrates that in this process marked character defects may be operative, including evasions of personal responsibility with serious repercussions for patients and families that doctors are willing to accept.

Brody (1992) rightly pushes past the "comforting" excuse that "mistakes sometimes happen" (22) to expose doctors' hermeneutical self-deception and show how self-transparency should be enhanced, to the good of the clinical tie. But he neglects to draw the requisite conclusion about human fallibility respecting character (what this study has called "ethical" fallibility) as distinct from cognitive or intellectual

---

[33] See especially chap. 7.

[34] Cf. 122–23, 136, 160–63, 178. Veatch's own discussion suggests a belief in absolutism ("the underlying moral reality," 184; cf. "the moral reality," 182). For emphasis on epistemic limits, see also Veatch (1981, 123, 313), whose handling of sin apropos of Catholic and Protestant theologies (43, 314) stresses the fallibility of human reason. Veatch (1981, 320) mentions fallible character but concentrates on epistemic limits.

[35] Guttentag (1979, 110) too notes the importance of doctors' self-knowledge.

[36] Cf. Veatch (1981, 223).

failings.[37] Regarding character, Brody asserts that "somewhere in our more primitive depths is a lust . . . to use whatever power we might have to victimize others less powerful, *and to enjoy it*" (21; italics in original).[38] Doctors have unique authority to "brand something as evil" (ibid.). Moreover (88), "some physicians take an almost perverse pleasure in pointing out that it is just as easy to manipulate patients with full disclosure as with incomplete disclosure, so long as one subtly emphasizes the right points."[39] Given such comments, it is surprising that character flaws as such are absent from Brody's list of "limitations" creating or fostering "bad outcomes" (141), which concentrates instead on excusable and culpable cognitive mistakes. The incongruity of this omission is enhanced by Brody's complaint that bioethics fails to address adequately "emotional and psychological factors" (147). These include doctors' "emotional distortions . . . that might interfere with rational analysis" (156), as when "an ideology of personal happiness," which is as such not "a rational belief . . . feeds [medical experts'] temptation" to use their authority "for social control or . . . personal gain" (227–28). While Brody's account has many strengths, its failure to address character flaws head-on is a salient omission, on which ground alone it stops well short of the *Laws*' treatment of human fallibility.

A failure to recognize more fully the nature and implications of human limitations involving insight and character (i.e., epistemological and ethical constraints), particularly the latter, has contributed to an ongoing provision of agonistic-style approaches. These give fixed primacy to one member of the clinical tie as surpassing the other (1) in understanding and/or (2) where pertinent values are concerned such that the parties seem at times to belong to different worlds. My claim is not that ethical shortcomings within medicine have received no emphasis. Thus far, however, ethical limitations have been attended to most in documents, such as the Nuremberg Code, Declaration of Helsinki, and Belmont Report, that acknowledge heinous abuses involving experimentation on human subjects, further incidence of which they aim to forestall. Such work is, of course, all to the good. My point here is that since, as Plato saw, ethical fallibility is intrinsic to human existence, it should be more deeply acknowledged as potentially operative in medicine, including clinical care from the dramatic to the routine.

---

[37] Brody's use of "ethical" is sometimes ambiguous between "anything of bioethical import involving human capacities" and ethics à la "character" (i.e., Greek *êthos*). Thus, it is unclear (28) whether doctors' self-deception about their reliance on patients' expressed "gratitude" is a matter of ethics just in the former sense or also reflects a character failing. Due to his account's limitations apropos of character, Brody's attention to medical education and doctors' education of patients (91, 110–11, 119, 199, 200) is less powerful than it might otherwise be.

[38] Cf. 29–30; 139 (doctors' "rescue fantasy" is called "a power trip").

[39] See also Gray (1991, 168).

Regarding fallibility qua error commission and proper responses thereto, our current approach is tied closely to the Institute of Medicine's 1999 report *To Err Is Human*, which identifies system failures as the source of "most human errors" (65).[40] As Sharpe (2004, 10) points out, before the rise to prominence of a "systems approach" to medical error, the focus was on "individual actors and their individual actions."[41] Current thinking is that attending to systemic flaws will help to redress an earlier overemphasis on individuals. When handling these flaws, we must detach an occupation with individuals from a narrow focus on discrete actions so that we do not, as Morreim (2004, 228n6) proposes, make it inessential that individuals be singled out as accountable.

While Merry and Smith (2001) stop short of Morreim here and rightly attend to broader contexts, including complex systems, their framework tends to weaken individual accountability. Merry and Smith take as fundamental a distinction between errors, which are "entirely involuntary" (98), and "violations," which are "a matter of choice" involving "a deliberate . . . deviation from those practices appreciated by the individual as being required by regulation" (101).[42] Due to errors' intrinsic involuntariness, culpability is precluded (101, 244). While Merry and Smith attribute their own binary to Aristotle (244), they overlook his key distinction between acting "in" and "due to" ignorance (*NE* III.1, 5). The result, here and elsewhere, is that they do not clearly single out the large class of actions that are for Aristotle neither involuntary—a highly restricted category—nor voluntary but instead nonvoluntary.[43] Merry and Smith thus remove culpability for some errors that Aristotle would classify as nonvoluntary, hence as involving, like voluntary actions, moral responsibility.

From a moral-psychological standpoint, this is a highly important class of actions for Aristotle, as they reflect character defects in their performers. For instance, acts stemming from an otherwise forgivable ignorance of specific information become culpable if the agent lacks deep regret for what transpired (*NE* 1110b18–25, cf. 1111a19–20). Merry and Smith (2001, 131–32), in contrast, do not reclassify such an action if "remorse" post-error is lacking. Also relevant moral-psychologically is that Merry and Smith downplay without argument doctors' own pecuniary motives in favor of those emanating from people "in the boardroom" (242).

---

[40] For a summary of earlier literature, consult Appendix C of the report. See Leape and Berwick (2005) for an assessment of where things stood five years after the report appeared.

[41] Merry and Smith (2001) call this a "'snapshot' view of . . . errors" (135), which both they (47, 143, 218) and Liang (2004, 65) tie closely to the tort system.

[42] The italics in this last quote, provided by the authors to signal a definition, have been removed.

[43] Sharpe (2004, 26n6) also wrongly attributes to Aristotle the view that individuals are responsible just for voluntary acts.

Endorsing movement away from a rigid "shame and blame" (Liang 2004, 63) notion of culpability need not and should not foster neglect of character.[44] Moreover, if, as Banja (2005) suggests, error concealment and character (on his account, narcissism) are comingled, a systems focus vis-à-vis error that does not hold individuals accountable for character flaws makes an artificial detachment of one from the other and hence cannot produce fundamental change. We must acknowledge what is useful in existing approaches but move beyond them to develop for the first time a true virtue-based account, from within whose focus on character actions are interpreted and addressed.

Pellegrino (2004) rightly sees that attending to systemic defects is not opposed to but actually requires an occupation with individuals. For this reason, "even while systemic responses are being designed, it will be necessary to reaffirm the moral nature of medical error, and to retain the notions of blame, accountability, and responsibility" (84–85). Pellegrino's formulation suggests that, within a systems-style approach, one could robustly incorporate individual culpability. In his view, "every action of individual professionals and every organizational policy and regulation must be measured by [the] gold standard of traditional medical morality" (85). Pellegrino's case for individual accountability here is strengthened by his recognition, unlike Liang (2004, 61), that error stemming from defective "knowledge and skill . . . is morally blameworthy" (90). A good illustration is the unusually high mortality rate from cardiac surgical procedures on infants at the Bristol Royal Infirmary during 1991–95 when surgery there was typically limited to adults (Klein 1998). Here, "self-interest" absent pertinent skill markedly increased procedures on children despite the well-established presence of expertise therein at other venues (Klein 1998, 1742).[45] One should note that acknowledging that cognitive and moral failings may be interwoven is quite different from claiming that moral limitations are, here or elsewhere, reducible to cognitive ones.[46]

Plato's *Republic* foregrounds the intellectual and moral infallibility of a select few, philosopher-rulers, whose untrammeled agency, not law, enables individual and communal thriving. Little known by comparison is that in the *Laws*, he sees

[44] As Pellegrino (2004, 86) points out, one can make character attributions to institutions, too. Addressing this topic directly falls outside the present inquiry.

[45] Though locating subsystemic or individual responsibility within a given milieu may be challenging (a point made by Klein [1998, 1741] regarding Bristol), it should be done as thoroughly as possible.

[46] One might ask, if the line between cognitive and moral errors is not always clear, would not the need for doctors' input on the former mean that one cannot avoid also involving them on the moral plane? The answer is yes, but this does not count against the notion that the broadly human plane of values is overarching, with those values then applied to pertinent arenas, including medicine.

clearly that fallibility in both domains lies at the core of human nature (713c, 875b–d) and hence that even the best possess it (767e, 926c–928d, 945c–948a, 952a–b). The *Laws*' model of the "free" physician and patient, like all else in that dialogue's account of human thriving, assumes this stress on human limitation, unprecedented in his previous work. For Plato, the human—versus strictly professional—nature of the operative limits makes it pivotal that sociopolitical structures and institutions be established and monitored with them in mind. One might, with effort, draw a similar implication from Brody's account (1992) of human tendencies involving power when tailored to the medical sphere. Plato, however, makes the point foundational and draws the requisite consequence for all endeavors, including medicine.[47]

While the *Laws*' view of human nature is often deemed pessimistic, its account of our fallibility reflects a hard yet profound truth. Rather than being an insight freshly achieved and applied to each area of human activity, this truth is front and center when institutions for Magnesia are forged. Further, epistemic and ethical limits—again, "ethical" as derived from *êthos* (character)—are a given that informs people's self-understanding and their conception of reciprocal ties. Together with his demotion to fallible of those who are best, Plato's blinders come off regarding the intellectual and moral abilities of ordinary folk. He sees clearly in the *Laws* that failing to acknowledge and accommodate in institutions universal human fallibility necessarily precludes an openness by those with greater authority to others' contributions. Such rigidity and resistance is precisely what the *Laws* militates against.

As we have seen, in Kallipolis, everyone else is radically subordinate to a select, infallible few. Though it is philosophers rather than doctors who are autocratic there, what is important is that infallibility and authoritarianism fit closely together, with the former anchoring the latter. Due to its dramatic gap in native capacity, the *Republic*'s contention that there is a single human nature is not well illustrated there. Further, besides circumscribed coordination, as between philosophers and auxiliaries, Kallipolis' running does not involve collaboration. In the *Laws*, in contrast, Plato's insight that the nature of all human beings contains a susceptibility to intellectual and ethical shortcomings prompts him to embrace a collaborative model that includes strong complementarity across an array of practices. While philosopher-rulers routinely act unilaterally in Kallipolis, not even those on Magnesia's nocturnal council may inaugurate action on their own. In sum, unlike

[47] Notably, as is evident from the *Gorgias*' Archelaus and Callicles, and the tyrant of *Republic* IX, one occupied with power qua an untrammeled dominance of others is sure to construe desire in starkly appetitive terms.

Kallipolis, no one in Magnesia is trusted to serve unidirectionally as arbiter where values and associated conduct are concerned.

Pellegrino and Thomasma's stress on medicine's self-policing function (1993, 180) and role as the source of values enrichment inclines to an authoritarianism repudiated by the *Laws*.[48] Instead, their assertion that "what America . . . need[s] desperately is moral leadership and medical statesmanship" (47) calls the *Republic*'s autocratic philosopher-rulers to mind. Though Pellegrino and Thomasma note in passing doctors' fallibility (75), the extent to which this impacts their ideal versus reflecting how things currently are is unclear.

Pellegrino (2004, 85; cf. 98) is right to pointedly include organizations and individuals apropos of responsibility. I diverge, however, from his continued assertion that medical morality specifically is the crux of assessments. In my view, colored by Plato, Pellegrino's fruitful attention to individual accountability works against his insistence on said morality as the basis of pertinent valuation, because the latter is precisely the kind of self-policing that a recognition of human fallibility à la the *Laws* rejects. Though much in Pellegrino's account is promising, his insistence that medicine is the source and monitor of relevant values, as opposed to their being human and grasped extramedically, keeps his account from adequately handling both fallibility and accountability.

It is worth recalling here the *Gorgias*' contrasting of helmsmanship with medicine (511d–512b), which is unusual among human pursuits for its governance by self-originating views of *phusis* and *eudaimonia*. Practitioners' sense of overarching insight, illustrated through Eryximachus in the *Symposium*, fosters notions of the field's supremacy. This situation makes it harder for medicine than for many other fields to accept restrictions on the applicability of its vision to the clinical setting and human existence tout court. The reason this is hard is also what renders it urgent that those limitations be revealed. Contemporary debates about medicine's self-policing and its proper role in forging values that medicine applies make clear that Plato's observations remain apropos.

Veatch (2012) appears to supply what Pellegrino's account does not when he argues that "professionally generated oaths and codes are no longer an acceptable

---

[48] Overconfidence in medicine is reflected too in London (2000). The view that professionalism's intrinsic "dark side" renders self-policing morally unjustifiable is defended by Erde (2008, 9, 17). Buchanan (1996) rightly contends that the "burden of argument" (116) respecting the legitimacy of medicine's self-policing—at the mere suggestion of the need for which some bristle (122)—lies squarely with the medical profession (116). Physicians' demonstrated shortcomings in altruism (123–24), along with medicine's wide-ranging failure to shoulder "the responsibility for effective collective self-regulation" (130), indicate that continued self-policing is untenable. Veatch's (2012) argument that doctors have no special claim to grasp the values that ought to guide medicine itself precludes the field's self-policing, which stance he also voices (184).

basis for medical morality" (4).[49] Instead, physicians' "role-specific duties must be derived from those ethical norms that have their foundation outside the profession" (6), "in favor of [which] commitments of the professional grounded outside the profession" medical-professional oaths should be "abandoned" (80). Although his claim about medical oaths goes perhaps too far, Veatch rightly contends that one errs in thinking that having medical knowledge necessarily makes one "an expert on the value choices, including the moral choices, about medical practice" (26). Since "on average, there is no reason to assume" that professionals surpass laypeople here, if a doctor happened to excel "at making these choices," it would not be qua physician that he did so (ibid.). Veatch's three mentions of Plato (17, 30, 41) are unrelated to my thesis about his pertinence. That said, Plato of the *Laws* would find congenial Veatch's claim that specific areas of human endeavor are rightly steered by encompassing values.[50] As we will see in Section 11, however, in other respects Plato and Veatch are importantly at odds.

7. PARITY AND *PAIDEIA*

Balint and Shelton (1996, 888) find Magnesia's model of the doctor-patient tie paternalistic. I contend, in contrast, that divergence on optimal medical practice exists already within antiquity. Although the Hippocratic Oath displays paternalism, Plato's *Laws* does not.[51] Far from being paternalistic, the *Laws* reminds us that one with authority may want the best for another in his care but not be aware of what that comprises (687d–e) or know what is required but act on a countervailing motivation

---

[49] "No longer" is a reference to the Hippocratic Oath. Veatch (2012) conflates the oath—which, following Edelstein's assertion of its Pythagorean source, he claims to be "a religious document" (2012, 12)—with ancient medical writings tout court. Hence, Veatch's insistence that the oath be scrapped slides without comment into a contention that Hippocratic praxis should be rejected. If the oath reflects "an initiation ritual into a kind of Greek cult" (10), this renders more intuitively plausible his critique of its extremity. If extremity is its pedigree, however, as Edelstein (1987a, 39) claims, the oath cannot (at least absent much argumentation) be taken as representative of Hippocratic medicine as such. Edelstein's view is contested by Staden (1996). I will not rehearse here the territory spanned by this debate, noting only that while I suspend judgment on whether the source is Pythagorean specifically, one has good reason for separating the oath from the Hippocratic mainstream.

[50] Similarly, he would approve Callahan's (2012, 153) linking the queries, "just what should those of us in [bioethics] be trying to do, and what kind of person ought we be in order to best do it?"

[51] While Entralgo (1969) notes that Greek views of the doctor-patient tie were not univocal (16), he wrongly opts for uniformity when considering the concept of *technê* (22). Though I broadly concur with Hofmann (2003) that recourse to ancient medicine is useful from our standpoint (404) and that there was not "one general and consistent conception of medicine in antiquity" (408), our approaches diverge. Notably, Hofmann assumes Plato's stance to be uniform throughout the corpus; in addition, his single reference (422n6) to the *Laws* (889c–d) reflects the standpoint of sophistic atheism repudiated by Plato.

(928b–d). While bioethical accounts that reference the *Laws* usually focus on Book IV (720a–e),[52] in Book IX we find Plato's highly significant comment that the free doctor's discussions with patients encompass "the source of the disease" and beyond that "the whole nature of the body" (857d2–4). Plato conveys here both his respect for what good doctors know and that physicians' *logoi* about the body and health are comprehensible to the patient. Further, patient and doctor's *exchanging logoi* (i.e., rational accounts; 720c–d, 857d) assumes a high level of reciprocity. The patient need not be a medical specialist for this bidirectionality—based on shared *human* aptitudes—to obtain.[53]

Aiming to counter a frequent, unjustified underestimation of patients' capacity for apprehension, Katz (1984, 92) observes that "the complexity of professional knowledge . . . does not necessarily suggest . . . that this knowledge cannot be communicated to, or understood by, patients."[54] This meshes with the stance of Plato, for whom the fact that the patient likely will not come in understanding everything needed for the encounter with his doctor does not mean that he is incapable of that understanding. The patient's education from childhood on, while not conveying specifically this, has prepared him intellectually and ethically to receive the apprehension bearing on health that the doctor conveys. A salient element of Plato's approach stemming from his epistemology and allied *technê* theory is that the patient's capacity not merely for information acquisition but for insight is strong, and indeed sufficient to enable his grasp of the doctor's diagnosis and account (*logos*) of how possible treatments foster health.

Plato's use of a parent-child analogy (*Laws* 720a) when noting the authority that doctors have might lead one unreflectively to attribute paternalism to him. As analogies' efficacy hinges on their provision against a backdrop of difference, one must consider both what this one stresses and where it breaks off. A parent's reason substitutes for that of a child because, developmentally speaking, the latter cannot be brought up to speed at the juncture in question. As to adults, philosophers' reason may stand in for that of producers in Kallipolis (*Republic* 590c–d). This measure is needed and paternalistic because the cognitive gap disadvantaging producers is

---

[52] An exception is Entralgo (1969, 36); as previously noted, however, he simply assumes that the *Laws* and *Republic* convey a uniform stance.

[53] Cf. the claim of Annas (2000, 118) that the *Laws*' doctor-patient tie "could serve Plato as an example of a cooperative relation between expert and nonexpert," which view of the tie she traces to "the [ancient] model of health as overall balance of bodily elements."

[54] According to Tumulty (1970), the doctor "formulates a reasoned explanation" (21) so that the patient "understands fully what is wrong" (22). While this sounds promising, Tumulty's actual account of patients' abilities is quite deprecatory (23).

firm and bears no temporal limitation. *Republic* X's restrictions on adults' access to poetry are also paternalistic, since they assume the fundamental inability of virtually all to reach the plane of insight and character needed to grasp that dramatic portrayals are representations, not models for their own experience (595a–b, 604d–605c, 606c–d).[55]

In the *Republic*, the sole individuals who act paternalistically are philosopher-rulers, while doctors number among producers, the largest group in society, who address citizens' material and physical needs (apart from safety, the province of auxiliaries). Doctors' classification there reflects ordinary views, which locate the doctor squarely in the category of craftsmen (Edelstein 1987b, 87). Far from being ultimate authorities themselves, doctors' medical judgments in Kallipolis will be overruled by philosophers if they are deemed to be at odds with what justice requires (409e–410a); less often, physicians' recommendations may be rejected by patients (406c–d).

Though Magnesian patients' verbal contributions will largely bear on their conditions, patients' *logoi* need not be limited to this. We see this by recalling that Magnesia contains no philosopher-rulers and that the patient typically has a fuller grasp of human values than the physician. He is therefore better poised to relate the doctor's offerings to *eudaimonia*. As we saw in Chapter 6, free doctors' patients in the *Laws* may instruct them about values in a twofold way. In this dialogue, Plato no longer views people's merit simply through their circumscribed occupational roles. Where doctors are prone to glean people's merit via their specific function (e.g., that of general or guardian of the law), citizen patients will have occasion to remind them that human value is not so narrowly restricted. Patients' input here serves as a hedge against undertreatment.

Second, patients may instruct their doctors on the content of goods' hierarchy (psychic, bodily, material), including intragroup relations as pertinent. The *Laws* places health (*hugieia*) atop the second class (631c). But here, as in the *Gorgias* and *Republic*, for the unjust, nonpsychic goods become "a curse, every one of them, from health all the way down" (661b). While free doctors will be sufficiently aware of virtue to help maintain communal unity, their occupational focus on a bodily good makes it likely that they will sometimes be prone to favor ailments' addressing where, from a comprehensive vantage point, health should be subordinated. Although the details are not the same, doctors' gleaning merit and options through a medical lens is not an historically circumscribed inclination. On Veatch's (1981, 121)

[55] This topic is discussed insightfully by Nehamas (1982; 1988).

formulation regarding the contemporary scene, doctors are likely to "give special weight to the value of their sphere of expertise."[56] In the following section of this chapter, I revisit Plato's conviction that a good on a higher tier is never rightly subordinated to one on a lower plane.

As we saw in Chapter 6, though the *Laws*' patient typically surpasses his metic-doctor regarding values tout court, noncitizens receive *paideia* (i.e., broad values education), not merely training directly required for the performance of their crafts. The play of all children in Magnesia aims to direct rightly their "pleasures and desires" (643c), which is the heart of formational *paideia* (653b-c), and is expressly directed toward character formation (792d–794c). This is strikingly at odds with Kallipolis, most of whose members will lack the childhood values education of *Republic* II–III and get training in their crafts alone. Moreover, from childhood all Magnesians participate in choruses, in whose activity all are to "find perpetual pleasure" (665c). Kallipolians en masse, in contrast, hear at most traditional-style hymns and encomia on notable civic occasions.[57]

Crucially, while citizen patients in the *Laws* generally surpass their physicians in their grasp and application of values tied to the soul, the free doctor's specialized grasp of health must be combined with the virtue of self-control (*sôphrosunê*) for him to be admitted into Magnesia as a metic (850b). Metics' role in setting their own profit margins (920b–c) suggests that this self-control is not insubstantial. Further support comes from the fact that their *sôphrosunê* renders metics receptive to communal honor, not remuneration, as the reward for nonoccupational activity that fosters thriving (881b). More generally, noncitizens' grasp of Magnesia's telos of virtue-based unity suffices for their assistance in the fostering of justice.

What of parity in the clinical tie? The *Laws*' stress on the patient's giving and apprehending *logoi* assumes in him a capacity to attain the highest plane of collaboration accessible to expert and layman. The *Laws*' free doctor assumes that his patient can be brought up to speed in a timely fashion on factors involving diagnosis and treatment, including rationales from the standpoint of health, through a series of reciprocal exchanges. The physician represents the parent in Plato's analogy at 720a due to his medical expertise—this is, after all, what led the patient to consult him[58]—not because patients are categorically inferior in epistemic gifts and values apprehension. On the contrary, having received more extensive *paideia*, patients will

---

56 Medicine is not unique here, of course, as the same applies, mutatis mutandis, to other professions (e.g., law).

57 For further discussion see Levin (2001, 162–66).

58 Unlike Veatch (2009), whose stress on patients' governance of deliberation and decision making goes too far, Kelley (2005, 197; cf. 193) rightly attends to the "inequality of expertise [that] is inherent in any skill-based profession."

typically surpass doctors in their broad cognitive attainment and capacity to locate health-related exchanges in the wider setting of *eudaimonia*.

Importantly, unlike many asymmetrical constructions favoring the doctor, what the patient contributes here is not simply what issues from privileged access to his own preferences and needs (see, e.g., Katz 1984, 102). This is a limited superiority not bearing within itself the seeds of its own broader application. Plato's citizen patient, in contrast, surpasses the doctor in his grasp of values tout court. The patient's typical superiority in the sphere of human values thus complements the doctor's medical knowledge, itself adequately expressible to patients through their reciprocal exchange of *logoi*. The resulting orientation is a modality that Chapter 6 dubbed a functionally complementary and ultimately balanced asymmetry.

The *Laws* shows that use of a parent-child analogy need not make the doctor-patient tie paternalistic in the sense that prompted a vociferous negative reaction in the 1960s and 1970s, helping to fuel bioethics' shift toward autonomy in the first place. Instead, in Plato's view, the parties are united by their ability to give and receive *logoi* even as they take precedence within the relation from distinct, albeit complementary, standpoints. Reflection on Plato thus suggests that while Pellegrino and Thomasma (1993) rightly note an intrinsic asymmetry of some kind favoring the doctor, they have not accurately pinpointed where it lies. Hence, they have not gone as far as possible toward parity between patient and doctor. Pellegrino and Thomasma too hastily propound a values contrast *essentially* favoring the doctor, leaving out of account the possibility of patients' frequent (or, as Plato would have it, usual) superiority respecting *eudaimonia*.

If one approaches the issue through the *Laws*, it becomes evident that recognizing doctors' medical knowledge need not negate the headway that greater attention to patient autonomy has wrought[59]—though it would preclude extreme notions thereof as reflected in the Emanuels' "informative" model (Emanuel and Emanuel 1992, 2221) and in Veatch (2009). In both instances, once doctors have provided patients with the information and other materials "relevant" to the situation, decision making is lodged squarely in patients' hands so that they may "exercise control" (Emanuel and Emanuel 1992, 2221). While subordinated from the broader standpoint of human values, Plato's free doctor is not in danger of being reduced to superfluity, the prospect of which is noted in connection with unmodulated patient autonomy (Erde 2008, 6).

---

[59] Cf. Kelley (2005, 193).

8. *PAIDEIA* AND MEDICAL SCHOOL: ISLAND OR WAY STATION?

According to the *Laws*, though human limits cannot be surpassed, they can be tempered through education so as to minimize unsalutary motivations and chances for their enactment. Pellegrino and Thomasma's (1993, 157) confidence in the transformative power of medical education vis-à-vis character is undiminished even where individuals' prior moral instruction has been flawed. Unlike Plato, who stresses upbringing and education from one's earliest days as the crux of good character's formation, Pellegrino and Thomasma pin their hopes largely on medical pedagogy as the route to the correction of shortcomings like too-generous constructions of "legitimate self-interest" (145). Though they concede that "the whole task of character formation cannot be left" to this venue (157), they still insist that "the most effective instruments of character formation are the professionals who teach in medical . . . schools" (158).[60]

Pellegrino and Thomasma's claim is problematized by their recognition that "intelligence is not enough. Character and virtue must precede it in human affairs" (178). Though ambiguous in this statement, "precede" vis-à-vis this topic properly encompasses both "undergird and direct decision making" and "come first developmentally." Regarding the latter, since, as Plato stresses, character's roots well antedate the advent of reason (*Laws* 653b–c, 672c; cf. *Republic* 402a), moral education must begin quite early. Appearances to the contrary notwithstanding, it may be the most promising natures—including those Pellegrino and Thomasma hope will become moral leaders in medicine—that wreak the most havoc when *paideia* is defective (*Republic* 491d–e). In any case, they do not leave one confident that faulty moral upbringing can be dramatically redressed during medical school with any steadiness, particularly since they wish to avoid a scenario in which people act rightly solely for fear of bad results issuing from others' discovery of their wrongdoing. This deep-seated human inclination is powerfully illustrated by the *Republic*'s tale of Gyges, a man who obeyed the law up to his discovery of a ring that made him invisible at will, at which point, straightaway, he committed grave offenses (359c–360d). Since "one fashions one's self-image as a physician over a whole lifetime" (Pellegrino and Thomasma 1993, 181; cf. 182), it is highly artificial, and humanly inaccurate, to place the doctor's existence prior to her direct pursuit of that professional goal in a separate

---

[60] Having depreciated the view that doctors' conduct hinges on moral orientations forged prior to medical school (1982, 203), Gorovitz stresses the import of right motivation (194) and of "who [those students] are at the outset," by which point "much of their ultimate character is already shaped" (206). Though virtue's promotion in medical school would necessitate that "the entire medical education culture . . . internally evolve" (Doukas 2004, 19), even that would not suffice if undesirable traits had already formed.

compartment.[61] As Pellegrino and Thomasma (179) insist, exemplary people, specifically doctors on their account, must do the right thing *because* it is right. Yet sound motivation is far more difficult to forge than habitual action of a certain sort, as Plato and his student Aristotle clearly saw.

Pellegrino and Thomasma's account of what is needed so that those entering medical school emerge as virtuous doctors contains a deep inconsistency, one that may not be resolvable from within their theory as it stands. On the one side, featuring Aristotle as does their account requires human values' forging from a young age, there being a single trajectory here from childhood to the end of life. On the other, for Pellegrino and Thomasma, what medical students learn is *medicine's* morality. This, combined with their *phronimos*-style notion of the profession's values expertise, suggests a self-containment, even self-sufficiency, of medical pedagogy—a view in keeping with their notion, treated in Section 2, that values enrichment fruitfully proceeds from the venue of medicine outward to other professions and society tout court.

My intent is not to deny that the knowledge base and "clinical skills" acquired in medical school are critical to the kind of practitioner one becomes[62] but rather to set that experience in a far wider pedagogical setting as regards human values, whose presence in oneself is both deepened and applied to medicine during that advanced educational sojourn.[63] Based on his philosophical work with children, Matthews (1994) argues that they are not "merely proto-people" (122), being instead to a degree "partners in inquiry" (14). While Plato would not go as far as Matthews here, he would concur that "most of us never lose the paradigms we first assimilated in

---

[61] More in line with Plato is the stance of Culver et al. (1985, 253): "We believe that the basic moral character of medical students has been formed by the time they enter medical school." As Rentmeester (2008, 41) observes, deficient prior education may leave "young practitioners and students . . . ill-prepared to discern differences between good and poor patterns of perception that are modeled by their mentors." Cf. Veatch (2012, 68): "It is absurd to think that four years of medical school should convert entire classes from their basic moral systems to one that they would suddenly come to adopt." On the all but absent teaching of medical ethics up to the early 1970s, see Callahan (2012, 61), who notes that ten years later "most medical schools had some kind of program or course" (ibid.). While now all do, "and many have good-sized centers and programs" (145), "one does not have to scratch far below the surface in most medical schools to find either indifference, or even some hostility, to ethics . . . taken to be soft and mushy against the transcendent value of hard scientific knowledge" (150–51).

[62] The quoted phrase is drawn from http://med.stanford.edu/md/curriculum.

[63] My own expansive view of values education was enriched several years ago through a collaborative effort, with a colleague in Education and Child Study at Smith College and a fourth-grade teacher at our Campus School, to explore the concept of friendship with the fourth graders; for instance, what differentiates friendship from other kinds of ties (e.g., that between siblings or parent and child, and relationships with pets)? Students' perceptiveness, including their thoughts on how one ought to treat friends past and present as a matter of principle, was stunning.

childhood" (65). Crucial is Matthews' finding that not a few children "act with some kind of understanding that what they are doing is a good thing to do because . . . it will help someone out, or comfort someone, and not just that it might be a way to avoid being punished or a way to get rewarded" (58).

The foregoing, combined with our prior discussions of Plato, strongly supports the view that an inclination to do the right thing because it is right is not formed as a matter of course. If children's ability to act thus is not engaged from early on, it is wont to become permanently dwarfed by whatever less salutary value structures are instilled. Even if one could subsequently regulate those adults' behavior via inducements, this is far different from transforming their moral orientations so that they consistently acted well for the right *reasons*. The latter outcome, however, is what Pellegrino and Thomasma (1993) and others present as attainable via medical school, perhaps combined with fitting undergraduate preparation.[64]

9. *PAIDEIA* AND (IM)MORAL INCENTIVES

As I have argued, if one seeks to cultivate doctors with the requisite motivation, one must construe education broadly to include the forging, refinement, and reinforcing of human values through the life cycle from childhood on. Given the notion's centrality to character and conduct, children would learn of qualitatively different classes of goods *(agatha)* that, as truly incommensurable, cannot be reciprocally exchanged. This view would then be applied to all their subsequent endeavors, including medicine. Adopting this lens shows that consideration of incentives has a strong values dimension tying it to character.

As Menzel (1983, 221, 227–28) observes, the medical profession is remarkable for the extent to which its setting of financial terms has been unfettered.[65] The rise of managed care, which includes far more than just HMOs (Peeno and Leopold 2003, 23), constricts doctors' freedom somewhat while at the same time offering new paths to revenue production.[66] Not only that, "payment systems that are *premised on* health care providers' responsiveness to economic incentives have been widely implemented" (Gray 1991, 322).[67] Peeno and Leopold (2003, 24) point out

[64] For attention to complementary ethical instruction in undergraduate and medical curricula, see Emanuel (2006).

[65] This should be distinguished from what happened in Magnesia, where metics' input on their profit margins fell well short of their being arbiters.

[66] For extensive discussion, see Gray (1991).

[67] Emphasis added. For Gray, who addresses trends in American health care, "in many different ways the profit motive . . . has come to shape the behavior of all parties. An ethos that emphasizes trust . . . is being replaced by undisguised self-interest, commercialization, competition, and the management of care by third parties" (xi).

that pecuniary rewards may be offered for under- or overtreatment. This is so not just sequentially—the latter on the older fee-for-service model and the former under managed care—as multiple pecuniary goals may foster both defects regarding individual patients (ibid.).

Although some tout "pay for performance" (P4P) as a promising remedy for both extremes, Brody (2009) rightly cautions us to avoid plunging headlong into its embrace as a justified application of current evidence-based medicine (66–67). Under P4P (66), a health-care venue (1) uses the best available data to frame "practice guidelines," (2) determines how individuals' and hospitals' success vis-à-vis those guidelines will be assessed, and (3) generates a grid that calibrates compensation to assessment outcomes under item (2). A supporter of evidence-based medicine, Brody rejects P4P at present for its lack of evidential backing (66–67, 75). He later suggests, however, that his objection to P4P is not contingent but foundational, since its "basic assumption," which he rejects, "is that physicians respond to financial incentives and, for all practical purposes, only to financial incentives" (80). While it falls outside Brody's project here to divide "perverse" from "virtuous" incentives (81), he argues persuasively that "this is a debate of substance . . . worth having. At present I see no signs of anyone engaging in this debate. And I am aware of no contributions that bioethics is making to identifying the debate as one worth pursuing" (ibid.). From Plato's standpoint, this neglect is perilous.

For medicine and in broader human terms, remuneration's increased use to shape doctors' behavior is harmful not just for its sending the flawed message that health (on Plato's second-highest tier of goods) and remuneration (on his third and lowest plane) are commensurate but for what it reveals more generally about our priorities. Key to human success is psychic goodness, hence Plato's lodging it at the pinnacle of *ta agatha* (literally, "the things that are good"). With that goodness, namely virtue, in view, one must act (or refrain from acting) due to the rightness of operating thus. From this perspective, Leape and Berwick's (2005) account displays a twofold mismatch: they require shifts in beliefs and intentions (i.e., inner states concerning benefits' promotion, 2390) yet propose to attain these through pecuniary prods and deterrents to action (2389). Activity regulated through procedures like "prohibitions, disclosure requirements, and utilization review and management" (Gray 1991, 197) is not functionally equivalent to, and hence cannot replace, one's possession of exemplary traits. Salutary action can foster virtuous conduct, particularly before character is fixed. What Leape and Berwick propose, however, is antithetical to that path. In addition, insofar as maximizing compensation is itself the object of desire, like Greek rhetoricians one risks tethering "right" conduct to governing parameters irrespective of whether they benefit those reliant on one's care. Even if interests happen to coincide, no built-in stability exists, since the policies whose following maximizes today's remuneration may not do so next week.

London (2000) is more restrained than Leape and Berwick (2005), but he too allows pecuniary rewards that do not seem to generate conflict between doctor and patient "for the same scarce resources" (143, cf. 144).[68] The size of what is offered should not, however, strictly determine what is permitted. As Beauchamp and Childress (2013) observe concerning manufacturers of pharmaceuticals and medical devices, "even small gifts . . . influence physicians' prescribing behavior. Moreover, gift relationships, however small, create a variety of temptations, dependencies, friendships, and forms of indebtedness" (329–30). In the words of "Gifts to Physicians from Industry," whose source is the American Medical Association (AMA)'s own Council on Ethical and Judicial Affairs (American Medical Association 1990, 193), "when a physician receives a gift from a company's sales representative, the physician may associate his or her feelings about the gift or the sales representative with his or her feelings about the company's products . . . even when the gift is a small one." From the side of industry, the large sums deployed in gifts' provision testify to a "conviction that such promotional activities are effective" (Beauchamp and Childress 2013, 347n81).

Hafferty (2004, 30) stresses organized medicine's substantive neglect of financial conflicts of interest: though it "has labeled 'improper' activities such as referring patients to . . . sites owned by the referring physician . . . all too often statements of proscription or prescription are labeled 'suggestions' or 'guidelines' and thus are formally identified as something open to individual discretion." The AMA's current Code of Medical Ethics allows doctors significant latitude involving sources of conflict that it deems relatively minor: for instance (Opinion 8.061), "individual gifts of minimal value are permissible as long as the gifts are related to the physician's work"; doctors and medical societies have notable discretion concerning financial gifts made by industry in their honor to charities, medical schools, and those very societies; individual doctors decide whether acceptance of gift certificates offered at events is appropriate; and medical consultants should determine whether subsidies for spouses' accompaniment of them on trips are "modest," hence also covered.

Though I have focused here on remuneration, one should recall Plato's lodging of a desire for financial gain with the Big Three under the appetitive aspect of soul (*Republic* 580e–581a), hence like them naturally insatiable (*Gorgias* 493a–494a). London (2000) fails to see that continuing to permit "incentives of various kinds"

---

[68] Cf. Brody (2009, 81), who, as previously observed, leaves room for unspecified "virtuous" as distinct from "perverse" incentives.

(149), central among them pecuniary, undermines just the deemphasis on remuneration that he aims to promote.[69] Interestingly, London concedes (152n15) that he "would . . . like to hold out the possibility of finding a set of effective incentives that do not appeal to a physician's financial interests at all." In my view, this should be taken straightaway as one's regulative ideal. As Relman (1985, 751), then editor of the *New England Journal of Medicine*, observes, "physicians serve their patients' interests best when they divorce themselves from financial interests in the medical marketplace," hence pertinent "financial arrangements . . . ought to be avoided."[70]

While the conflict was less overt in 1847 than it is now, a similar tension appears in the AMA's original Code of Medical Ethics, which stresses the profession's healing mission and associated virtues as categorically superior to other goods, especially remuneration: "To decline attendance [on one who is gravely ailing] . . . would be sacrificing to fanciful delicacy and mistaken liberality, that moral duty, which is independent of, and far superior to all pecuniary consideration" (94; cf. 98, 100). At the same time, the code is quite occupied with proper remuneration both in the clinical setting (e.g., cases where "at least a double honorarium may be reasonably expected," 102; cf. 99, 104) and when doctors assume public roles (e.g., autopsies, 105; cf. 106). Moreover, a concern with profit alone offers a sufficient impetus for "visit[ing] an individual who is under the direction of another practitioner" (102). Overall, the document militates against the success of its own quest to show that doctors are categorically different from businesspeople.[71]

What was missing in 1847, and threatens to become rampant now, is the pointed provision of financial incentives to intensify or reduce measures under the head of

[69] This is significant given his essay's attention to Plato's segregation of a money-making craft in *Republic* I, which pertains to the topic at hand but which vantage point, combined with the *Gorgias*' view of appetite's nature, supports the disallowance of wiggle room regarding pecuniary incentives. A similar risk attends the account of Gray (1991), which does not find problematic as such "commercial and entrepreneurial aspects of medicine" (181). Gray rests his case on what I view as a problematic distinction between care determined as needful directly by patients and that specified by doctors themselves (184–85).

[70] An identical level of strictness should apply to incentives directed toward patients. I thus diverge from Loewenstein, Brennan, and Volpp (2007), whose "asymmetric paternalism" allows financial incentives for patients' circumscribed behavior of restraint (2417). Like Plato, they focus on a trio of *epithumiai* where, however, smoking replaces sex in his Big Three (2415). Schmidt (2009, 23–25), too, supports such incentives. From Plato's standpoint, this procedure is wrong (1) due to the incommensurability of relevant *agatha* and (2) because it all but concedes the impossibility of doing the fundamental thing, which is not to punish or encourage based strictly on actions but rather to target motivation across pedagogical settings. Regarding *epithumiai* themselves, the overarching goal should be maximal cultivation of *sôphrosunê*. Though I believe that attending to patients' responsibilities is both useful and important, as my focus is on doctors, I limit myself to these comments.

[71] See also Gray (1991, 179), who, observing that "tensions between the physician as professional and as businessman are perhaps as old as the practice of medicine," cites the code of 1847; Veatch (2012, 55).

care (e.g., tests), whether or not the shifts harm patients, and to improve doctors' behavior without concern for whether relevant qualities (e.g., self-control, courage) belong to the agents themselves. Of course, medicine's greater pecuniary occupation is not an isolated event. It is likely, for instance, that prominent scientists' shift by the late 1970s into "economic entrepreneurship" (Callahan 2012, 90) contributed. More generally, "the embracing of market values in health care reflects a change in society as a whole. Because individualism and competition are increasingly celebrated, the principles of the marketplace now permeate our personal lives and even capture our judgment" (Kassirer 1995, 51).[72] The notion that "economic wealth is . . . both necessary and sufficient for permanent human happiness" appears as well in utopian visions lodged under posthumanism (Hauskeller 2012, 40).[73]

If goods are not cross-categorically translatable, and we wish to foster virtue, the core reward for right conduct and attitudes by doctors should not be monetary but something more in keeping with the tier of good reflected thereby, such as appreciative expressions visible to the community (e.g., in Plato's case, seats of honor at athletic games; *Laws* 881b). Our awards, built on Plato's insight, could be more substantive than this. Honors would spotlight human excellence displayed in medicine, including recognition for expressly and constructively addressing an acknowledged human limitation. One might, for example, recognize an exemplary doctor by calling a prize awarded to a student—even at the primary level—after that physician (e.g., the Sally Smith Prize for the Integrated Promotion of Human Values or the Frank Jones Award for Bravery and Humility under Challenging Conditions).[74] The specific content of each award, given to a student who showed appreciable promise or attainment regarding the pertinent trait, could be tailored to each one's situation,

---

[72] On greed as a societal trend impacting medicine, see Lundberg (1997, 1704). Koch (2012) indicts bioethics itself for capitulating straightaway to, then furthering, a societal emphasis on economic interests. Medical researchers are also criticized (208). Doctors who are not research-oriented, however, are often grouped with patients as victims (233–34, 253, 256) rather than viewed as themselves strongly motivated by the deleterious vision that has "reduced [the practice of medicine] to a commercial transaction" (253).

[73] Callahan (2012, 183) notes as "idiosyncratic" the United States' occupation with wealth and profit in medicine: "American physicians are the highest paid in the world, with a dominance of subspecialty physicians who command the highest fees. American medical students have overwhelmingly gone into those specialties in recent years . . . [in part] because their income will be more than if they went into primary care" (ibid.). Further, U.S. medicine "and the health care system of which it is a part are heavily commercial in their values and aspirations" (184).

[74] Schwab (2012) rightly notes the salience of doctors' disclosing their uncertainty, a "constant" feature of clinical practice (29), to patients (37, 40–42). While attending to "epistemic humility" (29) is useful, Schwab's argument for its precedence as "a characteristic of claims" (ibid.) over humility as a human trait (30) is weak: (1) he conflates "epistemic humility" with humility as a character trait; (2) contra Schwab, it is not the case that a focus on character here is salutary only if "perfection" (ibid.) is the operative norm, as the ideal is fruitfully viewed as regulative; and (3) his claim that epistemic humility may yield better results in certain cases is purely contingent.

comprising, for instance, a collection of books, hands-on experience at a nonprofit, or a "shadowing" and conversational opportunity with the award's eponym.

The idea is not to eschew direct awards to medical students or practicing physicians but rather to ensure that these too befit the nature of the good being acknowledged. Such honors should not comprise by default funds issued directly to the recipient. One might, for example, use relevant funds instead to support a project, loosely modeled on Phi Beta Kappa's Visiting Scholar Program,[75] whereby recipients visit colleges, universities, or high schools on an annually shifting list. Here, as with prizes honoring physicians but issued directly to students, supplanting remuneration with awards in keeping with the nature of the recognized asset would be a salient move toward fruitful consistency.[76] Unlike remuneration, such modes of honoring would, it is hoped, contribute directly to virtue and insight, the highest goods of the highest good, namely, soul.

Invocation of Plato, particularly his bedrock views of goods' incommensurability and appetites' natural insatiability, suggests why accounts treating problems of self-interest as centrally new—attending, say, the prominence of managed care and increasing for-profit ventures—fail to arrive at the root of the problem. The last thing we should do at a time when "the behavior of both providers of health care and third-party purchasers is driven more and more by the dollar" (Gray 1991, 5) is institutionalize measures that intensify gratification of the desire for financial gain. Though his account does not cover antiquity, Gray's assertion of "the declining plausibility of trust *and self-restraint* as shapers of the behavior of health care providers" (343) is quite telling from the standpoint of Platonic *sôphrosunê* as addressed in the present study.[77]

Interestingly, Gray's account suggests a close tie between a strengthened desire for financial gain and rising agonism within the health-care setting (e.g., 165, 210, 322, 331). In addition, though one might think that steady monitoring and procedural "safeguards"—which include the setting of remuneration—promote doctors' genuine occupation with their own patients, where character and act-character linkage are deemphasized, they may actually lower doctors' "sense of personal responsibility for patient care decisions" (308). On Pellegrino's (2004, 96; cf. 88) formulation, "blaming the system may diffuse accountability so widely that no one feels responsible." Both of these developments are the opposite of what we should seek.

[75] See http://www.pbk.org/programs/visitingscholars.aspx.

[76] Though not comprising an award, from this vantage point The Arnold P. Gold Foundation's nonpecuniary "Gifts for Rising Third Year Students" in medical schools (http://www.humanism-in-medicine.org/index.php/programs_grants/gold_foundation_programs/student_clinicians_ceremony#Gifts) are a worthwhile measure. My emphasis here is on bringing a nonpecuniary focus to awards themselves.

[77] Emphasis added.

Although certain historical trends are new, *epithumiai* and their insatiable nature are not. One begins to see more fully why the make-or-break virtue for metics, including doctors, entering Magnesia was *sôphrosunê*. From antiquity to the present day, the same inner tensions, translated to and from the outer world, have perforce been with us. Given their inherence and destructive potential, central facets of human agency and motivation operate to our detriment when veiled from the light of day, as Brody's (1992) account of power shows.[78]

10. TRANSPARENCY AND ACCOUNTABILITY: THE WHO AND WHAT OF KNOWING

Let us turn now to condition (4) noted in Section 5, which is transparency involving criteria (1)–(3). The *Laws* is Magnesia's core pedagogical text from childhood to the end of life, which means that from early on, instructed by their metic teachers (804d, 808d, 811c–812a), children are thoroughly exposed to Plato's stance regarding values (i.e., to his objectivism). The *Laws*' account of the optimal community, which features interwovenness, allows one to see how the doctor-patient tie is embedded therein.[79] Koppelman-White (2009, 455) rightly observes that "health and flourishing . . . are generated and sustained within communities (as opposed to individually) and physicians should be considered active members of the communities within which these values are nurtured and take shape."[80] The insight she directs us to here, often ignored nowadays, permeated Plato's *Laws* two and a half millennia ago.

Since Magnesians' exposure to the *Laws* is unrestricted (see Bobonich 2002, 106–7), not only will they be cognizant of Plato's proposals, including the full range of checks and balances, they will also be privy to how he reached his conclusions about human capacities and how his measures address human assets and limitations. Further, Magnesians glean that human values are overarching and get

[78] This is a central place where philosophical hermeneutics, particularly in Nietzsche, Heidegger, Gadamer, and Habermas, is quite helpful; though he does not discuss this material, much of what Brody (1992) says about transparency, centrally including enhanced self-knowledge and accountability (172, 183, 233, 237, 255), meshes with that tradition. Oddly, Brody's concerted handling of transparency invokes it to ground a transition from morality to law, i.e., to show how the "conversation model" can be effectively incorporated legally (115; see more generally 115–19). Though Plato would concur with Brody's focus on power, he would supplant Brody's notion of "[the] same power" (36, cf. 55) differently aimed with the existence of divergent claims about what genuine power is.

[79] Cf. Entralgo (1969, 41), according to whom shared membership in "the human community" is the core motivator for "Plato's ideal physician."

[80] For emphasis on embedment, see also Entralgo (1969, 11, 222–23). According to Rothman (1991, 108), following World War II the "social process [of detachment] . . . reached its culmination. . . . Doctors became a group apart . . . from their society."

rich indications of how those values apply to specific forms of human engagement. In sum, the *Laws'* being Magnesia's core educational text for all throughout the life cycle means that the foundation of all dealings is a transparent, generally accessible account of the city's guiding parameters and specific provisions, and why these were arrived at. Interestingly, despite elaborate webs of checks and balances, relations within and across Magnesian groups will typically be less adversarial than what obtains in Kallipolis between producers and the rest. Transparency, fostered through an education uniting people across sociopolitical and occupational lines, is key to weakening oppositionality and fostering collaboration.

Not coincidentally, in bioethics as in Plato, authoritarian stances (including but not limited to paternalism) and obfuscation—contra transparency as a salient value—go hand in hand. As we have seen, a presumption that medicine is the arbiter of its own ethics reaches back to the AMA's original code of 1847. This includes self-policing, to which that code is unabashedly committed (93).[81] Over a century later, medicine's early "skepticism [about the Hastings Center's founding] stemmed from the belief that if medicine had some ethical problems, these would best be handled within the profession" (Callahan 2012, 52). Work after the center's founding, including Pellegrino and Thomasma's (1993), displays the same attitude with its associated reluctance to give up medicine's self-regulation.[82] As one's views on transparency and accountability are closely related, one must not only ask, *who* should be in the know? but also consider afresh, transparency about *what*?

Although Brody (1992) does not directly tackle medicine's self-policing, he shows clearly that transparency fosters accountability, including a greater likelihood of timely "self-correction" (43).[83] I assume a higher bar for transparency than one's merely naming a supposed warrant, which can be anything from a metaphysical source to a hospital or clinical policy that has come to take on a life of its own.

[81] The original code also valorized the restricted conveyance of information to patients. For the persistence of that view, see Oken's discussion (1961) of doctors' pronounced tendency to withhold cancer diagnoses. Regarding self-policing's integral place in medical codes generally, as Veatch (1981, 82–83) observes, "a true professional ethic . . . includes the claim that only the profession itself is capable of adjudicating ethical disputes related to professional conduct and, moreover, that it bears a responsibility for imposing ethical discipline on its members" (cf. 91). Even where professionals concede the need for a broader foundation, they believe that only they can ascertain what the right grounding is (97–98, 107).

[82] Despite their rejecting "the old ideal of the authority," McIntyre and Popper (1983, 1922) opt for medicine's continued self-policing to avoid "an adversarial context" and foster instead the profession's "full cooperation." Similarly, Irvine (1997) does not question medicine's self-regulation, arguing instead for "a wider vision" of the parties involved (1541). On a purely practical level, the increasingly complex ways in which the health-care industry permeates society (on which see Gray 1991) make it less plausible to treat the medical profession as self-contained.

[83] On the need for greater transparency to foster assessment and accountability, see Gray (1991, 264, 311, 315, 318, 342).

What one provides here verges on tautology: one either relies without explanation on privileged access to that source or dissociates oneself as an individual from a policy that, even if one contributed to its formation (which, given bureaucracies, is increasingly unlikely), one sees as largely detached from oneself through its institutionalization.[84] While proclamations express where authority lies, they do not deepen understanding of authority structures themselves.

Intensified calls for "transparency" (e.g., doctors' disclosure of financial interests)[85] are broadly promising. They fall short, however, if rendering something transparent involves merely providing information, which differs markedly from the conveyance of understanding via *logoi* (i.e., rational accounts), as Plato's *technê* theory of the *Gorgias* makes clear.[86] Following Plato, one may argue that transparency worthy of the name goes beyond the supplying of information to involve real epistemic disclosure, as in Magnesia's legislative preludes and reciprocal provisions of *logoi*. Where transparency is thin at best, one is tethered to symbolic or diffuse accountability, with the result that agonism is built in and genuine collaboration impossible. It is precluded, too, if agonism qua mutual suspicion and perceived clashes of self-interest spiral out of control, since this opens the way to a theoretically infinite

---

[84] Institutionalization centrally includes the mutual dependence of practices and policies; for an example, see Gray (1991, 192). As Schauer (1995) observes, "reasons are what we typically give to support what we conclude precisely when the mere fact that we have concluded is not enough. And reasons are what we typically avoid when the assertion of authority is thought independently important" (637). In contrast, "when decisionmakers ... expect respect for decisions because the decisions are right rather than because they emanate from an authoritative source, then giving reasons becomes a way to bring the subject of the decision into the enterprise" (658).

[85] See, for instance, Mariner (1995, 242); Brennan et al. (2002, 521); Snyder and Neubauer (2007, 793). For a typology of financial incentives, see Rodwin (1993, 56, 136), who, drawing helpfully on the law, observes that the locution "potential conflict of interest" is self-contradictory since "conflicts of interest have the capacity to cause harm; the injury may not yet have occurred. To label such situations as merely *potential* would mitigate the very real risk involved" (9; italics in original). Similarly, Beauchamp and Childress (2013, 330–31) underscore the disvalue of attempts to parse "whether a conflict is *actual*, *potential*, or *merely apparent* ... since the potential or merely apparent conflict often constitutes a real conflict-of-interest situation" (italics in original).

[86] Moravcsik's stress (1992, 11–45) on the distinctiveness of Platonic understanding is useful here. As Thompson (1993, 575) points out, one shortcoming of disclosure is that patients may lack "reasonable alternative courses of action in the circumstances.... Disclosing a conflict only reveals a problem, without providing any guidance for resolving it." For helpful discussion, see also Rodwin (1993, 199, 215–19). The AMA's Code of Medical Ethics places excess weight on information's mere provision: e.g., "when physicians enter into arrangements that provide opportunities for self-referral they must ... disclose their financial interest in the facility, product, or equipment to patients; inform them of available alternatives for referral; and assure them that their ongoing care is not conditioned on accepting the recommended referral" (Opinion 8.0321); see also 8.047, 10.01. At times disclosure sounds reactive: "Physicians must *be prepared to discuss* with patients any financial arrangements [involving capitation] which could impact patient care" (Opinion 8.051; emphasis added); see further 8.054, 8.063.

regress of accountability structures as monitors increasingly distant from the agent, hence obscure, are forged to stem conduct that is not desired.[87]

The *Laws* showcases that transparency is essential to real, versus semi-emblematic or nebulous, accountability and that accountability is itself requisite for collaboration. Processes for holding transgressors responsible are credible just so far as they are premised on the illegitimacy of individuals' hiding behind societal roles and stature of whatever kind. Any party in Magnesia, irrespective of his current plane of officialdom or sociopolitical role, may—indeed, must—bring another party to justice. This framework centrally includes high officials' being reciprocally subject to review. Crucially, in Magnesia one is not simply told on what authority something is said. One learns why, based on the relevant subject matter, a practice or vantage point is defensible. This learning comes through the *Laws*' being Magnesia's core educational text. Regarding the constitution more specifically, it stems from the fact that the city's legislation includes preludes versus its comprising proclamations alone, whose embrace is insisted on merely because founding authorities happened to put those measures in place to steer Magnesia's administration.

According to Emanuel (1997), notwithstanding the diverse venues and vantage points involved, the accountability of all—doctors, managed care organizations, employers, investors, private payers, the government, and, "last but not least," patients (53)—is best promoted if there is "one party with broad responsibility for setting standards. Professional associations—whether national, state or county, specialty, licensing, or accrediting—are the natural parties to articulate tangible standards for professional accountability. Almost by definition, there are no other entities that have such ability and extensive responsibility to be the guardians of health care values—for the medical profession and for society" (53–54). Accountability "procedures" may include "a moral disposition, with only an internal conscience for monitoring accountability" (54).

While such an approach may lead to improvements, Plato would not favor making each subdomain of health care's provision the arbiter of its own practice. If less is reciprocally known, with transparency operating within more strictly delimited bounds, gains within subspecialties may be attenuated if not offset by liabilities elsewhere. In addition, Emanuel's (1997) approach is at odds with Plato's stress on reciprocal oversight of all, including high officials. In fact, far from promoting said reciprocity, implementing her proposal might seed medicine's power expansion,

---

[87] Cf. Gray (1991, 331). On agonism as built into the tort paradigm for handling medical malpractice, see Sharpe (2004, 17); Levine (2004, 47); Dauer (2004, 197, 200). In addition, that system stresses opacity (on which see, e.g., Levine 2004, 47), which is antithetical to the notion of accountability permeating the *Laws*' virtue ethic.

since medical associations in aggregate are the origin of relevant standards, including those for "good" patients. Moreover, by allowing "moral disposition" to enforce accountability in certain (unspecified) settings, Emanuel further ignores human fallibility in favor of what is essentially medicine's self-policing in a now expanded kingdom.

Interestingly, if one substitutes medicine for philosophy, Plato's *Republic* corresponds roughly to a scenario—not unlike that represented by Eryximachus in the *Symposium*—where medicine distinctively grasps values and uses that insight both to conduct its own profession and to oversee others. In Kallipolis, philosopher-rulers—to whom alone reality is known—are accountable to no human venue but rather strictly to their own metaphysical vision of the real, or divine, qua Forms. Plato's confidence in ordinary folk there is low enough overall that instead of openly explaining and defending to Kallipolis' citizens human nature's tripartition, he offers the so-called myth of the metals, according to which, subterranean in origin, humans literally contain qualitatively different metals hierarchically arranged (415a–c). Plato of the *Republic* thought that only on such a model, including minimal transparency across the city, was accountability ensured. Under such conditions, real collaboration among human beings is precluded.[88]

In the *Laws*, heralded by the *Statesman*, Plato sees that the moral buck's not stopping at a single spot does not of itself attenuate responsibility. Since all are raised on the text of the *Laws*, all have open, ongoing access to the same truths, which co-understanding is needed for true accountability. As Plato also sees in the *Laws*, reciprocal accountability both within and across milieux is essential to collaboration. This comparison of the *Republic* and *Laws* helps to illustrate why it is instructive to look not exclusively at the latter but also at the progression of thought by which Plato reaches this outcome. Above all, studying the trajectory of Plato's thought shows just how much difference deep acknowledgment of human fallibility can make to one's reflections in other foundational respects.

II. VEATCH AND BRODY ON LAYPEOPLE'S VALUES CONTRIBUTIONS

In *A Theory of Medical Ethics* (1981), Veatch introduces a three-tiered grid of values (a so-called triple contract, 108) that moves from the most general plane to specific clinical relationships. The foundational tier comprises moral principles and guidelines for human beings, while the second forges those for medicine against this

[88] Kallipolis' tiny group of philosopher-rulers may constitute an exception. Since, however, one philosopher suffices (*Republic* 540d4), these figures' collaboration cannot be requisite for the city's thriving.

backdrop. Finally, particular doctor-patient duos adjust details of their tie (e.g., how much information does this patient want?) within the parameters set by more general standards already forged (e.g., honesty as a human value figuring importantly in medicine).

Beyond their involvement on the third tier, how do patients (i.e., laypeople) figure in Veatch's account? Veatch wants principles on tiers 1–2 to be apprehensible (1981, 88, 91–92, 99, 134, 138) and "acceptable" (113) to ordinary folk. As to principles' formulation, he both envisions "reasonable laypeople coming together with reasonable members of the profession" (159) and stresses positions he views as right, for instance, not killing even aggressors (233–34) and precluding all "merciful killing" (239).

Veatch's "standard of the reasonable [lay]person" (182–83, 200, 203) included in deliberations about these levels is highly selective and divergent from the low opinion reflected in his claim (268) that "laypeople, generally grossly unequal to providers in income, educational, and social class, are unable to communicate their system of beliefs and values to the provider standing in a radically different tradition. A moral bond between such a layperson and physician is impossible." Veatch's reliance (e.g., 130–31; cf. 134, 241) on Rawls' *A Theory of Justice* suggests that at bottom he has in view "hypothetical" (130–31) "reasonable" people, not, as he claims, "real-life, fallible" (291) ones.[89] Veatch admits as much when endorsing "full participation by all who can approximate the role of reasonable people capable of taking the moral point of view" (327).

While a virtue-based stance also foregrounds a descriptive-normative gap, Veatch's level of desire and confidence respecting laypeople's contributions on tiers 1–2, including whether and how one might better prepare them for such, is unclear. In contrast, one can say assuredly that laypeople are centrally involved on level 3, where values parameters for individual duos' dealings are negotiated. At this point in Veatch's scheme, however, all the intellectual heavy lifting has been done. Moreover, this stance, far from being new, is in line with existing scenarios that focus on patients' values contributions qua subjective preferences. As Katz (1984, 102) puts the point, doctors "know more about disease. Patients know more about their own needs."

Veatch's leaning away from ordinary folk concerning values' framing on the broadest plane is more pronounced in *Hippocratic, Religious, and Secular Medical Ethics: The Points of Conflict* (2012). He remains staunchly committed to the view that "it is impossible to know the ends of medicine without looking outside medicine to some worldview" (88), where human values on tier 1 in the earlier work

---

[89] See Rawls (1999) on the "veil of ignorance," which he deems "purely hypothetical" (19), and contractors' "rationality" (123–30).

reside.[90] What differs is his express commitment to the view that professionals—albeit nonmedical ones—are distinctively poised to apprehend them: "One needs a claim to authority on the foundation or grounding of morality in order to claim expertise in matters of ethics. That is precisely what religions and philosophical schools of thought claim" (100). This assertion of expertise is warranted, with the result that "sources grounded in religion and philosophy" are the loci to which "laypeople as well as those who [happen] to be medical professionals" should "turn ... for establishing an ethic for lay-professional relations in health care" (66). Only on this broad foundation can we address "more narrow questions about how those who adopt a particular worldview understand how particular social roles like physician or patient should be governed" (138). Veatch's pointed distinction of religious and secular philosophical venues from "professional sources" (66) is misleading since his own emphasis, like that of Pellegrino and Thomasma (1993), is on professionals, in his case religious and philosophical ones who are laypeople strictly from a medical standpoint.[91]

Like Veatch, Brody (1992), whose confidence in patients is loosely reminiscent of the *Laws*' reciprocal provisions of *logoi*,[92] is concerned with values falling beyond the clinical tie narrowly construed, in particular with those in medicine (i.e., Veatch's second tier). Brody does, however, tie this plane to that of values tout court when claiming that "the types of power attributed to the physician ... arise less from the essential nature of medical practice and more from the fact that that practice has to be carried out by human beings in a particular social and cultural context. ... Medical practice is a social enterprise" (63, cf. 82). Further, doctors must "defend publicly [their] judgments as to who the good and the bad are" (229). Again a linkage of broad and medical values is forged: in casuistry, which Brody supports, "the mode of reasoning and the morally relevant features of the case are products of the whole culture" (241).

Brody's combining a focus on broader values and relative confidence in patients is important. He does not, however, unite these features to defend a more substantive values role for laypeople beyond the clinical setting, aligning himself instead with Pellegrino and Thomasma's (1993) claim that medical ethics should be formulated from within the medical profession (Brody 1992, 171n10, 176, 201, 271). Moreover,

---

90 On medicine's wider contextualization, cf. Koch (2012, xix), whose own study locates bioethics thus (22) and critiques it from that broader standpoint.

91 Cf. Koch (2013, 346).

92 For relative confidence see, e.g., Brody (1992, 35, 114, 116–17, 128, 155). As for similarities to the *Laws*, he speaks of "frank negotiation and persuasion," albeit "to redirect the patient's power toward the best outcome" (65); patients themselves may have occasion to persuade doctors (128).

insofar as Brody embeds the values guiding medicine in societal commitments, he might be thought to imply that doctors have a modicum of distinctiveness there. The foregoing discussion of Veatch (2012; 1981) and Brody (1992) shows that even where contemporary accounts focus on broader values and strive to acknowledge laypeople's abilities beyond what has often prevailed, they may not clearly ground and accommodate values roles for layfolk outside of specific clinical ties.[93]

Brody's account in *The Future of Bioethics* (2009) is more promising for its clear recognition that "any community dialogue process is quite capable of correction and refinement to an indefinite degree" (93).[94] He favors a model of public discussion that allows nonspecialists in bioethics to "collaborate in determining what questions the process ought to address" (99). Brody rightly sees that such undertakings involve education (regarding health care, at any rate) and that fresh ideas and perspectives can emerge from practically any source in the general public (ibid.). While he does not specify where laypeople are equipped to operate, including whether and how far experts, however identified, would themselves guide the undertaking, Brody's steps in this recent book to moderate what has been a heavily uneven playing field point in a promising direction.

12. CONCLUSION

Although he does not mention Plato, Brody (2009) stresses a greater need for clear-sighted attention to the history of ethics that bears on medicine (27–29). I contend that as we move forward from here to discern, defend, and pursue our aims, we can benefit by attending to Plato. I concentrate first on the clinical tie, then address the broader social context in which that relation is embedded.

If all we had was the *Republic*, Plato would not suggest a fruitful approach to the clinical tie or its social embedment. While the *Laws* has garnered more attention from specialists in recent decades, it remains understudied by comparison with the earlier dialogue. Not only is there no univocal Greek view of medicine, but Plato's own stance is far more nuanced than interpreters have previously observed. Though he is cited in contemporary treatments of the optimal doctor-patient tie, the promise of Plato—above all, the *Laws*, his final work—has so far been nearly untapped. Bioethical proposals striving for alternatives to paternalism and autonomy often fail

---

[93] Myser's (2004) "community-based participatory research" falls on Veatch's second plane. Daniels and Sabin's procedural model for allocation decisions (1998) is justifiably critiqued by Sabik and Lie (2008, 82–83) for its limitation to the content of Veatch's third tier (here, appealing decisions already made) versus its involving patients on the second level (i.e., at the point of coverage principles' formulation).

[94] Cf. 88–104, 226.

to preserve the delicate balance between authority and parity needed of the healing tie. I have argued that the *Laws*' dynamic involving doctor and patient prompts one to consider afresh whether these threads can helpfully coexist.

The *Laws*' conception of the physician-patient tie—including Plato's simultaneous provision of a parent-child analogy and avoidance of paternalism—may seem paradoxical, if not incoherent, at first blush. Yet this appearance is fruitful insofar as its probing helps to show how seemingly incompatible threads may intermingle in a rich account of what optimal medical practice involves. A designation for Plato's stance based on the *Laws* cannot be encompassed by a single term, as with "paternalism" or "autonomy." As previously suggested, one might, for starters, identify it as a functionally complementary and ultimately balanced asymmetry. As indicated in Section 5, my claim is not that the *Laws* itself fully realizes all salient criteria. That said, it is exciting indeed to think that antiquity provides us with an illustration of how one might acknowledge asymmetry of a kind without capitulating to the oppositional modalities of paternalism and autonomy.

On the clinical tie's social embedment, though Plato surpasses Veatch in his firm recognition of laypeople's gifts, Magnesians grasp what obtains but do not also coformulate it. Of course, no Magnesian, including higher officials, is thus involved, as the *Laws* is framed as an exercise in forging a constitution for a soon-to-be-established Cretan colony (702a–d).

While limited in this way, the *Laws* intermingles valuable threads whose substance, when recognized in current accounts, is often handled discretely. Key features of Plato's properly expansive approach are values' foundational nature; his account of human fallibility; a general confidence in human abilities; values' requisite transparency; his conviction of the efficacy of values *paideia* as a lifelong enterprise spanning formation, enrichment, and maintenance; reciprocal accountability within and across levels and kinds of activity; and such accountability's being requisite for collaboration.

As we have seen, Plato sees clearly just how far human fallibility extends, even in those who are best. Quite importantly, his notion equally covers intellectual and ethical (i.e., character-based) restrictions. Plato's deep recognition of human fallibility, thoroughgoingly built into Magnesia, opens his eyes to ordinary people's abilities, including the fact that people's rational and ethical capacities truly fall on a single continuum. Due to their native gifts, combined with extensive *paideia*, Magnesians will apprehend not only what the provisions are but their rationales. They are also crucially involved in the application of the city's legal code, which embodies reason. In addition, the citizen body must approve all permissible legal revisions. Moreover, ordinary citizens are eligible for most posts, including higher ones, and constitute citizen juries that render sophisticated decisions involving justice—ones that philosopher-rulers would have reached unilaterally in Kallipolis. Last but not least, the fact that the *Laws* is itself Magnesia's core educational text shows Plato's confidence in people's ability to appreciate the metalevel (i.e., the broadest plane of human values), since, for the first and only time in the dialogues, ordinary folk are allowed "backstage": they do not glimpse outcomes alone without underlying rationales, as in Kallipolis; instead, they are privy not merely to legislative preludes, already a huge improvement, but also to overarching structural discussions among the Stranger, Cleinias, and Megillus about how best to proceed, what to avoid, and why.

The *Laws* defends fallibility without excuses, which may seem like a paradox, but which Plato shows is not. Accepting our limitedness is essential if we are to build the best possible individual and collective existence. Knowing this, we should, for instance, make it integral to our deliberations as individuals and communities to ask not only what we should do but why we wish to do this or that, including whether our motives are mixed in such a way that a countervailing impact on our good intentions might be operative or take effect.

Grasping our fallibility and needed checks to minimize its harms, with those things' being in our power, means that we have nowhere to hide if we slip up. This is different from saying that we must be perfect at all times and from the get-go—a worry sometimes expressed about current notions of medical accountability.[95] Providing reasons for what we have done is fundamentally different from proffering excuses. For Plato, the latter reflect irrational attempts at justifying what will lack an exculpatory warrant (unless, of course, a capability for improvement toward virtue is lacking, as with insanity). Where the *Laws*' legal provisions focus on action, they do so with character in view. Whether we realize a failing on our own or have it pointed out, the cause of a culpable error may be a defect in character that has shown up in action. Because it permeates accountability, structural reciprocity characterizes opportunities for improvement: where A might point out B's shortcoming on one occasion, another time the situations could well be reversed.[96]

In addition to being reciprocal, accountability is exceptionless inasmuch as no one venue (e.g., medicine over against the rest of society) or intracontextual agency (within medicine, the AMA or a specially created professional body) is the ultimate arbiter, that is to say, where the evaluative buck always stops. Not only does accountability operate within and across levels, but anyone, irrespective of official or sociopolitical role, can be an agent through whom shortcomings are brought to light. These factors,

---

95 On the harm wrought by "perfectionistic demands" under the aegis of professionalism, see Fochtmann (2004, 39); cf. Ginsburg and Stern (2004, 15).

96 Cf. McIntyre and Popper (1983), except that their scenario is largely restricted to health-care practitioners and medical students.

taken together, could likely mitigate a sense of arbitrariness and the adversarial tone that might otherwise permeate relevant structures. Plato's insistence on oversight within and across levels has promise if we care to generate sound buffers against unchecked expressions of cognitive and ethical fallibility. While the detailed whole of what the *Laws* commends would likely create a blanketing effect beyond what our own democracy allows, there is a democratizing cast to the *Laws*' view of human capabilities and balanced oversight structures.[97]

Since the ultimate aim of human existence, irrespective of societal roles, is *aretê*, the overall purpose of legal measures in Magnesia is not retaliation but perpetrators' psychic improvement via *paideia*, which, as we have seen, is a lifelong affair.[98] Hence, wrongdoers are typically not separated from the community but aided from within it based on the values and parameters guiding everything that transpires. A sense that all truly are together in the enterprise of promoting *eudaimonia* is most likely fostered thereby.[99] That said, from the *Gorgias* through the *Laws*, Plato does not shy away from acknowledging that the vice of some may be irremediable, in which case detachment of them from the community is requisite. If all attempts at enhancement via *paideia* fail, this suggests that the relevant human capabilities are present either not at all or so dimly that those individuals' continued presence in the community is insupportable. As to medicine specifically, Plato's approach to rehabilitation and removal—generous in its way, yet firm—supports a harder line across a spectrum of acts and offenders than has typically operated under the aegis of medical boards and organizations.[100]

---

[97] See also Woozley (2010, 388–89, 392).

[98] In health care specifically, the aim is not to slight continuing medical education (CME) focused on knowledge and skills but rather to stress the salience of ongoing values pedagogy of the kind discussed here.

[99] Cf. Pellegrino (2004, 97), whose account of medicine here is broadly *Laws*-like, albeit without mentioning that dialogue.

[100] The notion of a broader spectrum applies not just to individual practitioners' assessment but also to venues' identity, with greater attention to what Hafferty (2004, 30) calls "professional deviance," i.e., "unprofessional behavior at the organizational level," which medicine has historically "insisted . . . was virtually nonexistent." A study of the Ohio State Medical Board's handling of complaints leaves Jost et al. (1993) concerned about medical boards' response to "problems concerning the clinical competence of their licensees (and thus ultimately the problem of medical error) through disciplinary interventions" (335). Further, the authors doubt that as things stand, "medical licensure boards are capable of systematically identifying incompetent practitioners, and that board interventions can address the problems caused by such practitioners" (336). According to Jung, Lurie, and Wolfe (2006), "although criminal activity by physicians is of great concern . . . state medical boards vary in their monitoring and discipline of criminal activities by licensed physicians" (336), including "often-modest sanctions by state medical boards even after" criminal convictions (344). Not all such bodies "consider a felony conviction related to the practice of medicine to be sufficient grounds in and of itself for a board review, hearing or action," and they "do not consistently conduct criminal background checks on all physicians applying for a medical license" (336). A study of state boards' "rate of serious disciplinary actions" (Wolfe 2012, 1) for 2009–11 grounds the conclusion

Finally, the very same conviction about human abilities undergirding Magnesia can support extending laypeople's contributions to metalevel reflections on topics including how best to balance "individual good and common good, ethics and the law . . . universal ethical principles and cultural particularities . . . essentialist and nonessentialist notions of human nature and human dignity, and the right and the good" (Callahan 2012, 157). As Veatch (2012; 1981) maintains, one rightly moves from the overarching plane of values to their medical application. Here, too, ordinary citizens' gifts warrant their involvement in formulatory work.[101]

Two caveats are in order. First, I am not committed to the view that all people's values contributions on the two planes will be, or even can be, equal in content or merit—a point that applies whether comparisons are intraprofessional or cross-populational. This was not a commitment of Plato's, nor should it be a goal of ours if we seek the richest possible deliberations. Second, I do not claim that experts are irrelevant on either level. While their involvement is fully expected, it is key that experts' participation avoid undue restriction of others, centrally including pronounced limitation from the get-go on what count as legitimate offerings. I worry

---

that "most states are not living up to their obligations to protect patients from doctors who are practicing medicine in a substandard manner. . . . Action must . . . be taken, through legislation and through pressure on the medical boards themselves, to increase the amount of discipline and, thus, the amount of patient protection. Without adequate legislative oversight, many medical boards will continue to perform poorly" (3). In 1994, the Federation of State Medical Boards asked its own Legislative and Legal Advisory Committee to consider "gaps in the oversight of residents" (Winn and Fuqua 1996, 160). The resulting "Report on Licensure of Physicians Enrolled in Postgraduate Training Programs" laid out an oversight scheme to place every resident from the outset "under the jurisdiction of [his or her] state medical board" (Legislative and Legal Advisory Committee 1996, 163). Apart from the fact that the report has the status of a recommendation, not a requirement, one might worry that existing defects in boards' oversight of physicians would simply carry over to their monitoring of an expanded medical population. From the side of the medical profession as reflected in organizations, "there is a marked difference between the formalized reaction . . . to a failed board exam and . . . responses to a breach of ethics. . . . The profession has been loath to discipline its own members and has opposed external regulation as intrusive into areas it considers its autonomous domain. In contrast to the proactive stance it assumes with respect to competency, organized medicine has generated only relatively passive [ethical] codes, which . . . have no teeth" (d'Oronzio 2002, 361–62).

101 Though they do not go far enough (notably, the broadest values plane is neglected), recent discussions of "public deliberation" are a good beginning: see Blacksher et al. (2012); Solomon and Abelson (2012); Goold et al. (2012); Abelson, Warren, and Forest (2012). While he does not cite Plato, Jennings (2001) makes valuable reference to Greek and Roman antiquity when speaking of "urban bioethics" as covering "political deliberation concerning the ends of life and the nature of human flourishing, including health and well-being" (102); Jennings' account calls to mind the *Laws'* view that the *ergon* of Magnesian citizens is being such. Recent occupation with medical "professionalism," which dates to the 1980s (Hafferty 2004, 28), also risks attending inadequately to the tier of human values. While discussions under that head include important material, this limitation in subject matter goes hand in hand with the term "professionalism," which reinforces the notion that the pursuit of ethics in and for medicine is a largely if not entirely self-contained affair—a stance toward values that was critiqued in Section 2. For similar worries regarding "professionalism," see Hester and Kovach (2004); Dudzinski (2004).

about just this in O'Doherty et al.'s (2012) account of discussions' "framing" by adepts, where

> to frame an issue means to select and highlight the aspects of it that will be presented in the deliberative forum and the ways in which problems, arguments, information, and positions will be presented. Appropriate framing is critical to ensure the legitimacy of a deliberative forum. Without it, the topics selected and the questions or tasks posed may place undue emphasis on a subset of considerations. . . . Appropriate framing involves clarifying and presenting the range of available perspectives. The framing of questions involves deciding how much leeway to give participants to define issues for themselves versus giving them specific questions to discuss. (21)

Although Callahan's (2012, 182) claim that "ethics is something that is grasped by everyone" may not be true as things stand, human intellectual and ethical attainment rendering us able to critique ideas and commit to proposals may be cultivated. To maximize the participatory abilities of all even as we remain attuned to abiding human limits, *paideia* (i.e., values education) from childhood on is key. Further application of these points to bioethics is a project for another time. What I hope to have shown here is that Plato's work, especially the *Laws*, attunes us to human concerns that we would do well to heed going forward, and thus that it merits fuller inclusion in bioethical accounts of medicine and its social embedment than it has heretofore received.

BIBLIOGRAPHY

Abelson, J., M.E. Warren, and P.-G. Forest. 2012. "The Future of Public Deliberation on Health Issues." *Hastings Center Report* 42/2: 27–29.

Adomėnas, M. 2001. "Self-Reference, Textuality, and the Status of the Political Project in Plato's *Laws*." *Oxford Studies in Ancient Philosophy* 21: 29–59.

Allen, J. 1994. "Failure and Expertise in the Ancient Conception of an Art." In *Scientific Failure*, 81–108. Ed. T. Horowitz and A.I. Janis. Lanham, Md.: Rowman and Littlefield.

American Medical Association. 1847. *Code of Medical Ethics*. http://www.ama-assn.org/resources/doc/ethics/1847code.pdf. Accessed May 18, 2013.

———. 1990. House of Delegates Proceedings, 165–96. 44th Interim Meeting, Report of the Council on Ethical and Judicial Affairs. http://ama.nmtvault.com/jsp/viewer.jsp?doc_id=House+of+Delegates+Proceedings%2Fama_arch%2FHOD00001%2F00000131&query1=&recoffset=200&collection_filter=All&collection_name=House+of+Delegates+Proceedings&init_width=640&sort_col=date. Accessed July 3, 2013.

———. 2013. *Code of Medical Ethics*. http://www.ama-assn.org/ama/pub/physician-resources/medical-ethics/code-medical-ethics.page. Accessed June 7, 2013.

Amundsen, D.W., and G.B. Ferngren. 1977. "The Physician as an Expert Witness in Athenian Law." *Bulletin of the History of Medicine* 51: 202–13.

Anagnostopoulos, G. 2000. "Euthanasia and the Physician's Role: Reflections on Some Views in the Ancient Greek Tradition." In *Bioethics: Ancient Themes in Contemporary Issues*, 251–90. Ed. M.G. Kuczewski and R. Polansky. Cambridge, Mass.: MIT Press.

Annas, J. 1981. *An introduction to Plato's* Republic. Oxford: Clarendon Press.

———. 2000. "Philosophical Therapy, Ancient and Modern." In *Bioethics: Ancient Themes in Contemporary Issues*, 109–27. Ed. M.G. Kuczewski and R. Polansky. Cambridge, Mass.: MIT Press.

Annas, J., and R. Waterfield, trans. 1995. Plato, *Statesman*. Cambridge: Cambridge University Press.

Anton, J.P. 1980. "Dialectic and Health in Plato's *Gorgias*: Presuppositions and Implications." *Ancient Philosophy* 1: 49–60.

Arnold P. Gold Foundation. 2010. "Student Clinician's Ceremony." http://www.humanism-in-medicine.org/index.php/programs_grants/gold_foundation_programs/student_clinicians_ceremony#Gifts. Accessed June 4, 2013.

Balint, J., and W. Shelton. 1996. "Regaining the Initiative: Forging a New Model of the Patient-Physician Relationship." *Journal of the American Medical Association* 275: 887–91.

Banja, J.D. 2005. *Medical Errors and Medical Narcissism*. Sudbury, Mass.: Jones and Bartlett.

Barker, E. 1960. *Greek Political Theory: Plato and His Predecessors*. London: Methuen.

Beauchamp, T.L., and J.F. Childress. 2013. *Principles of Biomedical Ethics*. 7th ed. New York: Oxford University Press.

Bentley, R.K. 2003. "Ruling Oneself: Platonic Hedonism and the Quality of Citizenship." *Polis* 20: 85–107.

Berman, S. 1991. "Socrates and Callicles on Pleasure." *Phronesis* 36: 117–40.

Blacksher, E., A. Diebel, P.-G. Forest, S.D. Goold, and J. Abelson. 2012. "What Is Public Deliberation?" *Hastings Center Report* 42/2: 14–17.

Bobonich, C. 1991. "Persuasion, Compulsion and Freedom in Plato's *Laws*." *Classical Quarterly* 41: 365–88.

———. 1995. "The Virtues of Ordinary People in Plato's *Statesman*." In *Reading the* Statesman: *Proceedings of the III Symposium Platonicum*, 313–29. Ed. C.J. Rowe. Sankt Augustin: Academia Verlag.

———. 1996. "Reading the *Laws*." In *Form and Argument in Late Plato*, 249–82. Ed. C. Gill and M.M. McCabe. Oxford: Clarendon Press.

———. 2001. "Akrasia and Agency in Plato's *Laws* and *Republic*." In *Essays on Plato's Psychology*, 203–37. Ed. E. Wagner. Lanham, Md.: Lexington Books.

———. 2002. *Plato's Utopia Recast: His Later Ethics and Politics*. Oxford: Clarendon Press.

Brennan, T., L. Blank, J. Cohen, and H. Kimball. 2002. "Medical Professionalism in the New Millennium: A Physicians' Charter." *Lancet* 359: 520–22.

Brickhouse, T.C., and N.D. Smith. 1997. "The Problem of Punishment in Socratic Philosophy." In *New Essays in Socratic Studies: Wisdom, Ignorance, and Virtue*, 95–107. Special issue of *Apeiron*, 30/4. Ed. M.L. McPherran. Edmonton, Alberta: Academic Printing and Publishing.

———. 2002. "Incurable Souls in Socratic Psychology." *Ancient Philosophy* 22: 21–36.

Brill, S.A. 2006. "Medical Moderation in Plato's *Symposium*." *Studies in the History of Ethics* 11: 1–28.

Brisson, L., and J.-F. Pradeau. 2007. *Les* Lois *de Platon*. Paris: Presses universitaires de France.

Brody, H. 1992. *The Healer's Power*. New Haven, Conn.: Yale University Press.

———. 2009. *The Future of Bioethics*. New York: Oxford University Press.

Brown, E. 2000. "Justice and Compulsion for Plato's Philosopher-Rulers." *Ancient Philosophy* 20: 1–17.

Buchanan, A.E. 1996. "Is There a Medical Profession in the House?" In *Conflicts of Interest in Clinical Practice and Research*, 105–36. Ed. R.G. Spece, D.S. Shimm, and A.E. Buchanan. New York: Oxford University Press.

Burkholder, P.M. 1978. "Plato's Treatment of Invalids in *Republic III*." *Tulane Studies in Philosophy* 27: 27–35.
Burnet, J., ed. 1901. Plato, *Opera*. Vol. 2. Oxford: Clarendon Press.
———, ed. 1903. Plato, *Opera*. Vol. 3. Oxford: Clarendon Press.
———, ed. 1907. Plato, *Opera*. Vol. 5. Oxford: Clarendon Press.
Bury, R.G., ed. 1932. *The* Symposium *of Plato*. 2nd ed. Cambridge: Heffer.
Bywater, I., ed. 1894. Aristotle, *Ethica Nicomachea*. Oxford: Clarendon Press.
Callahan, D. 2012. *In Search of the Good: A Life in Bioethics*. Cambridge, Mass.: MIT Press.
Capelle, W. 1922. "Zur hippokratischen Frage." *Hermes* 57: 247–65.
Carone, G.R. 2004. "Calculating Machines or Leaky Jars? The Moral Psychology of Plato's *Gorgias*." *Oxford Studies in Ancient Philosophy* 26: 55–96.
Carrick, P. 2001. *Medical Ethics in the Ancient World*. Washington, D.C.: Georgetown University Press.
Cherniss, H.F. 1965a. "The Philosophical Economy of the Theory of Ideas." In *Studies in Plato's Metaphysics*, 1–12. Ed. R.E. Allen. London: Routledge and Kegan Paul.
———. 1965b. "The Relation of the *Timaeus* to Plato's Later Dialogues." In *Studies in Plato's Metaphysics*, 339–78. Ed. R.E. Allen. London: Routledge and Kegan Paul.
Childress, J.F., and M. Siegler. 1984. "Metaphors and Models of Doctor-Patient Relationships: Their Implications for Autonomy." *Theoretical Medicine* 5: 17–30.
Cole, E.B. 1991. "Weaving and Practical Politics in Plato's *Statesman*." *Southern Journal of Philosophy* 29: 195–208.
Cooper, J.M., ed. 1997. *Plato: Complete Works*. Indianapolis: Hackett Publishing Company.
———. 1999a. "Plato's *Statesman* and Politics." In *Reason and Emotion: Essays on Ancient Moral Psychology and Ethical Theory*, 165–91. Princeton, N.J.: Princeton University Press.
———. 1999b. "Socrates and Plato in Plato's *Gorgias*." In *Reason and Emotion: Essays on Ancient Moral Psychology and Ethical Theory*, 29–75. Princeton, N.J.: Princeton University Press.
Cornford, F.M., trans. 1957. *Plato's Theory of Knowledge: The* Theaetetus *and the* Sophist *of Plato*. New York: Macmillan.
Craik, E.M. 2001. "Plato and Medical Texts: *Symposium* 185c–193d." *Classical Quarterly*, n.s., 51: 109–14.
Culver, C.M, K.D. Clouser, B. Gert, H. Brody, J. Fletcher, A. Jonsen, L. Kopelman, J. Lynn, M. Siegler, and D. Wikler. 1985. "Special Report: Basic Curricular Goals in Medical Ethics." *New England Journal of Medicine* 312: 253–56.
Daniels, N. 2008. *Just Health: Meeting Health Needs Fairly*. New York: Cambridge University Press.
Daniels, N., and J.E. Sabin. 1998. "Last Chance Therapies and Managed Care: Pluralism, Fair Procedures, and Legitimacy." *Hastings Center Report* 28/2: 27–41.
Dauer, E.A. 2004. "Ethical Misfits: Mediation and Medical Malpractice Litigation." In *Accountability: Patient Safety and Policy Reform*, 185–201. Ed. V.A. Sharpe. Washington, D.C.: Georgetown University Press.
Davidson, J.N. 1997. *Courtesans and Fishcakes: The Consuming Passions of Classical Athens*. New York: HarperCollins.
Diels, H. 1992. *Die Fragmente der Vorsokratiker*. Ed. W. Kranz. Vol. 1. 6th ed. Reprint, Zürich: Weidmann.
Dodds, E.R., ed. 1959. Plato, *Gorgias*. Oxford: Clarendon Press.

Dorion, L.-A. 2012. "*Enkrateia* and the Partition of the Soul in the *Gorgias*." In *Plato and the Divided Self*, 33–52. Ed. R. Barney, T. Brennan, and C. Brittain. Cambridge: Cambridge University Press.

Dorland's Illustrated Medical Dictionary. 2012. 32nd ed. Philadelphia: Elsevier.

d'Oronzio, J.C. 2002. "Practicing Accountability in Professional Ethics." *Journal of Clinical Ethics* 13: 359–66.

Dorter, K. 1969. "The Significance of the Speeches in Plato's *Symposium*." *Philosophy and Rhetoric* 2: 215–34.

Doukas, D.J. 2004. "Returning to Professionalism: The Reemergence of Medicine's Art." *American Journal of Bioethics* 4: 18–19.

Dover, K., ed. 1980. Plato, *Symposium*. Cambridge: Cambridge University Press.

———. 1989. *Greek Homosexuality*. Cambridge, Mass.: Harvard University Press.

Drabkin, I.E. 1955. "Remarks on Ancient Psychopathology." *Isis* 46: 223–34.

Dudzinski, D.M. 2004. "Integrity in the Relationship between Medical Ethics and Professionalism." *American Journal of Bioethics* 4: 26–27.

Dugdale, L.S., M. Siegler, and D.T. Rubin. 2008. "Medical Professionalism and the Doctor-Patient Relationship." *Perspectives in Biology and Medicine* 51: 547–53.

Duke, E.A., W.F. Hicken, W.S.M. Nicoll, D.B. Robinson, and J.C.G. Strachan, eds. 1995. Plato, *Opera*. Vol. 1. Oxford: Clarendon Press.

Edelstein, L. 1952. "The Relation of Ancient Philosophy to Medicine." *Bulletin of the History of Medicine* 26: 299–316.

———. 1987a. "The Hippocratic Oath: Text, Translation and Interpretation." In *Ancient Medicine: Selected Papers of Ludwig Edelstein*, 3–63. Ed. O. and C.L. Temkin. Baltimore, Md.: Johns Hopkins University Press.

———. 1987b. "The Hippocratic Physician." In *Ancient Medicine: Selected Papers of Ludwig Edelstein*, 87–110. Ed. O. and C.L. Temkin. Baltimore, Md.: Johns Hopkins University Press.

———. 1987c. "The Rôle of Eryximachus in Plato's *Symposium*." In *Ancient Medicine: Selected Papers of Ludwig Edelstein*, 153–71. Ed. O. and C.L. Temkin. Baltimore, Md.: Johns Hopkins University Press.

Emanuel, E.J. 2006. "Changing Premed Requirements and the Medical Curriculum." *Journal of the American Medical Association* 296: 1128–31.

Emanuel, E.J., and L.L. Emanuel. 1992. "Four Models of the Physician-Patient Relationship." *Journal of the American Medical Association* 267: 2221–26.

Emanuel, L.L. 1997. "Professional Standards in Health Care: Calling All Parties to Account." *Health Affairs* 16: 52–54.

England, E.B. 1921. *The* Laws *of Plato*. Manchester: Manchester University Press.

Entralgo, P.L. 1969. *Doctor and Patient*. Trans. F. Partridge. New York: World University Library.

Erde, E.L. 1997. "The Inadequacy of Role Models for Educating Medical Students in Ethics with Some Reflections on Virtue Theory." *Theoretical Medicine* 18: 31–45.

———. 2008. "Professionalism's Facets: Ambiguity, Ambivalence, and Nostalgia." *Journal of Medicine and Philosophy* 33: 6–26.

Eskin, C.R. 2002. "Hippocrates, *Kairos*, and Writing in the Sciences." In *Rhetoric and Kairos: Essays in History, Theory, and Praxis*, 97–113. Ed. P. Sipiora and J.S. Baumlin. Albany: State University of New York Press.

Finley, M.I. 1981. "The Elderly in Classical Antiquity." *Greece and Rome* 28: 156–71.
Fochtmann, L.J. 2004. "The Professionalism Movement: Pausing and Reflecting Are Essential." *American Journal of Bioethics* 4: 38–40.
Franklin, L. 2005. "*Technê* and Teleology in Plato's *Gorgias*." *Apeiron* 38: 229–55.
Frede, D. 2010. "Puppets on Strings: Moral Psychology in *Laws* Books 1 and 2." In *Plato's* Laws: *A Critical Guide*, 108–26. Ed. C. Bobonich. Cambridge: Cambridge University Press.
Fussi, A. 2000. "Why Is the *Gorgias* So Bitter?" *Philosophy and Rhetoric* 33: 39–58.
———. 2001. "The Myth of the Last Judgment in the *Gorgias*." *Review of Metaphysics* 54: 529–52.
Ginsburg, S., and D. Stern. 2004. "The Professionalism Movement: Behaviors Are the Key to Progress." *American Journal of Bioethics* 4: 14–15.
Golden, M. 2008. *Greek Sport and Social Status*. Austin: University of Texas Press.
Goold, S.D., M.A. Neblo, S.Y.H. Kim, R. De Vries, G. Rowe, and P. Muhlberger. 2012. "What Is Good Public Deliberation?" *Hastings Center Report* 42/2: 24–26.
Görgemanns, H. 1960. *Beiträge zur Interpretation von Platons* Nomoi. Munich: Beck.
Gorovitz, S. 1982. *Doctors' Dilemmas: Moral Conflict and Medical Care*. New York: Macmillan.
Gorovitz, S., and A. MacIntyre. 1975. "Toward a Theory of Medical Fallibility." *Hastings Center Report* 5/6: 13–23.
Gosling, J.C.B., and C.C.W. Taylor. 1982. *The Greeks on Pleasure*. Oxford: Clarendon Press.
Gould, C.S. 1994. "A Puzzle about the Possibility of Aristotelian *Enkrateia*." *Phronesis* 39: 174–86.
Gray, B.H. 1991. *The Profit Motive and Patient Care: The Changing Accountability of Doctors and Hospitals*. Cambridge, Mass.: Harvard University Press.
Groll, D. 2011. "What Health Care Providers Know: A Taxonomy of Clinical Disagreements." *Hastings Center Report* 41/5: 27–36.
Grube, G.M.A., trans. 1992. Plato, *Republic*. Rev. C.D.C. Reeve. Indianapolis: Hackett Publishing Company.
Guthrie, W.K.C. 1978. *A History of Greek Philosophy*. Vol. 5. Cambridge: Cambridge University Press.
Guttentag, O.E. 1979. "The Attending Physician as a Central Figure." In *Changing Values in Medicine*, 107–26. Ed. E.J. Cassell and M. Siegler. Frederick, Md.: University Publications of America.
Hafferty, F.W. 2004. "Toward the Operationalization of Professionalism: A Commentary." *American Journal of Bioethics* 4: 28–31.
Hall, R.W. 1971. "Techne and Morality in the *Gorgias*." In *Essays in Ancient Greek Philosophy*, 202–18. Ed. J.P. Anton and G.L. Kustas. Albany: State University of New York Press.
———. 2001. "Platonic Rule: Fiat or Law." *Polis* 18: 107–16.
Hamilton, E., and H. Cairns, eds. 1963. *The Collected Dialogues of Plato*. Princeton, N.J.: Princeton University Press.
Harrison, E.L. 1964. "Was Gorgias a Sophist?" *Phoenix* 18: 183–92.
Hauskeller, M. 2012. "Reinventing Cockaigne: Utopian Themes in Transhumanist Thought." *Hastings Center Report* 42/2: 39–47.
Heidel, W.A. 1941. *Hippocratic Medicine: Its Spirit and Method*. New York: Columbia University Press.
Heinimann, F. 1976. "Eine vorplatonische Theorie der *Technê*." In *Wege der Forschung*, vol. 187: *Sophistik*, 127–69. Ed. C.J. Classen. Darmstadt: Wissenschaftliche Buchgesellschaft.

Hester, D.M., and K. Kovach. 2004. "Trumping Professionalism." *American Journal of Bioethics* 4: 51–52.

Heyd, D. 1995. "The Medicalization of Health: Plato's Warning." *Revue Internationale de Philosophie* 49: 375–93.

Hoffmann, E. 1947. *Über Platons* Symposion. Heidelberg: Kerle.

Hofmann, B. 2003. "Medicine as *Techne*—A Perspective from Antiquity." *Journal of Medicine and Philosophy* 28: 403–25.

Holmes, B. 2010. *The Symptom and the Subject: The Emergence of the Physical Body in Ancient Greece.* Princeton, N.J.: Princeton University Press.

Hourani, G.F. 1949. "The Education of the Third Class in Plato's *Republic*." *Classical Quarterly* 43: 58–60.

Hude, C., ed. 1927. Herodotus, *Historiae*. Vol. 1. 3rd ed. Oxford: Clarendon Press.

Hunter, R. 2004. *Plato's* Symposium. New York: Oxford University Press.

Hunter, V. 2000. "Introduction: Status Distinctions in Athenian Law." In *Law and Social Status in Classical Athens*, 1–29. Ed. Hunter and J. Edmondson. Oxford: Oxford University Press.

Irvine, D. 1997. "The Performance of Doctors. I: Professionalism and Self Regulation in a Changing World." *British Medical Journal* 314: 1540–42.

Irwin, T.H. 1977. "Plato's Heracleiteanism." *Philosophical Quarterly* 27: 1–13.

———, trans. 1979. Plato, *Gorgias*. Oxford: Clarendon Press.

———. 1995. *Plato's Ethics*. New York: Oxford University Press.

Jaeger, W. 1986a. *Paideia: The Ideals of Greek Culture*. Vol. 2: *In Search of the Divine Centre*. Trans. G. Highet. New York: Oxford University Press.

———. 1986b. *Paideia: The Ideals of Greek Culture*. Vol. 3: *The Conflict of Cultural Ideals in the Age of Plato*. Trans. G. Highet. New York: Oxford University Press.

Jaspers, K. 1989. "The Physician in the Technological Age." *Theoretical Medicine* 10: 251–67.

Jennings, B. 2001. "From the Urban to the Civic: The Moral Possibilities of the City." *Journal of Urban Health: Bulletin of the New York Academy of Medicine* 78: 88–103.

———. 2007. "Autonomy." In *The Oxford Handbook of Bioethics*, 72–89. Ed. B. Steinbock. Oxford: Oxford University Press.

Jones, H.S., ed. 1942. Thucydides, *Historiae*. Vol. 1. Oxford: Clarendon Press.

Jones, W.H.S., trans. 1923a. *Hippocrates*. Vol. 1. Loeb Classical Library. Cambridge, Mass.: Harvard University Press.

———, trans. 1923b. *Hippocrates*. Vol. 2. Loeb Classical Library. Cambridge, Mass.: Harvard University Press.

———, trans. 1931. *Hippocrates*. Vol. 4. Loeb Classical Library. Cambridge, Mass.: Harvard University Press.

Jost, T.S., L. Mulcahy, S. Strasser, and L.A. Sachs. 1993. "Consumers, Complaints, and Professional Discipline: A Look at Medical Licensure Boards." *Health Matrix: The Journal of Law-Medicine* 3: 309–38.

Jouanna, J. 1961. "Présence d'Empédocle dans la Collection Hippocratique." *Bulletin de l'Association Guillaume Budé*, ser. 4: 452–63.

———. 1998. "The Birth of Western Medical Art." In *Western Medical Thought from Antiquity to the Middle Ages*, 22–71. Ed. M.D. Grmek. Cambridge, Mass.: Harvard University Press.

———. 1999. *Hippocrates*. Trans. M.B. DeBevoise. Baltimore, Md.: Johns Hopkins University Press.

Journal of the American Medical Association, Editorial. 1965. "Thomas Percival (1740–1804): Codifier of Medical Ethics." *Journal of the American Medical Association* 194: 1319–20.

Jung, P., P. Lurie, and S.M. Wolfe. 2006. "U.S. Physicians Disciplined for Criminal Activity." *Health Matrix: Journal of Law-Medicine* 16: 335–50.

Kahn, C.H. 1960. *Anaximander and the Origins of Greek Cosmology*. New York: Columbia University Press.

———. 1983. "Drama and Dialectic in Plato's *Gorgias*." *Oxford Studies in Ancient Philosophy* 1: 75–121.

———. 1987. "Plato's Theory of Desire." *Review of Metaphysics* 41: 77–103.

———. 1995. "The Place of the *Statesman* in Plato's Later Work." In *Reading the* Statesman: *Proceedings of the III Symposium Platonicum*, 49–60. Ed. C.J. Rowe. Sankt Augustin: Academia Verlag.

———. 1996. *Plato and the Socratic Dialogue: The Philosophical Use of a Literary Form*. Cambridge: Cambridge University Press.

———. 2004. "From *Republic* to *Laws*: A Discussion of Christopher Bobonich, *Plato's Utopia Recast*." *Oxford Studies in Ancient Philosophy* 26: 337–62.

———. 2010. "The Place of Cosmology in Plato's Later Dialogues." In *One Book, the Whole Universe: Plato's* Timaeus *Today*, 69–77. Ed. R.D. Mohr and B.M. Sattler. Las Vegas: Parmenides Publishing.

Kamtekar, R. 1997. "Philosophical Rule from the *Republic* to the *Laws*: Commentary on Schofield." *Proceedings of the Boston Area Colloquium in Ancient Philosophy* 13: 242–52.

———. 2006. "Plato on the Attribution of Conative Attitudes." *Archiv für Geschichte der Philosophie* 88: 127–62.

Karenberg, A., and H. Förstl. 2006. "Dementia in the Greco-Roman World." *Journal of the Neurological Sciences* 244: 5–9.

Kassirer, J.P. 1995. "Managed Care and the Morality of the Marketplace." *New England Journal of Medicine* 333: 50–52.

Kato, M. 1986. *Techne und Philosophie bei Platon*. Frankfurt am Main: Peter Lang.

Katz, J. 1984. *The Silent World of Doctor and Patient*. New York: Free Press.

Kelley, M. 2005. "Limits on Patient Responsibility." *Journal of Medicine and Philosophy* 30: 189–206.

Kennedy, G. 1963. *The Art of Persuasion in Ancient Greece*. Princeton, N.J.: Princeton University Press.

Kirk, G.S., J.E. Raven, and M. Schofield. 1983. *The Presocratic Philosophers: A Critical History with a Selection of Texts*. 2nd ed. Cambridge: Cambridge University Press.

Klein, R. 1998. "Competence, Professional Self-Regulation, and the Public Interest." *British Medical Journal* 316: 1740–42.

Klosko, G. 1981. "Implementing the Ideal State." *Journal of Politics* 43: 365–89.

———. 1984a. "The Refutation of Callicles in Plato's *Gorgias*." *Greece and Rome*, 2nd ser., 31: 126–39.

———. 1984b. "Provisionality in Plato's Ideal State." *History of Political Thought* 5: 171–93.

———. 1988. "The Nocturnal Council in Plato's *Laws*." *Political Studies* 36: 74–88.

———. 1993. "Persuasion and Moral Reform in Plato and Aristotle." *Revue Internationale de Philosophie* 47: 31–49.

———. 2006. *The Development of Plato's Political Theory*. 2nd ed. Oxford: Oxford University Press.

———. 2008. "Knowledge and Law in Plato's *Laws*." *Political Studies* 56: 456–74.

Koch, T. 2012. *Thieves of Virtue: When Bioethics Stole Medicine*. Cambridge, Mass.: MIT Press.

———. 2013. "The Ethicist as Language Czar, or Cop: 'End of Life.'" *HEC Forum* 25: 345–59.

Kohn, L.T., J.M. Corrigan, and M.S. Donaldson, eds. 2000. *To Err Is Human: Building a Safer Health System*. Report, Institute of Medicine, released November 1, 1999. Washington, D.C.: National Academy Press.

Konstan, D., and E. Young-Bruehl. 1982. "Eryximachus' Speech in the *Symposium*." *Apeiron* 16: 40–46.

Koppelman-White, E.R. 2009. "The Search for Reasons in a Unified Relationship." *Journal of Medicine and Philosophy* 34: 447–69.

Kraut, R. 1992. "The Defense of Justice in Plato's *Republic*." In *The Cambridge Companion to Plato*, 311–37. Ed. Kraut. Cambridge: Cambridge University Press.

———. 2010. "Ordinary Virtue from the *Phaedo* to the *Laws*." In *Plato's* Laws: *A Critical Guide*, 51–70. Ed. C. Bobonich. Cambridge: Cambridge University Press.

Kuczewski, M.G. 2000. "Can Communitarianism End the Shrill and Interminable Public Debates? Abortion as a Case-in-Point." In *Bioethics: Ancient Themes in Contemporary Issues*, 179–91. Ed. M.G. Kuczewski and R. Polansky. Cambridge, Mass.: MIT Press.

Kuczewski, M.G., and R. Polansky, eds. 2000. *Bioethics: Ancient Themes in Contemporary Issues*. Cambridge, Mass.: MIT Press.

Kurihara, Y. 2002. "Plato's Conception of Unhappiness in the *Gorgias*." *Skepsis* 13–14: 106–15.

Laks, A. 1990. "Legislation and Demiurgy: On the Relationship between Plato's *Republic* and *Laws*." *Classical Antiquity* 9: 209–29.

———. 1991. "L'utopie législative de Platon." *Revue philosophique* 181: 417–28.

———. 2000. "The *Laws*." In *The Cambridge History of Greek and Roman Political Thought*, 258–92. Ed. C. Rowe and M. Schofield. Cambridge: Cambridge University Press.

———. 2001. "In What Sense Is the City of the *Laws* a Second Best One?" In *Plato's* Laws *and Its Historical Significance*, 107–14. Ed. F.L. Lisi. Sankt Augustin: Academia Verlag.

Leape, L.L., and D.M. Berwick. 2005. "Five Years after *To Err Is Human*: What Have We Learned?" *Journal of the American Medical Association* 293: 2384–90.

Legislative and Legal Advisory Committee. 1996. "Report on Licensure of Physicians Enrolled in Postgraduate Training Programs." *Federation Bulletin: The Journal of Medical Licensure and Discipline* 83: 163–69.

Levin, S.B. 1996. "Women's Nature and Role in the Ideal *Polis: Republic* 5 Revisited." In *Feminism and Ancient Philosophy*, 13–30. Ed. J.K. Ward. New York: Routledge.

———. 2000. "Commentary on Osborne." *Proceedings of the Boston Area Colloquium in Ancient Philosophy* 15: 282–92.

———. 2001. *The Ancient Quarrel between Philosophy and Poetry Revisited: Plato and the Greek Literary Tradition*. New York: Oxford University Press.

———. 2008. "Platonic Metaphysics and Semantics: The *Cratylus*' Ties to the *Sophist* and *Politicus*." In *Logos and Language: Essays in Honour of Julius Moravcsik*, 73–98. Ed. D. Føllesdal and J. Woods. London: College Publications.

Levine, C. 2004. "Life but No Limb: The Aftermath of Medical Error." In *Accountability: Patient Safety and Policy Reform*, 43–48. Ed. V.A. Sharpe. Washington, D.C.: Georgetown University Press.

Levy, D. 2005. "*Technê* and the Problem of Socratic Philosophy in the *Gorgias*." *Apeiron* 38: 185–227.

Liang, B.A. 2004. "Error Disclosure for Quality Improvement: Authenticating a Team of Patients and Providers to Promote Patient Safety." In *Accountability: Patient Safety and Policy Reform*, 59–82. Ed. V.A. Sharpe. Washington, D.C.: Georgetown University Press.

Liddell, H.G., and R. Scott. 1996. *A Greek-English Lexicon*. Rev. H.S. Jones. Oxford: Clarendon Press.

Lidz, J.W. 1995. "Medicine as Metaphor in Plato." *Journal of Medicine and Philosophy* 20: 527–41.

Loewenstein, G., T. Brennan, and K.G. Volpp. 2007. "Asymmetric Paternalism to Improve Health Behaviors." *Journal of the American Medical Association* 298: 2415–17.

Loewy, E.H. 1986. "Physicians and Patients: Moral Agency in a Pluralistic World." *Journal of Medical Humanities and Bioethics* 7: 57–68.

London, A.J. 2000. "Thrasymachus and Managed Care: How Not to Think about the Craft of Medicine." In *Bioethics: Ancient Themes in Contemporary Issues*, 131–54. Ed. M.G. Kuczewski and R. Polansky. Cambridge, Mass.: MIT Press.

Longrigg, J. 1993. *Greek Rational Medicine: Philosophy and Medicine from Alcmaeon to the Alexandrians*. London: Routledge.

Lorenz, H. 2006. *The Brute Within: Appetitive Desire in Plato and Aristotle*. Oxford: Clarendon Press.

Lundberg, G.D. 1997. "The Business and Professionalism of Medicine." *Journal of the American Medical Association* 278: 1703–4.

MacDowell, D.M., ed. and trans. 1993. Gorgias, *Encomium of Helen*. Bristol: Bristol Classical Press.

Marchant, E.C., trans. 1923. Xenophon, *Memorabilia*. Loeb Classical Library. Cambridge, Mass.: Harvard University Press.

Mariner, W.K. 1995. "Business vs. Medical Ethics: Conflicting Standards for Managed Care." *Journal of Law, Medicine and Ethics* 23: 236–46.

Márquez, X. 2007. "Theory and Practice in Plato's *Statesman*." *Ancient Philosophy* 27: 31–53.

Marrou, H.I. 1982. *A History of Education in Antiquity*. Trans. G. Lamb. Madison: University of Wisconsin Press.

Matthews, G.B. 1994. *The Philosophy of Childhood*. Cambridge, Mass.: Harvard University Press.

Mayhew, R. 1997. *Aristotle's Criticism of Plato's* Republic. Lanham, Md.: Rowman and Littlefield.

———. 2007. "Persuasion and Compulsion in Plato's *Laws* 10." *Polis* 24: 91–111.

———. 2008. *Plato:* Laws *10*. Oxford: Clarendon Press.

———. 2010. "The Theology of the *Laws*." In *Plato's* Laws: *A Critical Guide*, 197–216. Ed. C. Bobonich. Cambridge: Cambridge University Press.

Mayo Clinic. 2011. "Ankylosing Spondylitis." http://www.mayoclinic.com/health/ankylosing-spondylitis/DS00483. Accessed August 19, 2013.

———. 2012. "Tongue-Tie (Ankyloglossia)." http://www.mayoclinic.com/health/tongue-tie/DS01200. Accessed August 19, 2013.

McCabe, M.M. 1997. "Chaos and Control: Reading Plato's *Politicus*." *Phronesis* 42: 92–117.

McIntyre, N., and K. Popper. 1983. "The Critical Attitude in Medicine: The Need for a New Ethics." *British Medical Journal (Clinical Research Edition)* 287: 1919–23.

McKirahan, R.D. 1994. *Philosophy before Socrates: An Introduction with Texts and Commentary*. Indianapolis: Hackett Publishing Company.

McPherran, M.L. 2006. "Medicine, Magic, and Religion in Plato's *Symposium*." In *Plato's* Symposium: *Issues in Interpretation and Reception*, 71–95. Ed. J.H. Lesher, D. Nails, and F.C.C. Sheffield. Washington, D.C.: Center for Hellenic Studies.

Megone, C. 2000. "Potentiality and Persons: An Aristotelian Perspective." In *Bioethics: Ancient Themes in Contemporary Issues*, 155–77. Ed. M.G. Kuczewski and R. Polansky. Cambridge, Mass.: MIT Press.

Menzel, P.T. 1983. *Medical Costs, Moral Choices: A Philosophy of Health Care Economics in America*. New Haven, Conn.: Yale University Press.

Merry, A., and A.M. Smith. 2001. *Errors, Medicine and the Law*. Cambridge: Cambridge University Press.

Meyer, S.S. 2003. "The Moral Dangers of Labour and Commerce in Plato's *Laws*." In *Plato's* Laws: *From Theory into Practice*, 207–14. Ed. S. Scolnicov and L. Brisson. Sankt Augustin: Academia Verlag.

Mishima, T. 1995. "Courage and Moderation in the *Statesman*." In *Reading the* Statesman: *Proceedings of the III Symposium Platonicum*, 306–12. Ed. C.J. Rowe. Sankt Augustin: Academia Verlag.

Montgomery, K. 2000. "*Phronesis* and the Misdescription of Medicine: Against *The* Medical School Commencement Speech." In *Bioethics: Ancient Themes in Contemporary Issues*, 57–66. Ed. M.G. Kuczewski and R. Polansky. Cambridge, Mass.: MIT Press.

Moravcsik, J.M.E. 1971. "Reason and Eros in the 'Ascent'-Passage of the *Symposium*." In *Essays in Ancient Greek Philosophy*, 285–302. Ed. J.P. Anton and G.L. Kustas. Albany: State University of New York Press.

———. 1973a. "Plato's Method of Division." In *Patterns in Plato's Thought*, 158–80. Ed. Moravcsik. Dordrecht: D. Reidel Publishing Company.

———. 1973b. "The Anatomy of Plato's Divisions." In *Exegesis and Argument*, 324–48. Ed. E.N. Lee, A.P.D. Mourelatos, and R.M. Rorty. New York: Humanities Press.

———. 1992. *Plato and Platonism: Plato's Conception of Appearance and Reality in Ontology, Epistemology, and Ethics, and Its Modern Echoes*. Oxford: Blackwell.

Morreim, E.H. 2004. "Medical Errors: Pinning the Blame versus Blaming the System." In *Accountability: Patient Safety and Policy Reform*, 213–32. Ed. V.A. Sharpe. Washington, D.C.: Georgetown University Press.

Morrow, G.R. 1939. *Plato's Law of Slavery in Its Relation to Greek Law*. Urbana: University of Illinois Press.

———. 1941. "The Status of the Alien in Plato's *Laws*." *Scientia* 70: 38–43.

———. 1953. "Plato's Conception of Persuasion." *Philosophical Review* 62: 234–50.

———. 1993. *Plato's Cretan City: A Historical Interpretation of the* Laws. Princeton, N.J.: Princeton University Press.

Moss, J. 2006. "Pleasure and Illusion in Plato." *Philosophy and Phenomenological Research* 72: 503–35.

———. 2007. "The Doctor and the Pastry Chef: Pleasure and Persuasion in Plato's *Gorgias*." *Ancient Philosophy* 27: 229–49.

Murray, J.S. 2001. "Plato on Power, Moral Responsibility and the Alleged Neutrality of Gorgias' Art of Rhetoric (*Gorgias* 456c–457b)." *Philosophy and Rhetoric* 34: 355–63.

Myser, C. 2004. "Community-Based Participatory Research in United States Bioethics: Steps toward More Democratic Theory and Policy." *American Journal of Bioethics* 4: 67–68.

Naddaf, G. 2000. "Literacy and Poetic Performance in Plato's *Laws*." *Ancient Philosophy* 20: 339–50.

Nails, D. 2002. *The People of Plato: A Prosopography of Plato and Other Socratics*. Indianapolis: Hackett Publishing Company.

Nails, D., and H. Thesleff. 2003. "Early Academic Editing: Plato's *Laws*." In *Plato's* Laws: *From Theory into Practice*, 14–29. Ed. S. Scolnicov and L. Brisson. Sankt Augustin: Academia Verlag.

Nehamas, A. 1982. "Plato on Imitation and Poetry in *Republic* 10." In *Plato on Beauty, Wisdom, and the Arts*, 47–78. Ed. J. Moravcsik and P. Temko. Totowa, N.J.: Rowman and Littlefield.

———. 1988. "Plato and the Mass Media." *Monist* 71: 214–34.

———. 1999. *Virtues of Authenticity: Essays on Plato and Socrates*. Princeton, N.J.: Princeton University Press.

Nehamas, A., and P. Woodruff, trans. 1989. Plato, *Symposium*. Indianapolis: Hackett Publishing Company.

Neiman, P. 2007. "The Practicality of Plato's *Statesman*." *History of Political Thought* 28: 402–18.

Nichols, M.P. 2009. *Socrates on Friendship and Community: Reflections on Plato's* Symposium, Phaedrus, *and* Lysis. New York: Cambridge University Press.

Nightingale, A. 1993. "Writing/Reading a Sacred Text: A Literary Interpretation of Plato's *Laws*." *Classical Philology* 88: 279–300.

———. 1999. "Plato's Lawcode in Context: Rule by Written Law in Athens and Magnesia." *Classical Quarterly* 49: 100–122.

Norlin, G., trans. 1929. *Isocrates*. Vol. 2. Loeb Classical Library. Cambridge, Mass.: Harvard University Press.

North, H. 1966. *Sophrosyne: Self-Knowledge and Self-Restraint in Greek Literature*. Ithaca, N.Y.: Cornell University Press.

Notomi, N. 1999. *The Unity of Plato's* Sophist: *Between the Sophist and the Philosopher*. Cambridge: Cambridge University Press.

Nussbaum, M.C. 1986. *The Fragility of Goodness: Luck and Ethics in Greek Tragedy and Philosophy*. Cambridge: Cambridge University Press.

O'Doherty, K., F.-P. Gauvin, C. Grogan, and W. Friedman. 2012. "Implementing a Public Deliberative Forum." *Hastings Center Report* 42/2: 20–23.

Oken, D. 1961. "What to Tell Cancer Patients: A Study of Medical Attitudes." *Journal of the American Medical Association* 175: 1120–28.

Olympic Movement. 2013. http://www.olympic.org/gymnastics-artistic. Accessed August 8, 2013.

Ostwald, M., trans. 1962. Aristotle, *Nicomachean Ethics*. New York: Macmillan.

Owen, G.E.L. 1953. "The Place of the *Timaeus* in Plato's Dialogues." *Classical Quarterly*, n.s., 3: 79–95.

Page, D., ed. 1972. Aeschylus, *Tragoediae*. Oxford: Clarendon Press.

Pangle, T.L. 1980. *The* Laws *of Plato*. New York: Basic Books.

Parry, R.D. 1996. *Plato's Craft of Justice*. Albany: State University of New York Press.

Peabody, F.W. 1927. "The Care of the Patient." *Journal of the American Medical Association* 88: 877–82.

Peeno, L., and T.J. Leopold. 2003. "When HMOs Put Profits over Patients." *Trial* 39/4: 18–25.

Pellegrino, E.D. 2001. "The Internal Morality of Clinical Medicine: A Paradigm for the Ethics of the Helping and Healing Professions." *Journal of Medicine and Philosophy* 26: 559–79.

———. 2004. "Prevention of Medical Error: Where Professional and Organizational Ethics Meet." In *Accountability: Patient Safety and Policy Reform*, 83–98. Ed. V.A. Sharpe. Washington, D.C.: Georgetown University Press.

Pellegrino, E.D., and D.C. Thomasma. 1993. *The Virtues in Medical Practice*. New York: Oxford University Press.

Penner, T. 1991. "Desire and Power in Socrates: The Argument of *Gorgias* 466A–468E that Orators and Tyrants Have No Power in the City." *Apeiron* 24: 147–202.

Phi Beta Kappa Society. 2013. "About the Visiting Scholar Program." http://www.pbk.org/programs/visitingscholars.aspx. Accessed June 5, 2013.

Phillips, J.-O. 2011. "Law, Compulsion and Community in Plato's *Republic*." *Polis* 28: 108–25.

Popper, K.R. 1963. "Back to the Presocratics." In *Conjectures and Refutations: The Growth of Scientific Knowledge*, 136–65. London: Routledge and Kegan Paul.

Potter, P., trans. 1988a. *Hippocrates*. Vol. 5. Cambridge, Mass.: Harvard University Press.

———, trans. 1988b. *Hippocrates*. Vol. 6. Cambridge, Mass.: Harvard University Press.

———, ed. and trans. 1995. *Hippocrates*. Vol. 8. Cambridge, Mass.: Harvard University Press.

———, ed. and trans. 2010. *Hippocrates*. Vol. 9. Cambridge, Mass.: Harvard University Press.

———, ed. and trans. 2012. *Hippocrates*. Vol. 10. Cambridge, Mass.: Harvard University Press.

Prior, W.J. 2006. "The Portrait of Socrates in Plato's *Symposium*." *Oxford Studies in Ancient Philosophy* 31: 137–66.

Rawls, J. 1999. *A Theory of Justice*. Rev. ed. Cambridge, Mass.: Harvard University Press.

Reeve, C.D.C. 1988. *Philosopher-Kings: The Argument of Plato's* Republic. Princeton, N.J.: Princeton University Press.

Relman, A.S. 1985. "Dealing with Conflicts of Interest." *New England Journal of Medicine* 313: 749–51.

Rentmeester, C.A. 2008. "Moral Damage to Health Care Professionals and Trainees: Legalism and Other Consequences for Patients and Colleagues." *Journal of Medicine and Philosophy* 33: 27–43.

Rettig, G.F. 1876. *Platons* Symposion. Halle: Waisenhaus.

Richards, I.A. 1936. *The Philosophy of Rhetoric*. New York: Oxford University Press.

Robin, L., ed. and trans. 1929. *Platon: Œuvres complètes*, vol. 4, pt. 2: *Symposium*. Paris: Société d'Édition "Les Belles Lettres."

Robinson, R. 1984. *Plato's Earlier Dialectic*. 2nd ed. Oxford: Clarendon Press.

Rodwin, M.A. 1993. *Medicine, Money, and Morals: Physicians' Conflicts of Interest*. New York: Oxford University Press.

Rosen, S. 1987. *Plato's* Symposium. 2nd ed. New Haven, Conn.: Yale University Press.

Rothman, D.J. 1991. *Strangers at the Bedside: A History of How Law and Bioethics Transformed Medical Decision Making*. New York: BasicBooks.

Rowe, C.J., trans. 1997. Plato, *Statesman*. In *Plato: Complete Works*, 295–358. Ed. J.M. Cooper. Indianapolis: Hackett Publishing Company.

———, ed. and trans. 1998. Plato, *Symposium*. Warminster: Aris and Phillips.

———. 1999. "The Speech of Eryximachus in Plato's *Symposium*." In *Traditions of Platonism: Essays in Honour of John Dillon*, 53–64. Ed. J.J. Cleary. Aldershot, U.K.: Ashgate.

Russell, D.C. 2005. *Plato on Pleasure and the Good Life*. Oxford: Clarendon Press.

Sabik, L.M., and R.K. Lie. 2008. "Principles versus Procedures in Making Health Care Coverage Decisions: Addressing Inevitable Conflicts." *Theoretical Medicine and Bioethics* 29: 73–85.

Sabine, G.H. 1973. *A History of Political Theory*. 4th ed. Hinsdale, Ill.: Dryden Press.

Samaras, T. 1996. "When Did Plato Abandon the Hope that Ideal Rulers Might Appear among Human Beings?" *History of Political Thought* 17: 109–13.

Saunders, T.J. 1962. "The Structure of the Soul and the State in Plato's *Laws*." *Eranos* 60: 37–55.

———. 1991. *Plato's Penal Code: Tradition, Controversy, and Reform in Greek Penology*. Oxford: Clarendon Press.

———, trans. 2004. Plato, *Laws*. London: Penguin Books.

Sayre, K.M. 2006. *Metaphysics and Method in Plato's* Statesman. New York: Cambridge University Press.

Schaffner, K.F. 1979. "Modeling Clinical Medicine: A Commentary on Mark Siegler." In *Changing Values in Medicine*, 43–58. Ed. E.J. Cassell and M. Siegler. Frederick, Md.: University Publications of America.

Schaps, G.D.-D. 2001. "The Economy: What Plato Saw and What He Wanted." In *Plato's* Laws *and Its Historical Significance*, 143–47. Ed. F.L. Lisi. Sankt Augustin: Academia Verlag.

Schauer, F. 1995. "Giving Reasons." *Stanford Law Review* 47: 633–59.

Schindler, D.C. 2007. "Plato and the Problem of Love: On the Nature of Eros in the *Symposium*." *Apeiron* 40: 199–220.

Schmidt, H. 2009. "Just Health Responsibility." *Journal of Medical Ethics* 35: 21–26.

Schofield, M. 1997. "The Disappearance of the Philosopher King." *Proceedings of the Boston Area Colloquium in Ancient Philosophy* 13: 213–41.

———. 2003. "Religion and Philosophy in the *Laws*." In *Plato's* Laws: *From Theory into Practice*, 1–13. Ed. S. Scolnicov and L. Brisson. Sankt Augustin: Academia Verlag.

———. 2006a. *Plato: Political Philosophy*. Oxford: Oxford University Press.

———. 2006b. "Law and Absolutism in the *Republic*." *Polis* 23: 319–27.

———. 2010. "The *Laws'* Two Projects." In *Plato's* Laws: *A Critical Guide*, 12–28. Ed. C. Bobonich. Cambridge: Cambridge University Press.

Schultz, D.S., and F.A. Carnevale. 1996. "Engagement and Suffering in Responsible Caregiving: On Overcoming Maleficence in Health Care." *Theoretical Medicine* 17: 189–207.

Schwab, A. 2012. "Epistemic Humility and Medical Practice: Translating Epistemic Categories into Ethical Obligations." *Journal of Medicine and Philosophy* 37: 28–48.

Scott, G.A., and W.A. Welton. 2008. *Erotic Wisdom: Philosophy and Intermediacy in Plato's* Symposium. Albany: State University of New York Press.

Sedley, D. 2009. "Myth, Punishment and Politics in the *Gorgias*." In *Plato's Myths*, 51–76. Ed. C. Partenie. Cambridge: Cambridge University Press.

Segvic, H. 2000. "No One Errs Willingly: The Meaning of Socratic Intellectualism." *Oxford Studies in Ancient Philosophy* 19: 1–45.

Sharpe, V.A., ed. 2004. *Accountability: Patient Safety and Policy Reform*. Washington, D.C.: Georgetown University Press.

Shuchman, P. 1963. "Comments on the Criminal Code of Plato's *Laws*." *Journal of the History of Ideas* 24: 25–40.

Sickinger, J.P. 2007. "Rhetoric and the Law." In *A Companion to Greek Rhetoric*, 286–302. Ed. I. Worthington. Malden, Mass.: Blackwell.

Siegler, M. 1981. "Searching for Moral Certainty in Medicine: A Proposal for a New Model of the Doctor-Patient Encounter." *Bulletin of the New York Academy of Medicine* 57: 56–69.

———. 1985. "The Progression of Medicine: From Physician Paternalism to Patient Autonomy to Bureaucratic Parsimony." *Archives of Internal Medicine* 145: 713–15.

———. 2000. "Professional Values in Modern Clinical Practice." *Hastings Center Report* 30/4: S19–S22.

Singpurwalla, R. 2010. "The Tripartite Theory of Motivation in Plato's *Republic*." *Philosophy Compass* 5: 880–92.

Skemp, J.B., trans. 1992. Plato, *Statesman*. Rev. M. Ostwald. Indianapolis: Hackett Publishing Company.

———, trans. 2002. Plato, *Statesman*. 2nd ed. Bristol: Bristol Classical Press.

Slings, S.R., ed. 2003. Plato, *Respublica*. Oxford: Clarendon Press.

Smith, W.D., ed. and trans. 1994. *Hippocrates*. Vol. 7. Loeb Classical Library. Cambridge, Mass.: Harvard University Press.

Snyder, L., and R.L. Neubauer. 2007. "Pay-for-Performance Principles that Promote Patient-Centered Care: An Ethics Manifesto." *Annals of Internal Medicine* 147: 792–94.

Solbakk, J.H. 2014. "The Whole and the Art of Medical Dialectic: A Platonic Account." *Medicine, Health Care and Philosophy* 17: 39–52.

Solomon, S., and J. Abelson. 2012. "Why and When Should We Use Public Deliberation?" *Hastings Center Report* 42/2: 17–20.

Sorabji, R. 1980. "Aristotle on the Role of Intellect in Virtue." In *Essays on Aristotle's Ethics*, 201–19. Ed. A.O. Rorty. Berkeley: University of California Press.

Sprague, R.K. 1976. *Plato's Philosopher-King: A Study of the Theoretical Background*. Columbia: University of South Carolina Press.

Staden, H. von. 1996. "'In a Pure and Holy Way': Personal and Professional Conduct in the Hippocratic Oath?" *Journal of the History of Medicine and Allied Sciences* 51: 404–37.

Stalley, R.F. 1980. "The Role of the Doctor: Technician or Statesman?" *Journal of Medical Ethics* 6: 19–22.

———. 1981. "Mental Health and Individual Responsibility in Plato's *Republic*." *Journal of Value Inquiry* 15: 109–24.

———. 1983. *An Introduction to Plato's* Laws. Indianapolis: Hackett Publishing Company.

———. 1994. "Persuasion in Plato's *Laws*." *History of Political Thought* 15: 157–77.

Stanford University, School of Medicine. 2013. "Stanford's Medical Curriculum." http://med.stanford.edu/md/curriculum. Accessed June 9, 2013.

Stauffer, D. 2006. *The Unity of Plato's* Gorgias: *Rhetoric, Justice, and the Philosophic Life*. New York: Cambridge University Press.

Taylor, C.C.W. 1997. "Plato's Totalitarianism." In *Plato's* Republic: *Critical Essays*, 31–48. Ed. R. Kraut. Lanham, Md.: Rowman and Littlefield.

Tenkku, J. 1956. *The Evaluation of Pleasure in Plato's Ethics*. *Acta Philosophica Fennica*, fasc. 11. Helsinki: Societas Philosophica.

Thanassas, P. 2005. "Beyond Legislation, Close to Philosophy: Plato's Last Critique of Writing in the *Laws*." *Philosophical Inquiry* 27: 45–56.

Thomasma, D. 2000. "Aristotle, *Phronesis*, and Postmodern Bioethics." In *Bioethics: Ancient Themes in Contemporary Issues*, 67–91. Ed. M.G. Kuczewski and R. Polansky. Cambridge, Mass.: MIT Press.

Thompson, D.F. 1993. "Understanding Financial Conflicts of Interest." *New England Journal of Medicine* 329: 573–76.

Tress, D.M. 2000. "Classical and Modern Reflections on Medical Ethics and the Best Interests of the Sick Child." In *Bioethics: Ancient Themes in Contemporary Issues*, 193–228. Ed. M.G. Kuczewski and R. Polansky. Cambridge, Mass.: MIT Press.

Tschemplik, A. 2008. "Callicles: From 'Here' to Hades." *Polis* 25: 79–93.

Tumulty, P.A. 1970. "What Is a Clinician and What Does He Do?" *New England Journal of Medicine* 283: 20–24.

Urmson, J.O. 1980. "Aristotle's Doctrine of the Mean." In *Essays on Aristotle's Ethics*, 157–70. Ed. A.O. Rorty. Berkeley: University of California Press.

Veatch, R.M. 1981. *A Theory of Medical Ethics*. New York: Basic Books.

———. 2009. *Patient, Heal Thyself: How the New Medicine Puts the Patient in Charge*. New York: Oxford University Press.

———. 2012. *Hippocratic, Religious, and Secular Medical Ethics: The Points of Conflict*. Washington, D.C.: Georgetown University Press.

Versényi, L. 1961. "The Cretan Plato." *Review of Metaphysics* 15: 67–80.

Vlastos, G. 1953. "*Isonomia*." *American Journal of Philology* 74: 337–66.

———. 1955. "A Review of F.M. Cornford, *Principium sapientiae: The Origins of Greek Philosophical Thought*." *Gnomon* 27: 65–76.

———. 1957. "Socratic Knowledge and Platonic 'Pessimism.'" *Philosophical Review* 66: 226–38.

———. 1978. "Justice and Happiness in the *Republic*." In *Plato: A Collection of Critical Essays*, 66–95. Vol. 2: *Ethics, Politics, and Philosophy of Art and Religion*. Ed. Vlastos. Notre Dame, Ind.: University of Notre Dame Press.

Walker, R.L. 2009a. "Medical Ethics Needs a New View of Autonomy." *Journal of Medicine and Philosophy* 33: 594–608.

———. 2009b. "Respect for *Rational* Autonomy." *Kennedy Institute of Ethics Journal* 19: 339–66.

Wardy, R. 2002. "The Unity of Opposites in Plato's *Symposium*." *Oxford Studies in Ancient Philosophy* 23: 1–61.

Wehrli, F. 1951. "Der Arztvergleich bei Platon." *Museum Helveticum* 8: 177–84.

Weiss, R. 1992. "Killing, Confiscating, and Banishing at *Gorgias* 466–468." *Ancient Philosophy* 12: 299–315.

———. 2007. "Wise Guys and Smart Alecks in *Republic* 1 and 2." In *The Cambridge Companion to Plato's* Republic, 90–115. Ed. G.R.F. Ferrari. New York: Cambridge University Press.

White, F.C. 1990. "The Good in Plato's *Gorgias*." *Phronesis* 35: 117–27.

Whitehead, D. 1977. *The Ideology of the Athenian Metic*. Cambridge: Cambridge Philological Society.

Winn, J.R., and D.R. Fuqua. 1996. "Licensure of Physicians in Postgraduate Training Programs in the United States." *Federation Bulletin: The Journal of Medical Licensure and Discipline* 83: 158–62.

Withington, E.T., trans. 1928. *Hippocrates*. Vol. 3. Loeb Classical Library. Cambridge, Mass.: Harvard University Press.

Wolfe, S.M., ed. 2012. "Ranking of State Medical Board Serious Disciplinary Actions, 2009–2011." *Public Citizen: Health Letter* 28/6: 1–6.

Wolfsdorf, D. 2008. "*Gorgias* 466a4–468e5: Rhetoric's Inadequate Means." *Classical Philology* 103: 109–34.

Woodruff, P., trans. 1982. Plato, *Hippias Major*. Indianapolis: Hackett Publishing Company.

———. 1990. "Plato's Early Theory of Knowledge." In *Companions to Ancient Thought*, vol. 1: *Epistemology*, 60–84. Ed. S. Everson. Cambridge: Cambridge University Press.

Woolf, R. 2000. "Callicles and Socrates: Psychic (Dis)Harmony in the *Gorgias*." *Oxford Studies in Ancient Philosophy* 18: 1–40.

Woozley, A. 2010. "Plato and the Need for Law." *Philosophical Quarterly* 60: 373–95.

Yunis, H. 2005. "The Rhetoric of Law in Fourth-Century Athens." In *The Cambridge Companion to Ancient Greek Law*, 191–208. Ed. M. Gagarin and D. Cohen. New York: Cambridge University Press.

INDEX LOCORUM

Page numbers followed by n indicate notes.

GENERAL INDEX

Page numbers followed by n indicate notes.

www.ingramcontent.com/pod-product-compliance
Ingram Content Group UK Ltd.
Pitfield, Milton Keynes, MK11 3LW, UK
UKHW020849150926
475595UK00003B/79

9 780199 919802